Evaluating Challenges and Opportunities for Healthcare Reform

Raj Selladurai
Indiana University Northwest, USA

Charlie Hobson
Indiana University Northwest, USA

Roshini Isabell Selladurai
In His Image Family Medicine Residency, Ascension St. John Medical Center, USA

Adam Greer
Ascension St. John Medical Center, USA

A volume in the Advances in Healthcare Information Systems and Administration (AHISA) Book Series

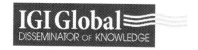

Published in the United States of America by
    IGI Global
    Medical Information Science Reference (an imprint of IGI Global)
    701 E. Chocolate Avenue
    Hershey PA, USA 17033
    Tel: 717-533-8845
    Fax: 717-533-8661
    E-mail: cust@igi-global.com
    Web site: http://www.igi-global.com

Library of Congress Cataloging-in-Publication Data

Names: Selladurai, Raj, 1954- editor. | Hobson, Charlie, 1952- editor. |
   Selladurai, Roshini Isabell, 1991- editor. | Greer, Adam, 1987- editor.
Title: Evaluating challenges and opportunities for healthcare reform / Raj
   Selladurai, Charlie Hobson, Roshini Isabell Selladurai, and Adam Greer,
   editors.
Description: Hershey, PA : Medical Information Science Reference, [2020] |
   Includes bibliographical references and index. | Summary: "This book
   explores and analyzes various challenges and opportunities in healthcare
   reform"--Provided by publisher.
Identifiers: LCCN 2019046432 (print) | LCCN 2019046433 (ebook) | ISBN
   9781799829492 (hardcover) | ISBN 9781799829508 (ebook)
Subjects: MESH: Health Care Reform--organization & administration |
   Organizational Case Studies | Models, Organizational
Classification: LCC RA771.5 (print) | LCC RA771.5 (ebook) | NLM WA 525 |
   DDC 362.1/0425--dc23
LC record available at https://lccn.loc.gov/2019046432
LC ebook record available at https://lccn.loc.gov/2019046433

This book is published in the IGI Global book series Advances in Healthcare Information Systems and Administration (AHISA) (ISSN: 2328-1243; eISSN: 2328-126X)

British Cataloguing in Publication Data
A Cataloguing in Publication record for this book is available from the British Library.

All work contributed to this book is new, previously-unpublished material.
The views expressed in this book are those of the authors, but not necessarily of the publisher.

For electronic access to this publication, please contact: eresources@igi-global.com.

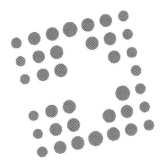

Advances in Healthcare Information Systems and Administration (AHISA) Book Series

ISSN:2328-1243
EISSN:2328-126X

Editor-in-Chief: Anastasius Moumtzoglou, Hellenic Society for Quality & Safety in Healthcare and P. & A. Kyriakou Children's Hospital, Greece

MISSION

The **Advances in Healthcare Information Systems and Administration (AHISA) Book Series** aims to provide a channel for international researchers to progress the field of study on technology and its implications on healthcare and health information systems. With the growing focus on healthcare and the importance of enhancing this industry to tend to the expanding population, the book series seeks to accelerate the awareness of technological advancements of health information systems and expand awareness and implementation.

Driven by advancing technologies and their clinical applications, the emerging field of health information systems and informatics is still searching for coherent directing frameworks to advance health care and clinical practices and research. Conducting research in these areas is both promising and challenging due to a host of factors, including rapidly evolving technologies and their application complexity. At the same time, organizational issues, including technology adoption, diffusion and acceptance as well as cost benefits and cost effectiveness of advancing health information systems and informatics applications as innovative forms of investment in healthcare are gaining attention as well. **AHISA** addresses these concepts and critical issues.

COVERAGE

- Virtual health technologies
- Telemedicine
- Clinical Decision Support Design, Development and Implementation
- IT security and privacy issues
- Management of Emerging Health Care Technologies
- E-Health and M-Health
- Decision Support Systems
- IS in Healthcare
- IT Applications in Health Organizations and Practices
- Measurements and Impact of HISA on Public and Social Policy

IGI Global is currently accepting manuscripts for publication within this series. To submit a proposal for a volume in this series, please contact our Acquisition Editors at Acquisitions@igi-global.com or visit: http://www.igi-global.com/publish/.

Titles in this Series

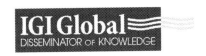

701 East Chocolate Avenue, Hershey, PA 17033, USA
Tel: 717-533-8845 x100 • Fax: 717-533-8661
E-Mail: cust@igi-global.com • www.igi-global.com

Editorial Advisory Board

Table of Contents

Section 1

Chapter 1

> *Raj Selladurai, Indiana University Northwest, USA*
> *Roshini Isabell Selladurai, In His Image Family Medicine Residency,*
> *Ascension St. John Medical Center, USA*

Chapter 2

> *Raj Selladurai, Indiana University Northwest, USA*
> *Roshini Isabell Selladurai, In His Image Family Medicine Residency,*
> *Ascension St. John Medical Center, USA*
> *George VandeWerken, Providence Bank, USA*

Chapter 3

> *Jeff Gourdji, Prophet, USA*
> *Scott M. Davis, Prophet, USA*

Section 2

Section 3

Detailed Table of Contents

Section 1

Chapter 1

Raj Selladurai, Indiana University Northwest, USA
Roshini Isabell Selladurai, In His Image Family Medicine Residency,
Ascension St. John Medical Center, USA

This chapter focuses on developing an enhanced US healthcare delivery system
model by learning from the "best" healthcare systems in the world and adapting
some of their best working principles to the existing US healthcare system. These
global systems include the Swiss healthcare system, which is considered one of
the best in the world, and some of the other leading healthcare systems such as the
German, the UK, French, Italian, and Singaporean. It would also explore, among a
few alternatives, the state innovation-based approach to healthcare reform. Major
concerns such as cost containment, affordability, flexibility, accessibility, feasibility,
and implementation-related issues have been addressed.

Chapter 2

Raj Selladurai, Indiana University Northwest, USA
Roshini Isabell Selladurai, In His Image Family Medicine Residency,
Ascension St. John Medical Center, USA
George VandeWerken, Providence Bank, USA

This chapter explores, discusses, analyzes, and presents some recommendations for new, innovative alternative healthcare models to the traditional insurance and healthcare models that currently exist. These include a revised and enhanced hybrid model of healthcare; healthcare cost-sharing faith-based model; healthcare cost-reduction corporate partnership model (for example, Amazon, Berkshire Hathaway, and JPMorgan Chase partnership); direct primary care model; and wellness program model including subscription type payment services, concierge medicine services, networks of primary care physicians providing patient retention, personalized medicine, and preventive care (MD VIP for example). Significant outcomes such as lowering healthcare costs, enhancing the quality and delivery of healthcare services, improving patient satisfaction, and promoting overall sustainability are addressed, including their implications for various stakeholders.

    Jeff Gourdji, Prophet, USA
    Scott M. Davis, Prophet, USA

In the face of government reform and competitive disruption, healthcare organizations are in need of consumer-centric transformation: transformation that will help them win when consumers shop for a doctor, plan, or medicine and engage them in their care to form a partnership that will improve outcomes and lower costs. The authors interviewed 70 senior executives at leading provider systems, health plans, and pharmaceutical manufacturers to understand their transformation agenda. Interviews asked such question as What initiatives and changes are underway? Where have they had success? What will come next? Where have they struggled?" And, most importantly, What can others learn from them? Davis and Gourdji uncovered five shifts and share practical advice and examples of what these leaders are doing to set them in motion.

Section 2

    Adam Greer, Ascension St. John Medical Center, USA
    Roshini Isabell Selladurai, In His Image Family Medicine Residency,
        Ascension St. John Medical Center, USA
    Andrea L. Pfeifle, Indiana University, USA
    Raj Selladurai, Indiana University Northwest, USA
    Charles J. Hobson, Indiana University Northwest, USA

The chapter focuses on high-performing people and effective teamwork in healthcare at accountable care organizations (ACOs). Studies have found that patients are more satisfied when they engage with providers who understand and express their 'soft-skill' competencies. The model presented will illustrate how teamwork training and innovative care, Leader-less Group Discussions, interprofessional education and communication, and leadership/top management support have been found to positively impact effective teamwork, which in turn would synergistically impact the quadruple aim of patient experience, quality of patient care, lower cost, and provider satisfaction. Patient satisfaction is closely linked to provider related outcomes such as employee performance, job satisfaction, and reducing costs.

The American healthcare system is vast and complex. An overview of the United States' healthcare system provides a view into the interrelated dynamics between three categories of factors: consumers, intermediaries, and providers. Consumers demand health inputs in order to produce health status that allows them to live productive lives. Intermediaries, such as insurance companies and government programs, reduce the direct cost of healthcare for consumers. Providers, such as hospitals and physicians, amongst others, have historically exhibited a degree of monopolistic power in the healthcare market. The modern trend towards managed care organizations, firms that vertically integrate multiple aspects of the healthcare market, aims to reduce costs imposed by such providers.

The Health Insurance Portability and Accountability Act of 1996 (HIPAA) was initially enacted as an administrative simplification to standardize electronic transmission of common administrative and financial transactions. The program also calls for implementation specifications regarding privacy and security standards to protect the confidentiality and integrity of individually identifiable health information or protected health information. The Affordable Care Act further expanded many of the protective provisions set forth by HIPAA. Since its implementation, healthcare organizations around the nation have invested billions of dollars and have cycled through numerous program attempts aimed at meeting these standards. This chapter reviews the process taken by one organization to review the privacy policy in place utilizing a maturity model, identify deficiencies, and lead change in order to heighten the maturity of the system. The authors conclude with reflection related to effectiveness of the process as well as implications for practice.

The healthcare system in the U.S. is very fragmented in its structure. It is generally agreed that it needs to be reformed. This chapter addresses this issue from an organizational point of view with specific reference to cancer, a disease termed "The Emperor of All Maladies." The basic tenet of this chapter is that any healthcare system should be designed so as to maximize the benefit to all the stakeholders involved, while incorporating the newer advances in technologies, but above all, must be patient-centered. Solving a complex adaptive problem requires different approaches compared to solving a simple technical challenge. Especially, when it comes to dealing with cancer—a very intelligent, continually adapting, rule breaking, self-sustaining disease—simple technical solutions are insufficient without an understanding of how to change the system. After discussing the current healthcare system in the U.S., a proposal is made as to how to reform the system.

Mapping opportunities and challenges of telemedicine adoption in an emerging economy has always been presumptive due to the scarcity of empirical evidence. Only recently the potential influencing factors of both issues in the rural context of emerging economies (using Bangladesh as a cases study) were investigated. Analysis of existing literature identified seven broad categories of challenges (e.g., deficient organisational commitment, inadequate technological infrastructure, insufficient resource allocations, deficient service quality, clinicians demotivation, patients' dissatisfaction, and patients' distrust) and six broad categories of opportunities (e.g., service usefulness, service assurance, secured patient privacy, adequacy of services, peer influence on use of services, and environmental conditions) concerning telemedicine adoption. Their significance is outlined. These findings contribute to the literature by distinguishing significant factors, which can positively favour or deter telemedicine implementation in developing countries and similar settings.

Section 3

Chapter 9

Interprofessionality: A Pathway to a More Sustainable National Healthcare
Chidiebele Constance Obichi, Indiana University Northwest, USA
April D. Newton, Indiana University, USA
Ukamaka Marian Oruche, Indiana University, USA

Preventable medical errors (PME) is the third leading cause of death in the United States with an incidence range of 210,000 to 400,000 deaths per year and an estimated cost of $19.5 billion to $958 billion per year. Despite advances in patient safety, PME persists across the nation. An unmarked extremity, a soft sponge, medication dose, poor communication, etc. are possible precursors of PME that may lead to death. Preventable medical errors such as wrong-patient or wrong-site surgery, botched transplants, and death from myocardial infarction or septic shock following a discharge from the emergency department are frequently reported. According to the Institute of Medicine, most PME in the healthcare system are caused by poor team collaboration and care coordination, particularly when patient care was provided by independent providers. Therefore, the healthcare workforce must work within interprofessional teams for safe, cost-effective, and quality care delivery significant to sustainable healthcare reform.

Chapter 10

Overview of Professionalism Competence: Bringing Balance to the Medical
Barry A. Doublestein, Regent University, USA
Walter T. Lee, Duke University Medical School, USA
Richard M. Pfohl, Leadership Peaks, LLC, USA

Lately, the term 'high-value care' has become a popular mantra among healthcare leaders and policymakers. These people claim that changes are necessary in healthcare to reduce costs, minimize overuse, and optimize outcomes. While few can argue that changes are needed in these areas, there is disagreement as to how to make the largest impact. The authors agree with those who believe that the greatest potential for success is found in professionalism improvements, not through payment or policy reforms. While medical education prides itself on producing highly competent and technically proficient physicians, it has generally neglected professionalism development considering these skills something to be acquired outside of formal medical education. The authors consider recent efforts to define professionalism competency and offer a useful model that brings parity to physician training. If professionalism is the bedrock of high-value care, the time has come to provide physicians with the skills to excel.

The existing medical education paradigm is not structured in a way that prepares future physicians with knowledge or the skill set to excel in professionalism. The authors provide information in the form of a case study of a professionalism competency development program that was undertaken in the Duke University Medical School Division of Head and Neck Surgery and Communications Sciences, barriers found that impede development, and offer five reforms that are necessary in order to bring about the movement toward high-value care. The authors propose to 1) prioritize professionalism competency training in medical education, 2) make curricular revisions to promote professionalism competency training across the continuum, 3) revise selection criteria for entrance to the profession that deals with basic professionalism skills, 4) institute new prerequisite requirements for entrance to the profession centered on professionalism competency, and 5) require professionalism competency training as part of certification and re-certification processes.

Foreword

The complexity and super specialization of the United States health care system complicates and prevents high quality health outcomes that should occur based on the number of dollars spent. The editors and authors have presented options and opportunities for reformation that should encourage innovation and improved health care. We as leaders in health care delivery and design must move forward the ideas brought by the authors and others to engage and change our system allowing improvement in the health of all Americans.

Douglas W. Curran
Lakeland Associates, USA & UT Health Athens, USA

Douglas W. Curran, *who practices at Lakeland Associates and at UT Health Athens, pushed for the passage of Texas' groundbreaking medical liability reforms in 2003; fought for sweeping patient-rights protections including holding managed care insurance companies accountable for their actions; supported legislation to improve the Children's Health Insurance Program (CHIP) and Medicaid; and fought to protect patients from unsafe care. He has testified before legislative committees countless times, and visits regularly with Texas and Washington lawmakers to push for a better health care system. Dr. Curran has been very active in his 38 years in TMA. He is the immediate past-chair of the TMA Board of Trustees and a member of TMA's Select Committee on Medicaid, CHIP, and the Uninsured. He chaired TMA's Select Committee on National Health System Reform, served on the TMA PracticeEdge Board of Managers; was district vice chair of TEXPAC, the association's political action committee; and a member of the board of the philanthropic TMA Foundation. Dr. Curran also has represented the Henderson County Medical Society in the TMA House of Delegates, the association's policymaking body, for more than 20 years. He is a past president of the Texas Academy of Family Physicians (TAFP); has chaired two of the group's commissions, and served on the TAFP Board of Directors. Dr. Curran also has served in the American Academy of Family Physicians and its Commission for Governmental Advocacy. The family physician has received many awards and accolades, including the Rural Health Champion Award from the Texas Rural Health Association in 2017. Dr. Curran and his wife, Sandy, have been married for 49 years. They have a daughter, Cortney, and a son, Chris, and daughter-in-law, Britne. Dr. Curran enjoys serving his church, visiting with friends and neighbors, and dancing to a "good Texas swing band" when possible. The country doctor lives on a ranch just outside of Athens and tends to 221 head of cattle. Doing so connects him to the roots of his upbringing in Arkansas, where he attended medical school at the University of Arkansas for Medical Sciences. He completed his residency at The University of Texas Southwestern Medical School Family Medicine Residency Program at John Peter Smith Hospital in Fort Worth.*

Preface

Hope is a psychological need that universally impacts every human heart. Perhaps it is the most dominant of all psychological, spiritual, and medical needs. Dr. McNair Wilson stated in his autobiography, *Doctor's Progress*, "Those who require heart surgery need hope. Hope is the medicine I use more than any other – hope can cure nearly anything" (Wilson, 1938). Dr. Wilson's inspirational comments on hope are still so appropriate today for all our physicians and medical professionals in healthcare to remember and emulate as they serve their patients in the world!

The purpose of our book, *Evaluating Challenges and Opportunities for Healthcare Reform*, focuses on our continual hope that it would add value to our nation's healthcare system reform. Though complicated as it may be, healthcare reform needs continuous improvement toward developing a more optimal, sustainable healthcare system to benefit all the stakeholders in the US. Among some unique aspects of this book, one that stands out is that several authors have written chapter/s from their very own personal experiences, perspectives, and interactions with our healthcare system in the US. Although the US healthcare system is not the perfect system, yet it is considered as one of the largest and one of the best in the world today (America Next, 2014). It is considered to be the source for several amazing innovations, especially in the medical fields, and provides the best, high-quality care for those who need it at the right time. The US has some of the best physicians, nurses, researchers, and healthcare provider systems in the world. People from all over the world, including leaders and influential people, when needing critical lifesaving treatments, services, and surgeries, come to the US. "It is here, in America, where treatments are discovered, methods are improved, and diseases are cured" (America Next, 2014, p. 3). Overall, the US healthcare system is remarkably resilient, indeed. It continues to thrive despite all the dynamic factors that impact our healthcare systems, such as the number of stakeholders, complexity of healthcare, large size of the country, costs and quality-related issues, and partisan groups' conflicting priorities, views, and perspectives.

Healthcare Reform in the United States is a significant, actively debated issue facing the nation since the early 1900s through current times. Despite the recently developed Affordable Care Act and several existing healthcare plans, the country is continually attempting to improve, revise, develop a more optimal, sustainable, and comprehensive healthcare system resulting in a win-win for all key stakeholders. The American Medical Association's (AMA) leader Steven Stack (2016) has discussed the several challenges and opportunities related to creating a more sustainable healthcare system. He asks all American physicians the question, "How can we best adapt to change?" (p. 156). All stakeholders need to ask the question, "For a win-win for all, how best can we all adapt to changes leading us toward an optimal sustainable healthcare system for our nation?

In this book project, we have attempted to explore, analyze, discuss, and present various challenges and opportunities in healthcare reform. Also, we would be discussing and evaluating some potentially new, revised, and improved models such as direct primary care (DPC), accounting care organizations (ACO), corporate partnerships models, and other optimal patient care related models. Further, based on finding common ground and by integrating the various models and approaches, we plan to develop rational, feasible policy recommendations toward a more sustainable national healthcare system.

The objectives of our healthcare reform book include:

- To present comprehensive coverage of healthcare reform in terms of various challenges and opportunities.
- To develop new models of healthcare system/s toward sustainable, optimal healthcare.
- To present the views and perspectives of key stakeholders, including scholars, academicians, physicians, dentists, physician assistants, nurses, healthcare leaders, and practitioners from a variety of fields – medical, healthcare-related, private, public, academic, business, and other areas.

IMPACT

Our book project would add significant value to the current healthcare reform debate and discussions in a variety of settings, including in the U.S Congress and state legislative levels, medical and healthcare fields, business, academia, and industry, etc. It would have a significant impact on healthcare policy development toward a more sustainable optimal healthcare system.

The target audience would include all key stakeholders in the U.S interested in healthcare. These would consist of scholars, physicians, healthcare leaders, academicians, and practitioners from a variety of fields – academic, business, industry, medical, healthcare-related, private, public, and others. Our book would be useful to the general public, too, who will be most impacted by the current and future healthcare plans for them and their family members. It would also be beneficial to government leaders and policy-makers such as the U.S Congress, state legislatures, and other government agencies. Physicians and other healthcare personnel would use the book to understand better the "big picture" of why many changes are necessary and implemented, especially to improve quality and decrease costs. The book would be used to help all interested key stakeholders and policymakers to make better-informed decisions related to healthcare reform and policy development for the United States and to help all individuals and families in their decisions related to choices of optimal healthcare plans.

Out healthcare reform book is divided into three sections. Section 1 explores some innovative, new, enhanced healthcare models, including the latest shifts in healthcare toward patient-centricity and emerging transformations in the healthcare field.

Authors Raj Selladurai and Roshini Selladurai in Chapter 1, titled "An Enhanced Healthcare Delivery System Model for the US: Adaptation of Principles from the 'Best,'" focused on developing a bipartisan, enhanced US healthcare delivery system model. This new model includes five different plans to choose from by learning from the "best" healthcare systems in the world and adapting some of their best working principles to the existing US healthcare system. These global systems include the Swiss healthcare system, which is considered one of the best in the world, and some of the other leading healthcare systems such as the German, British, French, Italian, and Singaporean. It would also explore, among a few healthcare alternatives, the state innovation-based approach to healthcare reform. Major concerns such as cost containment, affordability, flexibility, accessibility, feasibility, and implementation related issues have been addressed.

In Chapter 2, "Exploring Innovative, Alternative Healthcare Models in the US," the authors Raj Selladurai, Roshini Selladurai, and George VandeWerken explored, discussed, analyzed, and present some recommendations for new, innovative alternative healthcare models to the traditional insurance and healthcare models that currently exist. These include a revised and enhanced hybrid model of healthcare; healthcare cost-sharing faith-based model; healthcare cost-reduction corporate partnership model (for example, Amazon, Berkshire Hathaway, and JPMorgan Chase partnership); direct primary care model, and wellness program model including subscription type payment services, concierge medicine services, networks of primary care physicians providing patient retention, personalized medicine, and preventive care (MD VIP for example). Significant outcomes such as lowering healthcare costs, enhancing the quality and delivery of healthcare services, improving patient satisfaction, and promoting overall sustainability are addressed, including their implications for various stakeholders.

Similarly, authors Jeff Gourdji and Scott Davis focused on the new shifts in healthcare, government reform, and competitive disruption in Chapter 3. Healthcare organizations need consumer-centric transformation, a transformation that will help them win when consumers shop for a doctor, plan, or medicine, and engage them in their care to form a partnership that will improve outcomes and lower costs. The authors interviewed 70 senior executives at leading provider systems, health plans, and pharmaceutical manufacturers to understand their transformation agenda. Interviews asked such questions as What initiatives and changes are underway? Where have they had success? What will come next? Where have they struggled? And, most importantly, What can others learn from them? The authors have uncovered five shifts in healthcare and shared practical advice and examples of what these leaders are doing to set them in motion.

In Section 2, we have addressed some of the challenges and opportunities that emerge in the discussions and decision-making deliberations of healthcare reform.

In Chapter 4, "Effective Teamwork and Healthcare Delivery Outcomes," the authors Adam Greer, Roshini Selladurai, Andrea Pfeifle, Raj Selladurai, and Charlie Hobson have focused on high-performing people and effective teamwork in healthcare at Accountable Care Organizations (ACOs). Studies have found that patients are more satisfied when they engage with providers who understand and express their 'soft-skill' competencies. The authors concluded that effective teamwork and communication were found to positively impact the quadruple aim of patient experiences, high quality and safe delivery of patient care, lower costs, and provider satisfaction.

Next, in Chapter 5 titled, "The Economics of Health: An Overview of the American Healthcare System," the authors Sean Michael Haas, Sanjana Janumpally, and Brendan Lamar Kouns presented an overview of the United States' healthcare system. It provides a view of the inter-related dynamics between three categories of factors: consumers, intermediaries, and providers. Consumers demand healthy inputs to produce health status that allows them to live productive lives. Intermediaries, such as insurance companies and government programs, reduce the direct cost of healthcare for consumers. Providers, such as hospitals and physicians, amongst others, have historically exhibited a degree of monopolistic power in the healthcare market. The modern trend towards managed care organizations, firms that vertically integrate multiple aspects of the healthcare market, aims to reduce costs imposed by such providers.

In Chapter 6, "Maturing an Information Technology Privacy Program: Assessment, Improvement, and Change Leadership," authors Mike Gregory and Cynthia Roberts have discussed the implications of the Health Insurance Portability and Accountability Act of 1996 (HIPAA). It was initially enacted as an administrative simplification to standardize the electronic transmission of everyday administrative and financial transactions. The program also calls for implementation specifications regarding privacy and security standards to protect the confidentiality and integrity of individually identifiable health information or protected health information. The Affordable Care Act further expanded many of the protective provisions set forth by HIPAA. Since its implementation, healthcare organizations around the nation have invested billions of dollars and have cycled through numerous program attempts aimed at meeting these standards. This chapter reviews the process taken by one organization to review the privacy policy in place utilizing a maturity model, identify deficiencies, and lead change to heighten the maturity of the system. The authors concluded with reflection related to the effectiveness of the process as well as implications for practice.

Subsequently, in Chapter 7, titled "Healthcare Reform: A Dire Need to Retool the System," author Abburi Anil Kumar shared his recent personal experience with the healthcare system in terms of his undergoing treatment and recovery from cancer. He discussed the healthcare system in the U.S. and its very fragmented structure. It is generally agreed that the healthcare system in the U.S. needs to be reformed. The basic tenet of this paper is that any healthcare reform in a capitalist society should be designed to maximize the benefit to all the stakeholders involved, while incorporating the newer advances in technologies, and above all, must be patient-centered. As always, solving a complex adaptive problem requires different approaches than solving a simple technical challenge. Especially when it comes to dealing with cancer – a very intelligent, continually adapting, rule-breaking, self-sustaining disease – simple technical solutions are insufficient without an understanding of how to change the system. After discussing the current healthcare system in the U.S., a proposal is being made as to how to reform the system.

In the following chapter, "Telemedicine Adoption in the Developing World: Opportunities and Challenges," authors Khondker Zobair, Louis Sanzogni, Kuldeep Sandhu, and Md Islam have studied the use of telemedicine in healthcare. Mapping opportunities and challenges of telemedicine adoption in an emerging economy have always been presumptive due to the scarcity of empirical evidence. Only recently, the potential influencing factors of both issues in the rural context of emerging economies (using Bangladesh as a case study) were investigated. Analysis of existing literature identified seven broad categories of challenges (e.g., deficient organizational commitment, inadequate technological infrastructure, insufficient resource allocations, deficient service quality, clinicians demotivation, patients' dissatisfaction, and patients' distrust) and six broad categories of opportunities (e.g., service usefulness, service assurance, secured patient privacy, adequacy of services, peer influence on use of services, and environmental conditions) concerning telemedicine adoption. Their significance is outlined. These findings contribute to the literature by distinguishing significant factors, which can positively favor or deter telemedicine implementation in developing countries and similar settings.

In Section 3, we have made some recommendations related to interprofessionality, professionalism competence, and continuous improvement in the US medical education continuum.

In Chapter 9, "Interprofessionality: A Pathway to a More Sustainable National Healthcare System," the authors Chidiebele Obichi, April Newton, and Ukamaka Oruche have shown the positive effects of interprofessionality on healthcare outcomes such as cost-effective, quality patient care. Preventable medical errors (PME) is the third leading cause of death in the United States with an incidence range of 210,000 to 400,000 deaths per year and an estimated cost of $19.5 billion to $958 billion per year. Despite advances in patient safety, PME persists across the nation. An unmarked extremity, a soft sponge, medication dose, poor communication are possible precursors of PME that may lead to death. Preventable medical errors such as wrong-patient or wrong-site surgery, botched transplants, and death from myocardial infarction or septic shock following discharge from the emergency department are frequently reported. According to the Institute of Medicine, most PME in the healthcare system is caused by poor team collaboration and care coordination, particularly when patient care was provided by independent providers. Therefore, the healthcare workforce must work within interprofessional teams for safe, cost-effective, and quality care delivery significant to sustainable healthcare reform.

Chapter 10 focuses on professionalism competence in medical education continuum. The authors Barry Doublestein, Walter Lee, and Richard Pfohl in their chapter, "Overview of Professionalism Competence: Bringing Balance to the Medical Education Continuum," discussed the term, 'high-value care,' which has become a popular mantra among healthcare leaders and policymakers. These people claim that changes are necessary for healthcare to reduce costs, minimize overuse, and optimize outcomes. While few can argue that changes are needed in these areas, there is disagreement as to how to make the most significant impact. The authors agree with those who believe that the greatest potential for success is found in professionalism improvements, not through payment or policy reforms. While medical education prides itself on producing highly-competent and technically-proficient physicians, it has generally neglected professionalism development, considering these skills something to be acquired outside of formal medical education. The authors consider recent efforts to define professionalism competency and offer a useful model that brings parity to physician training. If professionalism is the bedrock of high-value care, the time has come to provide physicians with the skills to excel.

In Chapter 11, authors Barry Doublestein, Walter Lee, and Richard Pfohl have shown the practice and application of professionalism competence via a case study. They contend that the existing medical education paradigm is not structured in a way that prepares future physicians with the knowledge or the skill set to excel in professionalism. The authors provide information in the form of a case study on a professionalism competency development program that was undertaken in the Duke University Medical School – Division of Head and Neck Surgery and Communications Sciences. They found barriers that impede development, and offer five reforms that are necessary to bring about the movement toward 'high-value care.' The authors propose: 1) prioritize professionalism competency training in medical education; 2) make curricular revisions to promote professionalism competency training across the continuum; 3) revise selection criteria for entrance to the profession that deals with basic professionalism skills; 4) institute new prerequisite requirements for entrance to the profession centered on professionalism competency; and, 5) require professionalism competency training as part of certification and re-certification processes.

In conclusion, our book is a comprehensive, updated effort to explore, analyze, discuss, and present various challenges and opportunities in healthcare reform that would impact millions of stakeholders in the US. It includes scholarly and pragmatic perspectives from a variety of key stakeholders such as scholars, academicians, physicians, dentists, physician assistants, nurses, healthcare leaders, and practitioners from a variety of fields – medical, healthcare-related, private, public, academic, business, and other areas. We believe that such a synergistically produced compilation of chapters on healthcare reform in this book project would make an exceptional contribution to sustainable and optimal healthcare reform in the United States.

Our editorial team would like you our readers to join us and participate in this vital process of discussions and deliberations on healthcare reform for the US. We welcome your input, opinions, thoughts, and suggestions as we attempt to add value to healthcare reform and assist our leaders and policymakers in developing an optimal, sustainable healthcare system to benefit all the stakeholders in the US. Please feel free to connect with us at healthcarereform2020@gmail.com

We look forward to hearing from you! Thank you.

Raj Selladurai
Indiana University Northwest, USA

Charlie Hobson
Indiana University Northwest, USA

Roshini Selladurai
In His Image Family Medicine Residency, Ascension St. John Medical Center, USA

Adam Greer
Ascension St. John Medical Center, USA

REFERENCES

America Next, . (2014). *The freedom and empowerment plan: The prescription for conservative consumer-focused health reform*. Alexandria, VA: America Next.

Stack, S. J. (2016). Health Care Reform in the United States: Past, Present, and Future Challenges. *World Medical Journal, 62*(4), 153–157.

Wilson, M. (1938). *Doctor's Progress*. Retrieved from https://www.amazon.com/Doctors-progress-reminiscences-McNair-Wilson/dp/B00085YUEY

Acknowledgment

I like to thank my co-editors, Dr. Charlie Hobson, Dr. Roshini Selladurai, and Dr. Adam Greer, for all their advice, recommendations, help, and support for this book. It was indeed a rewarding academic and professional experience working with them on this healthcare book project. I wish to acknowledge my dean, Dr. Cindy Roberts, for her encouragement and support of my research interests and efforts in healthcare management and this healthcare project.

I like to acknowledge every author who made a valuable chapter contribution and added value to our book project. Also, I wish to thank all the Editorial Advisory Board members for their wisdom, advice, and guidance given toward this project. I like to thank all our reviewers for taking the time to review and evaluate the various chapters in our book.

I like to thank my wife, Revathi Rebecca, my daughter Roshini Isabell, and my son Roshan Isaac for their total, continually growing love, patience, support, and encouragement.

Above all, I would like to thank my Lord Jesus for everything, and I wish to dedicate this book to Him all for His glory – Colossians 3:17, 23-24.

Raj Selladurai
Indiana University Northwest, USA

I fully endorse the acknowledgments of our Senior Editor, Dr. Raj Selladurai. I would only add that without his inspirational leadership, this project would have never been conceived or completed. I truly appreciate everything he has done to complete the book.

Charles J. Hobson
Indiana University Northwest, USA

Acknowledgment

I'm grateful to my Heavenly Father for giving me such a brilliant and innovative earthly father who created the concept for this book and has carried it to completion. I've seen the long hours my dad (Dr. Raj Selladurai) has poured into this book, his encouragement to the various authors, his persistence in facilitating conversations on this topic, and his desire to do his part to make this world a better place--this time through writing a textbook on the business of medicine. I'd like to acknowledge and celebrate all of his hard work, as well as the contributions of all involved in this project--including my co-editors, the various authors, advisory board members, and chapter reviewers. Thank you also to my wonderful mom who is the master encourager, my brother who keeps us all laughing, and my dogs Houston and Winston for always entertaining us. As a physician, I want the best for my patients—I hope this book helps us all continue to improve our healthcare system to provide excellent medical care.

Roshini Selladurai
In His Image Family Medicine Residency, Ascension St. John Medical Center,
USA

First of all I would like to thank Jesus for being the reason I could have ever made my way through medical school at Oklahoma State University and In His Image Family Medicine residency to be in a position to be an editor for a book on healthcare reform, and especially have to thank my wife Hillary for sticking with me through it all. I have enjoyed my experience working with my co-editors, authors, and editorial advisory board on this project and hope that it will be beneficial as the US healthcare system is in a complicated state of flux and significant change at this moment. I appreciate Ascension St. John allowing me to participate helping paint several possible ways forward in the healthcare arena and hope that we can use the concepts presented here to significantly improve the quality of care for every American moving forward.

Adam Greer
Ascension St. John Medical Center, USA

Section 1

Chapter 1
An Enhanced Healthcare Delivery System Model for the US:
Adaptation of Principles From the "Best"

Raj Selladurai
 https://orcid.org/0000-0003-4126-4160
Indiana University Northwest, USA

Roshini Isabell Selladurai
In His Image Family Medicine Residency, Ascension St. John Medical Center, USA

ABSTRACT

This chapter focuses on developing an enhanced US healthcare delivery system model by learning from the "best" healthcare systems in the world and adapting some of their best working principles to the existing US healthcare system. These global systems include the Swiss healthcare system, which is considered one of the best in the world, and some of the other leading healthcare systems such as the German, the UK, French, Italian, and Singaporean. It would also explore, among a few alternatives, the state innovation-based approach to healthcare reform. Major concerns such as cost containment, affordability, flexibility, accessibility, feasibility, and implementation-related issues have been addressed.

DOI: 10.4018/978-1-7998-2949-2.ch001

INTRODUCTION

The focus of this chapter is to develop an enhanced US healthcare delivery system model by learning from some of the other "best" healthcare systems in the world, including Switzerland, Germany, the UK, France, Italy, and Singapore, and adapting some of their best working principles toward the enhanced US healthcare delivery system model. The objectives include to present a background, based on a review of the literature, some of the powerful features of the best healthcare systems in the world, and then to develop an enhanced healthcare system model for the US by adopting and adapting these best principles to the US healthcare system model. Also, the chapter would evaluate the enhanced hybrid healthcare model and other related models in terms of outcomes such as cost containment, affordability, flexibility, accessibility, feasibility, and implementation issues.

BACKGROUND

Healthcare reform involves challenges and complexities due to the very nature of the subject – that all people have access to and receive useful, reasonable quality healthcare, which is an essential part of human life. Further, especially as one gets older, healthcare becomes more of a critical necessity for a good quality of life. Questions such as do we use public or private insurance plans, employer-provided plans, or some other group or organizational provided plans have to be addressed. Is healthcare a federally administered program, or should it be handled and managed at the state levels by each state, respectively? What about people who may not be employed or those who are self-employed, or those who may not be offered or are ineligible for healthcare from their employer/s?

And why did/does the US need healthcare reform in the first place? The current healthcare system in the US is one of the largest and the best in the world (America Next, 2014). It is considered to be the source for several amazing innovations, especially in the medical fields, and provides the best, high-quality care for those who need it at the right time. The US has some of the best physicians, nurses, researchers, and healthcare provider systems in the world. People from all over the world, including leaders and influential people, when needing critical lifesaving treatments, services, and surgeries, come to the US. "It is here, in America, where treatments are discovered, methods are improved, and diseases are cured" (America Next, 2014, p. 3).

However, despite having the best healthcare system in the world, the US still has to address and manage several continuing problems, complexities, high costs, universal access, universal coverage, and other related issues. Before the passage of the Affordable Care Act (ACA), several estimates showed that approximately 50 million Americans were not insured; healthcare costs were increasing tremendously; and about 50% of the American adult population suffered from chronic problems such as diabetes, blood pressure, and heart-related conditions and diseases. Hence the healthcare system in the US was not optimally sustainable, and some form of healthcare reform became very necessary to address these problems. After multiple series of heated discussions and controversial debates in the US Congress related to healthcare, the Affordable Care Act (ACA) was passed in 2010. It was supposed to have been a more sustainable healthcare system and was designed primarily to address the lack of healthcare insurance coverage for the uninsured millions of Americans in the country. But several years later, despite providing expanded coverage for millions of Americans, the ACA faces significant serious challenges and shortcomings. Studies showed that many people still are unable to get access to affordable healthcare insurance, that the costs of healthcare are skyrocketing in many states and regions of the country, and several insurance companies are exiting from unprofitable markets, leaving millions stranded to fend for themselves (Stack, 2016).

MAIN FOCUS OF THE CHAPTER

The main focus of this chapter is the development of a bipartisan, enhanced healthcare delivery system in the US-based on the "best" principles from some of the global healthcare systems that have been adapted to fit the US healthcare delivery system.

Issues, Controversies, Problems

Healthcare reform has been a contentious issue for many years and went through several controversial debates over the years. After much planning, collaborating, having lengthy discussions, and involving in collaborative deliberations in various settings, including the US Congress, the Affordable Care Act (ACA) healthcare bill was passed in 2010. It was considered to be the right, first step in making healthcare more affordable and accessible for the lower and moderate-income segments of the US population (Jost & Pollack, 2018). However, many scholars and experts believe that this healthcare bill was unconstitutional. It was considered more a tax bill legislation (as confirmed by Justice Roberts in the Supreme Court) and as so should have originated in the House of Representatives, but it did not, and originated instead in the Democratic majority led Senate (McCarthy, A, 2013). It was then passed in the House of Representatives, and subsequently, it was signed as an executive order by President Barack Obama in 2010 (McCarthy, A, 2013). Also, one of the critical factors/promises of the new ACA health care package proposal was that if American

3

citizens "wished to keep their plans, keep their doctor" they could. This promise also did not fully materialize as intended, and so further plans and discussions about repealing, modifying, revising, and enhancing the current healthcare have emerged. One such concerted effort over several weeks resulted in a narrow unsuccessful vote in the US Senate in 2018. However, this ACA healthcare law continues to be controversial, and the whole healthcare issue is expected to gain momentum again in the 2020 election year. Studies show that in the US around 177 million Americans (more than half of the country) pay for and rely on private health insurance from their jobs provided by their employers or some group or organization, or by insurance companies. And Gallop polls have shown that most Americans (around 70 percent) positively rated the quality of their private healthcare plans, and therefore would like to continue keeping their individual healthcare plans (McCarthy, J., 2018).

ANALYSIS

"Best Models" and Adaptable Lessons

The following section, based on a review of the literature, highlights the key attributes of the major European systems, including Switzerland, Germany, the UK, France, Italy, and others like Singapore, that make up the leading global healthcare systems. Some of the lessons learned from these global systems are analyzed and presented, and how these lessons and principles may be adapted to enhance the US healthcare system.

Swiss Healthcare System

Why is the Swiss healthcare system considered by many scholars and experts as the best in the world?

One of the significant strengths of the Swiss healthcare systems is the universal coverage provided for all of its citizens at an optimal cost. Hence, it is remarkable indeed considering the Swiss government spends only about 2.7 percent of GDP on healthcare, which is the lowest among the developed countries. Compared to the Swiss, the US government spends 7.4 percent of GDP on healthcare, and if the US were to cut its healthcare costs about 50% to spend more closely to what the Swiss government spends, the US would benefit tremendously from more than 700 billion savings a year (Roy, 2011). Also, the Swiss ensure an individual mandate system where insurance coverage is mandatory for every individual, with the Swiss government providing subsidies for the needy; one-third of all the insured citizens have received subsidies for their healthcare ("United States: Swiss health system offers key lessons," 2008). Other features that make the Swiss healthcare the best in the world are that the Swiss have access to the latest healthcare technology and healthcare services, just as the American citizens do, have comparably efficient patient care services, and low waiting times for appointments, services, and procedures. Further, the Swiss people are considered to be among the healthiest in the world, with a focus on wellness programs, eating healthy, fitness and exercise, etc., and their average life expectancy is the second-best in the world, next to Japan, which has the highest life expectancy potential for its people in the world.

Interestingly, unlike in the US, the majority of Swiss citizens buy their healthcare insurance for themselves -- private insurance plans; they do not have any government-sponsored or employer-provided plans. Hence, prices and cost optimization choices are critical, transparent elements to the consumer beneficiary (Roy, 2011). The Swiss government determines the minimum benefit package for all of the citizens, and the citizens have to pay a certain percentage of the healthcare costs in terms of deductibles and coinsurance. Hence, their healthcare system motivates the citizens to be more conscious and thrifty in choosing the customized healthcare services relevant to their needs and paying the best optimal prices for healthcare.

For the poor citizens or those who cannot afford it, the Swiss government subsidizes healthcare on a graduated basis to ensure that no more than ten percent of their income is spent toward healthcare. If they wish to get supplemental coverage, they may do so by paying out of pocket themselves. Almost 100 percent of all Swiss citizens have health insurance coverage; they may choose from about 100 private insurance companies, who compete effectively by providing optimal services and prices to win and maintain their loyal Swiss customers. Citizens may freely choose their doctors, and appointment waiting times are relatively low, similar to those in the US.

The Swiss have a unique healthcare system in which the citizens can consume healthcare in value and cost-conscious ways. It is a healthcare system that includes a private, consumer-choice program to buy healthcare insurance from one of many private insurance providers, but it is also regulated by the Swiss government that defines the minimum benefit package and other related mandates. In the US, a majority of the citizens receive their healthcare coverage through their employer-sponsored programs or the government, and only 10 percent of Americans buy private insurance for themselves. In Switzerland, however, 100 percent of the citizens purchase insurance for themselves.

Lastly, the critical driving force for the universal healthcare system in Switzerland is the political bipartisanship solution – it pleases the liberal policy-makers' interests of universal healthcare coverage, and regulated insurance market, and also it wins support from the conservatives in terms of low government healthcare expenditures and privately managed healthcare.

German Healthcare System

Unlike the Swiss healthcare system, the German state is not responsible for managing and controlling healthcare programs and expenses. Professional, regional, and local healthcare funds manage healthcare programs and expenses. The Allgemeine Ortkrankenkassen (AOK) handles the private companies; Betriebskrankenkassen (BKK) manages the large companies including Krupp and Bayer; for corporations, tradesmen, and craftsmen, the Innungkrankenkassen (IKK) manages the healthcare; and for farmers, the Landwirtschaftliche Krankenkassen (LKK) takes care of their healthcare programs (Simonet, 2010). These various local organizations operate nationally, are both autonomous (they fix the premiums, manage all their resources, fees, and costs, but they are regulated as patient contribution rates are decided by a committee bi-annually. The premiums and health services are monitored by the law, which ensures stability in the health care system and protects the most vulnerable – the older pensioners. The public-private partnership in the German healthcare system involves the federal government to control and manage hospital planning and construction, whereas the health insurance funds finance the operating costs. Just like in Switzerland, universal health care is available for all Germans, and the patient can choose an insurance plan of his/her choice and the provider from the several 50+ private for-profit insurers. Several measures were introduced to encourage competition among insurance companies, which led to more equal premium rates for all the insured. In 2001, the government introduced insurance capitalization to replace traditional insurers. Employees directly received the employer's insurance contribution, which was then used by the employee to buy any private insurance plan. Though several decentralized measures to manage healthcare were introduced prior to the 1990s, subsequently and more recently, the German health care has become more of a centralized decision-making structure (Simonet, 2010). The German healthcare system today is a three-fold system – self-governed, private, social, not for profit, and public operator system. Among the healthcare providers, one-third of the hospitals are public, one-third is private and not for profit, and one third is private and for profit. Overall, it is still a private-public partnership that is responsible for providing healthcare in Germany.

The United Kingdom (UK) Healthcare

Unlike the US healthcare system, the UK healthcare system is based on a National Health Service (NHS) that is responsible to the British Parliament; and it is financed primarily from taxes (81 percent), national insurance contributions (15 percent), and some other sources. And like the Swiss and German healthcare systems, the UK healthcare system is also universal healthcare for all (Simonet, 2010). Similar to the German healthcare system, the UK system is also composed of decentralized healthcare services by dividing the Department of Health into geographic areas and districts. Though access to hospital services was free for all patients, the long wait to receive services led many to seek private providers and insurers. Waiting for hospital services in many cases was about three to six months for specialists' appointments and about six months for surgical procedures. Hence, private insurance was a much-needed alternative that was available with the NHS, and about four million British citizens bought their own private medical insurance (Richard, 1996). The healthcare system encouraged competition so that the General Practitioners (GP), acting on behalf of their patients, could choose and pay for most appropriate and optimal healthcare. They negotiated the best and cheapest treatment available (for example specialized services, medical screening exams, medicine prescriptions, etc.) directly with the private clinical staff and hospitals that they chose, emphasizing the highly competitive market that healthcare providers were competing in, to secure the lowest rates and improved service quality for their patients (Simonet, 2010).

In spite of some definite healthcare positives like new hospitals, a national cardiac disease campaign, and new openings for physicians, the NHS encountered much criticism and controversies. Costs of healthcare in the UK were much higher than the European Union countries; its budget is lower, and its deficit increased from £250 million in the early 2000s to £590 million in 2006 (Simonet, 2010). Long waiting lines, more deaths due to prescription errors committed in the hospital systems, nursing and medical staff shortages, wastage of resources including time, and many missed consultations over 17 million annually! So, although universal health care was a significant advantage of healthcare in the UK, private healthcare was a much better alternative to the federal healthcare system, and many British citizens were in favor of purchasing their own private insurance and healthcare services.

French Healthcare Networks

Unlike the German and some other European systems, the French healthcare system gave the government more authority on healthcare-related decisions and affairs. Managed care was not used in France due to patient freedom, little to no competition between healthcare insurance providers, and state-controlled lower prices that decreased the need for price competition amongst healthcare providers. The French healthcare system enjoyed a significant advantage in that it allowed patients the freedom to choose their own physicians. This choice of physicians is in sharp contrast to the apparent lack of continuing to keeping your prior physician/s, which is a compelling disadvantage and perceived weakness that is drawing heavy criticism in the US with its managed healthcare system, especially with the ACA federal healthcare program. The French healthcare system is also focused on strengthening healthcare networks (more than 300 currently) to improve communication and networking activities between healthcare professionals, developing complementing collaboration between general practitioners and specialists, and enhancing coordination among all healthcare providers and stakeholders, all of which are aimed to provide high-quality healthcare to their patients (Simonet, 2010).

Italian Healthcare System

Prior to the 1978 healthcare reform in Italy, workers' healthcare was managed at the national level. It did not cover everyone in the population even though the constitution considered healthcare as every citizen's basic right. Several smaller private insurance companies offered services then; however, the National Institute for Health Assistance (NIHA) was the dominant, significant insurer. It covered 75 percent of the Italian population and managed a healthcare provider national network. The NIHA also managed its own infrastructures and paid general practitioners a capitation fee (Simonet, 2010). However, dissatisfaction increased rapidly among citizens, public deficits grew, insurer indebtedness increased, and the new coalition in political power emerged to manage the country, all of which gave rise to the major healthcare reform in 1978. The Italian healthcare reform offered universal healthcare to all citizens but also encouraged decentralization, health services planning, and more delegation of authority by dividing the country into 600 local sanitary units, which were responsible for healthcare planning, evaluation of local provider effectiveness, and the allocation of healthcare-related resources. However, local management of healthcare ran into several problems of high costs, rising budget deficits, increased public indebtedness that reforms again became necessary in the 1990s. After the 1992 reform, about 200 small-scale local units provided healthcare to the local population with tighter management control. GPs were paid a capitation fee and acted as gatekeepers to make referrals of patients to specialists or hospitals. Overall, the patients had full access to healthcare, and they could choose their own healthcare providers, physicians, and hospitals, but they have to wait long for their healthcare services (Simonet, 2010).

Singapore And Mixed Economy

The mixed economy solution in healthcare in Singapore has unique challenges for implementation. The blending of both private and public providers, as well as high government regulation of policies, rules, and legal constraints, are best exemplified in the Singapore and Swiss healthcare economies (Bessard, 2008). The Singapore residents' high life expectancy (80 years) is similar to the Swiss life expectancy (82 years), and the infant mortality rates are lower; yet, it costs four times less per capita than the Swiss healthcare system. Singapore seems to make more optimal use of its resources –it has fewer (about 65 percent less) physicians per 10,000 residents than Switzerland and has a higher ratio of nurses to physicians. Also, in Singapore, 68% of healthcare expenditures are market-based, whereas it is 40% in Switzerland; and 94% of private spending is made through out-of-pocket cash against 76% in the Swiss healthcare system (Bessard, 2008). Singapore's successful healthcare system is due primarily to the high degree of consumer choice given to its citizens. The residents are encouraged to effectively take better care and control of their health to avoid or minimize unfavorable health and financial consequences. All healthcare decisions are made between the best parties to do so – patients with their physicians, rather than politicians and third-party vendors. For the small proportion of those unable to manage their own healthcare, the government provided tax-funded medical care through its public hospitals. Overall, Singapore residents have access to the full choice of providers and high-quality healthcare. Individuals taking responsibility for their own healthcare has been implemented effectively in Singapore, and the government has a subsidiary part. Medisave, a mandatory national healthcare savings system of individual accounts, has been set up by the Singapore government. Every month, a percentage of every employee's salary or self-employed individual's income is invested into a personal savings account, enabling the residents to build up a healthcare-related fund for healthcare expenses. All healthcare-related expenses for hospitalization, treatments, and outpatient treatment expenses can be paid from the owner's personal savings account or immediate family members' accounts. Medisave enables patients to pay for their own healthcare and depend less on government subsidies, so the government can channel the subsidies to the less wealthy and to those who need these more (Cheong, 2004).

In addition to Medisave, the Singapore government has set up MediShield, a supplementary voluntary health insurance program for cases of unexpected serious long term illnesses or/and hospitalization. Medisave accounts may be used to pay for MediShield, which has low, age-related premiums to encourage more participation. Residents have the choice to pay for and buy additional insurance coverage through government-approved private insurers for more health-related products and services as they see it. For about 10 percent of the population that cannot afford savings or insurance, the government has set up Medifund to help provide healthcare to these needy citizens.

The various incentive programs, the emphasis on individual responsibility, compulsory savings with limited use, withdrawal limits, co-payments, and the freedom of choice given to consumers have all led to favorable results. Residents have voluntarily chosen healthier lifestyles as prevention costs are better/lower than medical costs. Also, the Singapore government often offers extensive nutrition, exercise, anti-smoking, and anti-stress programs for its residents. And the results show that the percentage of overweight individuals and smokers is relatively lower in Singapore than in most countries, including Switzerland (Bessard, 2008). All these, together with more transparency required from providers to make available to their patients' information on charges and itemized billing listing for every service and amount, have led to better innovation and cost reduction outcomes.

Common Principles and Lessons

On the whole, the selected global healthcare systems all had some key principles in common. These included universal coverage for all citizens, and thus, they had to respond to political and social pressures from professionals and patients nationwide. The countries offered universal coverage to all their residents in different ways – in the UK, a national healthcare control system through the NHS, and Switzerland offered a comprehensive, universal coverage by mandating health insurance for all citizens, who could choose to buy their own healthcare insurance companies from several private companies, and the government was also subsidizing health insurance premiums. These countries also showed that universal coverage came with high healthcare outcomes. They also showed that the best of the healthcare systems had limitations. British physicians had limited bargaining power over providers (hospitals). The various partners and stakeholders in the healthcare system were not collaboratively organized to maintain optimal effectiveness, and so transaction costs were very high.

Similarly, in the Swiss healthcare system, rising patient empowerment to choose their insurer and to pay premiums directly to them, and more competition between insurers to sell patients their healthcare were all insufficient to minimize the healthcare costs. Further, several factors such as lack of control over physicians, lack of access to patient data due to confidentiality laws, etc. have prevented the reform of primary care physicians especially in France, Italy, and Germany, and thus cost control was difficult to implement (Simonet, 2010). Countries like Switzerland and Germany have less federal government control and more local control leading to more competition and better reforms; non-competition based healthcare like in France, which has substantial central government control, has slower reforms. Decentralization and more local levels of healthcare systems, especially in Germany, the UK, and Italy, which were intended to lower the cost of healthcare have not always materialized. Also, price competition is difficult to implement and sustain in healthcare, and the UK fund-holders could not get cheaper care for their patients, nor were the Swiss consumers willing to switch insurers to get lower premium rates (Dormant et al., 2007). A common thread across all these European countries' healthcare systems is that none of them supported the US managed type healthcare, although they may have shown some interest in it. Also, it is because EU healthcare systems are heavily regulated and must meet minimum mandatory principles and requirements. However, the US healthcare is more expensive than each of the other EU healthcare systems, but yet it has not been able to provide universal coverage; and also the EU countries' citizens are more likely to accept higher tax burdens to pay for their more generously funded public healthcare programs than their US counterparts.

Table 1 presents the key factors form the best global systems adaptable to suit the US market.

To summarize, the key factors from the best global systems that could be adapted for the US healthcare system and customized to suit the US market would include:

- Universal health coverage –healthcare for all citizens and residents
- Regulation of healthcare insurance programs and patient services
- Freedom to choose from several private insurance plans –privately managed healthcare
- Low, optimal private healthcare costs for individuals and overall low, optimal healthcare expenditures for the government
- Private and public collaboratively managed healthcare
- Individual responsibility-sharing for personal healthcare and well-being

SOLUTIONS AND RECOMMENDATIONS

This section would take some of the lessons learned from the global healthcare systems and present an analysis of how these lessons and principles may be adapted to the US healthcare system markets. Primary outcomes, such as cost containment, affordability, flexibility, accessibility, feasibility, and implementation issues, have been addressed.

Table 1. Key factors from the best global systems

Key factors	Switzerland	Germany	UK	France	Italy	Singapore
Universal health coverage	Yes	Yes	Yes	Yes	Yes	Yes
Regulations	Yes	Yes	Yes	Yes	Yes	Yes
Free choice	Yes	Yes	Yes	Yes	Yes	Yes
Low cost	Yes*	Yes*	Yes*	Yes*	Yes*	Yes*
Private and public managed healthcare	Yes	Yes	Yes	No	Yes	Yes
Individual responsibility	Yes	Yes	Yes	Yes	Yes	Yes

*Goal: low cost, but not always attainable; this is the case with all the healthcare systems, which are trying to lower costs and to maintain optimal sustainability.

Figure 1 presents the current US healthcare system model in the US.

Figure 2 presents the current US healthcare system model – it shows employer-sponsored healthcare plans, which are the most popular type of healthcare coverage and covering a majority of the US population. It also includes the federally sponsored healthcare plan (ACA). In addition to these, several other individual or group-based plans are currently offered to residents in the US. Several faith-based programs such as Medi-Share, Liberty Healthshare, Christian Healthcare Ministries, and Samaritan Ministries are becoming increasingly popular, and as of 2018, over one million

Figure 1. Current US healthcare system model

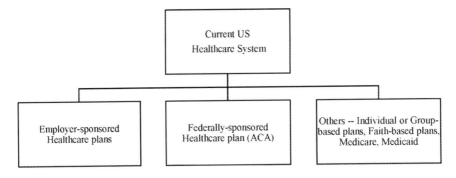

Figure 2. Proposed "Enhanced" US healthcare system model

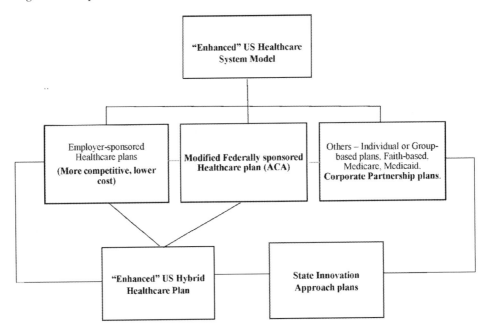

individuals are using these faith-based medical sharing programs (Zamosky, 2018). Further, the traditional and critical federal programs such as Medicare and Medicaid will continue to be offered in the US to all permanent residents and citizens.

In Figure 2, the authors are presenting a proposed "Enhanced" US healthcare system model that covers five different healthcare plan options.

"Enhanced" US Hybrid Healthcare Plan

Figure 3 shows one of the innovative "enhanced" healthcare plans, referred to as the "Enhanced" US Hybrid Healthcare Plan that is developed from the existing employer-sponsored plans and the current ACA plan. Currently, the nation has primarily two major options for healthcare – employer-sponsored private insurance healthcare plans, and the federally sponsored ACA public healthcare plan. The Republican lawmakers almost unanimously seem to support the first type, which is private insurance, and the Democratic lawmakers are wholly supportive of the latter, government-sponsored healthcare for all. Neither extreme solution appears to be the most optimal, sustainable one for the country. Instead, a third option – the "Enhanced" US Hybrid Healthcare Plan option – expected to be almost a wholly non-partisan acceptable plan, would be worth consideration. This option would include several significant features that would appeal to both Republican and Democratic lawmakers. The private insurance healthcare plans, which would consist of competitive options offered at lower, optimal, sustainable costs, sponsored by employers for their employees as job benefits, or privately self-funded plans for small business owners and others, would continue to be used by the majority of the US population for most healthcare-related services. However, for specialized care and expensive specialized treatments, the government plan/s should subside these services' costs. Government subsidies are necessary so that no family should be unnecessarily burdened and often financially wrecked because of some catastrophic illnesses or conditions; especially those that require specialized care and services such as some life-threatening, critical, and necessary cancer treatments, transplants, and other related surgical procedures. The healthcare premiums, co-pays, deductibles, etc. will continue to be paid by the individuals but on a sliding scale related to one's income level (Huckabee, 2019). Similar to most other global healthcare systems, for the less fortunate, more-needy segment of the population that cannot afford to pay for health insurance, the government must provide healthcare for them through subsidies from a safety net fund.

Modified Federal sponsored Healthcare Plan

Further, with the ACA, certain modifications are necessary to improve this healthcare plan. Keeping the positive aspects of the program, such as health insurance was available to millions of people, who did not have health insurance before, and improvements made in quality and efficiency of the healthcare system, revisions are necessary for controlling costs and making it more affordable for more people (Stack, 2016). The medical profession is taking a more active role in promoting healthcare for the country. The American Medical Association (AMA) is encouraging physicians to take the lead and initiative to influence the future healthcare vision for the country. The AMA is working with government officials to alleviate some of the problems that have emerged from the ACA – making it more affordable for people and lowering costs through financial assistance programs and cost-cutting, market-driven initiatives.

Other Plans

Further, promotional and marketing efforts must attract the younger, healthier people to participate in the healthcare programs to offset some of the healthcare costs incurred, necessarily so, by the older, health-challenged segments of the population. Also, several new corporate partnership healthcare plans, offering high-quality healthcare at optimal costs, are in the process of being developed and soon would be implemented in the healthcare markets. These include the Amazon-Berkshire Hathaway-JP Morgan corporate partnership model being developed under the leadership of a Harvard Medical School physician/surgeon to be first implemented for all the employees at the three corporate organizations (Snider, 2018), and subsequently will be offered to the other organizations and regions, and perhaps to the entire country. Such innovative healthcare programs focusing on high-quality healthcare offered at a lower cost to patients would compete and challenge existing healthcare companies and plans to become more cost-effective and sustainable.

State Innovation Approach Plans

An important option that may be worthy of attention and consideration is the State Innovation approach plan/s. In 2017, the Senate considered a State innovation-based approach to healthcare reform that was brought up as a legislative amendment by Senators Graham, Cassidy, Heller, and Johnson, which did not receive the necessary support in the Senate by a small margin at that time (Chen, 2018). However, the State innovation approach is likely to receive more attention in the 2020 elections as part of President Donald Trump's re-election campaign, especially as it was included in the fiscal year 2019 budget (Office of Management and Budget, 2019). The key incentives for state-managed healthcare plans are to lower healthcare costs and provide adequate coverage. Therefore, as in other types of insurance programs like auto, home, and life, state and local insurance managed programs can effectively encourage robust competition between insurance companies within the states. And state regulators, agencies, leaders, and healthcare providers can maintain lower, more optimal healthcare expenditures overall for the programs, and be able to offer lower, more optimal premiums for the consumers.

Further, to lower healthcare costs, offer adequate healthcare coverage, and expand access, another incentive to consider could be providing states with a grant pool of $100 billion over ten years to provide healthcare to their residents (America Next, 2014). Mandatory restrictions must include guaranteed access for those individuals with pre-existing conditions, lower healthcare premiums to make it more affordable, and price and quality transparency so patients can make better-informed choices, and the medical providers can improve their quality care services. Further, to continue protecting the most vulnerable groups in society, premium support, a bipartisan issue for more than 20 years, has to be enhanced for seniors with more health insurance choices, and by strengthening Medicare to become more financially solvent and sustainable for the future generations. Additionally, Medicaid reforms to strengthen these programs by giving them the flexibility to design solutions and meet changing needs must continue. Similarly, pro-life protections enacted by Congress annually since 1976 need to be reformed to make them permanent in law, and also to strengthen the conscience protections for businesses and medical providers without any negative repercussions. Also, state reforms to expand access through making changes to medical licensure and construction of new medical facilities would lead to a higher supply of healthcare providers, more options, and lower healthcare costs. States may use these funds to subsidize insurance coverage for those residents with pre-existing conditions and their lower-income residents (America Next, 2014).

State innovation plans would also focus on better access to individuals who may change employers to move into lower cost, individual health coverage options without forcing them first to exhaust the COBRA continuation coverage, which is a costly mandate on businesses and individuals. Also, allowing small businesses, groups, and associations to pool together to offer lower-cost health insurance options that their members may purchase health coverage that may be continued from job to job, if necessary. Further, state innovation plans that allow individuals to buy healthcare insurance across state lines would enable Americans to buy the optimal-cost healthcare plan that best suits their needs.

Other incentives to lower costs would be the health savings accounts (HSA) where individuals could use HSA funds to pay for their health insurance premiums, and allowing them more flexibility to design their benefits, thereby participating in the innovative state insurance plans and helping with lower costs. Further, ten states in the US would be offering health-based wellness programs as part of a Centers for Medicare & Medicaid Services (CMS) pilot program. These ten states may use incentives such as lower premiums for those residents that do achieve their health outcomes (HealthMarkets, 2019). Therefore, using more incentives for maintaining wellness, including tax-free incentives, would enhance healthy behavior, and may also increase efforts toward changing practices that can help lower the healthcare cost growth.

The objectives of state innovation-based programs, namely lowering healthcare costs, expanding access to specialized, nonstandard coverage options, and giving state and local leaders more freedom to make the best decisions related to their residents' healthcare needs have to be met. Other policy issues that such state innovation-based reforms need to address would also include providing state and local control of the healthcare programs and expanding the accessibility and affordability of health coverage for all residents in the states. Also, lowering premiums for all in the various states regardless of income, and giving freedom for state residents to choose their own private insurance provider and healthcare service providers would continue to be the goals. Further, any state innovation-based healthcare model/s to be pragmatic and feasible must continue to address the non-partisan features that would satisfy both parties' lawmakers. Features that would be of concern must include universal health coverage for all (including the lower-income and needy segments of the state/s), necessary regulations to ensure the optimal cost/services of healthcare insurance providers and patient services' providers; lower cost, optimal government healthcare expenditures, and privately managed healthcare (Chen & Troy, 2017).

FUTURE DIRECTIONS

Future research studies could focus on empirically testing these newly proposed healthcare models, when implemented, to measure their effectiveness and benefits in the long run. Research must also evaluate the potential impact on various stakeholders (including patients, physicians, the insurance company, healthcare providers, hospitals, and other healthcare-related organizations in terms of the new enhanced healthcare delivery model being more optimal, sustainable, and beneficial to them. Research studies would need to formulate strategies for improving existing and proposed healthcare models so that all US stakeholders will benefit from a comprehensive, sustainable healthcare system for the country. Further, research must explore if healthcare for the US should continue as a private employer-sponsored program, a federally-managed program, or state-managed program/s, or some combination of these.

CONCLUSION

This chapter focused on reviewing and evaluating the best principles from some of the leading global healthcare systems in the world, and integrating these best market-tested lessons and policies, and then adapting/customizing them to be applicable for the US healthcare delivery system. The authors have also presented recommendations toward a proposed "Enhanced" US healthcare delivery model that includes the five different healthcare plans to choose from to benefit all the stakeholders in the US.

REFERENCES

America Next. (2014). *The freedom and empowerment plan: The prescription for conservative consumer-focused health reform.* Alexandria, VA: America Next.

Bessard, P. (2008, December 22). Challenges of Mixed Economy Solutions in Healthcare: The Examples of Switzerland and Singapore. *Economic Affairs, 28*(4), 16–21. doi:10.1111/j.1468-0270.2008.00863.x

Chen, L. (2018, December). Getting Ready for Health Reform 2020: Republicans' Options before Improving upon the State Innovation Approach. *Health Affairs, 37*(12), 2076–2083. doi:10.1377/hlthaff.2018.05119 PMID:30444425

Chen, L., & Troy, T. (2017, February 2). *Trump wants health 'insurance for everybody.' Here's how the GOP can make it happen.* Retrieved from https://www.washingtonpost.com/opinions/trump-wants-health-insurance-for-everybody-heres-how-the-gop-can-make-it-happen/2017/02/02/284e51b0-e4f1-11e6-a547-5fb9411d332c_story.html

Cheong, L. (2004). *Medical savings accounts in Singapore: The impact of Medisave and income on healthcare expenditure.* Stanford, CA: Center for Primary Care and Outcomes Research, Stanford University.

HealthMarkets. (2019, October 1). *Healthcare Reform News Updates. CMS announces 10-state pilot wellness program for ACA marketplace.* Retrieved from https://www.healthmarkets.com/resources/health-insurance/trumpcare-news-updates/

Huckabee, M. (n.d.). *Free healthcare for everyone! Bad idea!* Retrieved from https://www.youtube.com/watch?v=4IacUBgGz7w

Jost, T. J., & Pollock, H. (2016). Making Healthcare Truly Affordable after Healthcare Reform. *The Journal of Law, Medicine & Ethics, 44*(4), 546–554. doi:10.1177/1073110516684785 PMID:28661251

McCarthy, A. (2013, October 5). Obamacare's unconstitutional origins. *National Review.* Retrieved from https://www.nationalreview.com/2013/10/obamacares-unconstitutional-origins-andrew-c-mccarthy/

McCarthy, J. (2018, December 7). Most Americans rate still rate their healthcare quality quite positively. *Well-Being.* Retrieved from https://news.gallup.com/poll/245195/americans-rate-healthcare-quite-positively.aspx

Office of the Management and Budget. (2018). *Budget of the US Government: FY 2019.* Washington, DC: Government Publishing Office. Available from: https://www.govinfo.gov/content/pkg/BUDGET-2019-BUD/pdf/BUDGET-2019-BUD.pdf

Richard, M. (1996). NHS waiting lists have been a boon for private medicine in the UK. *Canadian Medical Association Journal, 154*(3), 378–381. PMID:8564909

Roy, A. (2011, April 29). Why Switzerland has the world's best health care system. *Forbes.*

Simonet, D. (2010). Healthcare Reforms and Cost Reduction Strategies in Europe: The Cases of Germany, UK, Switzerland, Italy, and France. *International Journal of Health Care Quality Assurance, 23*(5), 470–488. doi:10.1108/09526861011050510 PMID:20845678

Snider, M. (2018, January 30). Amazon, Berkshire Hathaway, JPMorgan Chase to tackle employee healthcare costs, delivery. *USA Today (Online).* Retrieved from https://www.usatoday.com/story/money/americasmarkets/2018/01/30/amazon-berkshire-hathaway-jpmorgan-chase-tackle-employee-health-care-costs-delivery/1077866001/

Stack, S. (2016). Health Care Reform in the United States: Past, Present, and Future Challenges. *World Medical Journal, 62*(4), 153–157.

United States: Swiss Health System offers Key Lessons. (2008, July 5). *Oxford Analytics Daily Brief Service.*

Zamosky, L. (2018, Dec. 18). *Healthcare sharing ministries: A leap of faith?* Retrieved from https://www.healthinsurance.org/other-coverage/healthcare-sharing-ministries-a-leap-of-faith/

ADDITIONAL READING

Armour, S. (2017, October 17). *Conservatives make new push to repeal Affordable Care Act.* Retrieved from https://www.wsj.com/articles/conservatives-make-new-push-to-repeal-affordable-care-act-1529400721

Collins, S., & Blumenthal, D. (2016, February 24). *New federal survey shows gains in private health coverage and fewer cost-related problems getting care.* Retrieved from https://www.commonwealthfund.org/blog/2016/new-federal-survey-shows-gains-private-health-coverage-and-fewer-cost-related-problems

DeJulio, B., Firth, J., Kirzinger, A., & Brodie, M. (2016). *Kaiser health tracking poll.* Retrieved from https://www.kff.org/health-costs/poll-finding/kaiser-health-tracking-poll-january-2016/

Mayer, P., & Denz, M. (2000). Social change in the physician's role and medical practice caused by managed care in Switzerland. *Gesundheitswesen (Bundesverband der Arzte des Offentlichen Gesundheitsdienstes (Germany))*, *62*(3), 138–142. PMID:10815339

Raetzo, M. (2000). Continuing education, motivation for cost control, a Swiss experiment. *Gesundheitswesen (Bundesverband der Arzte des Offentlichen Gesundheitsdienstes (Germany))*, *62*(3), 143–147. doi:10.1055-2000-10486 PMID:10815340

Ratajcak, T. (1998). Approaches to managed care in Germany. *Medicine and Law*, *17*(4), 545–551. PMID:10396915

Reinhardt, U. (2004). The Swiss health system: Regulated competition without managed care. *Journal of the American Medical Association*, *292*(10), 1227. doi:10.1001/jama.292.10.1227 PMID:15353536

Simonet, D. (2008). The new public management theory and European health-care reforms. *Canadian Public Administration*, *51*(4), 617–635. doi:10.1111/j.1754-7121.2008.00044.x

KEY TERMS AND DEFINITIONS

Affordable Care Act (ACA): The federally sponsored healthcare plan (ACA) was signed into law by President Barack Obama in 2010. A major overhaul of the U.S. health-care system aimed to reduce the amount of uncompensated care the average U.S. family pays for by requiring everyone to have health insurance or pay a tax penalty.

Buy Own Health Insurance: One can buy one's own health insurance and not have to get coverage through his/her employer. Depending on where one works, one may have the option of getting employer-sponsored health insurance, called group coverage.

Employer-Sponsored Healthcare Plans: Healthcare insurance plans sponsored/ offered by the employer, which are currently the most popular type of healthcare coverage used by a majority of the US population.

"Enhanced" Healthcare Delivery System: Improved healthcare system, which includes five different plans/approaches/options to healthcare delivery in this context.

"Enhanced" US Hybrid Healthcare Plan: A combination of two or more existing healthcare plans by taking the best of each to form one new healthcare option plan.

Free Choice in Healthcare Insurance Plans: The "Freedom of Choice in Health Care Act" allows an individual to freely enter into contractual agreements with health care providers for health care services and coverage without a mandate or penalty, of any kind, from state legislatures.

Global Healthcare Systems: Healthcare systems that exist outside of the US. Examples include Swiss, German, the UK, French, and Singaporean.

Private and Public Healthcare: Private healthcare can be provided through "for-profit" hospitals and self-employed practitioners, and "not for profit" non-government providers, including faith-based organizations. Public health care is usually provided by the government through national healthcare systems.

Universal Healthcare Access: This usually means everyone in a given country has access to and can enjoy the protection of health insurance, whether the country has a single-payer system, socialized medicine, an insurance mandate, or relies on a set of subsidies and other incentives.

Universal Healthcare Coverage: All the residents in the country are included to receive and benefit from healthcare through some healthcare or insurance plan/s available.

Chapter 2
Exploring Innovative, Alternative Healthcare Models in the US

Raj Selladurai

https://orcid.org/0000-0003-4126-4160
Indiana University Northwest, USA

Roshini Isabell Selladurai
In His Image Family Medicine Residency, Ascension St. John Medical Center, USA

George VandeWerken
Providence Bank, USA

ABSTRACT

This chapter explores, discusses, analyzes, and presents some recommendations for new, innovative alternative healthcare models to the traditional insurance and healthcare models that currently exist. These include a revised and enhanced hybrid model of healthcare; healthcare cost-sharing faith-based model; healthcare cost-reduction corporate partnership model (for example, Amazon, Berkshire Hathaway, and JPMorgan Chase partnership); direct primary care model; and wellness program model including subscription type payment services, concierge medicine services, networks of primary care physicians providing patient retention, personalized medicine, and preventive care (MD VIP for example). Significant outcomes such as lowering healthcare costs, enhancing the quality and delivery of healthcare services, improving patient satisfaction, and promoting overall sustainability are addressed, including their implications for various stakeholders.

DOI: 10.4018/978-1-7998-2949-2.ch002

INTRODUCTION

The current healthcare system in the US is one of the largest and the best in the world (America Next, 2014). However, it seems to have so many problems and complexities, which necessitate the nation's leaders and lawmakers to continue exploring healthcare reform. Recent efforts in 2018 to change, modify, enhance, and reform the Affordable Care Act (ACA) federal healthcare program came close to being passed in the United States Senate but fell short by a few key votes. This chapter explores, discusses, analyzes, and presents recommendations for some new, innovative alternative healthcare models to the existing traditional insurance and healthcare models. These include a revised or enhanced hybrid model of healthcare; healthcare cost-sharing faith-based models; healthcare cost-reduction corporate partnership models (for example, Amazon, Berkshire Hathaway, and JPMorgan Chase partnership); direct primary care models, and wellness programs model including subscription type payment services, concierge medicine services including networks of primary care physicians providing patient retention, personalized medicine, and preventive care (MD VIP for example). Significant outcomes such as lowering healthcare costs, enhancing the quality and delivery of healthcare services, improving patient satisfaction, and promoting overall sustainability are addressed, including their implications for various stakeholders.

BACKGROUND

After many lengthy discussions and controversial debates in the US Congress related to healthcare, the Affordable Care Act (ACA) was passed in 2010. It was supposed to have been a more sustainable healthcare system and was designed primarily to address the lack of healthcare insurance coverage for the uninsured millions of Americans in the country. But several years later, despite providing expanded coverage for millions of Americans, the ACA faces significant serious challenges and shortcomings. Studies have shown that many people still are unable to get access to affordable healthcare insurance, that the costs of healthcare are skyrocketing in many states and regions of the country, and that several insurance companies are exiting from unprofitable markets, thereby leaving millions stranded to fend for themselves (Stack, 2016). Also, healthcare and healthcare reform in the US continue to be much-discussed but controversial topics and will likely be among the top issues on the agenda for both parties in the 2020 election year.

Among the current severe concerns facing the US healthcare system, the high cost of healthcare is perhaps the most significant detrimental factor that needs to be addressed. Healthcare costs in various healthcare areas are exorbitantly high and continuing to increase. National health expenditures (NHE) have skyrocketed over the years, from $27.2 billion in 1960 to $3,492 billion in 2017 (Centers for Medicare and Medicaid, 2018). Further, the NHE per capita amount has increased tremendously from $146 in 1960 to $10,739 in 2009 (Folland et al., 2013). Also, a Harvard School of Public Health research study showed that the cost of medical malpractice in the United States is about $55.6 billion a year and that a significant amount estimated to be $45.6 billion is spent toward defensive medicine practiced by physicians, attempting to avoid litigation and lawsuits (Mello, 2010).

Furthermore, a recent study showed that administrative costs accounted for about 25 percent of total hospital costs in the US -- more than $200 billion -- which was higher than all other nations with Canada and Scotland being the lowest. The US would have saved $150 billion in 2011 alone if US per capita spending was similar to Canada's or Scotland's lower spending levels (Himmelstein, 2014). In the another University of British Columbia and Harvard University joint study, researchers found that US healthcare spending far exceeds other countries, with hundreds of billions of dollars being spent on administrative costs rather than the quality of healthcare for patients or on goods or services related to them (Gottlieb & Shepard, 2018). Therefore, it would seem that the urgent goal and focus of new, innovative models should be on the development and implementation of high-quality healthcare options to be offered at optimal, low cost for all in the US.

MAIN FOCUS

The primary purpose and focus of this chapter are to explore and present some new, innovative models in healthcare as alternatives to currently available healthcare programs and options.

ACCESS AND FUNDING ANALYSIS

Cultural attitudes and expectations create societal healthcare expectations, some of which could be characterized as unrealistic and unsustainable. It could be argued that the culture seems to encourage egocentric behavior and expectations. Dr. Doug Curran, a nationally renowned physician with impressive healthcare leadership and administrative credentials, observes that many millennials and younger people today seem to be a "me too," "instant gratification" generation with a consumer-centric mentality. This mentality demands everything right here and now! The demand for "free healthcare for all" seems to be a natural expression of this mindset and one that expects the government to provide free healthcare because many individuals consider it a right or entitlement (Doug Curran, MD, personal communication, Aug. 16, 2019).

Of course, this demand for free healthcare is also driven by the challenge of healthcare access. The consequences of inadequate access are significant, putting increasing pressure on national leaders to solve this dilemma. So, to fix this problem, an appealing solution is to make health care access a right for all citizens. But this immediately raises the question of cost. If everyone has a right to healthcare services, how are these services to be paid for and by whom? The choices are limited. Consumers either pay as they go, or they borrow and force their progeny to pay in the future. Because devising a plan to pay as they go is so difficult, the habit in the United States has been to borrow to pay for current needs. However, if people are to avoid burdening future generations, they must find a way to pay as they go. It seems prudent and to make sure that current consumers of healthcare services pay for their healthcare.

In addition to looking at funding considerations, new models of healthcare service delivery may also offer solutions to issues of access, affordability, and quality. The authors now address some of the criteria, measures, and perspectives to consider in the process of developing new innovative models of healthcare.

Medicare for All

Kessler (2019) has discussed one of the several types of Medicare-for-all plans that is advocated by Senator Bernie Sanders, which would raise taxes to pay for this plan but which would be at a lower cost overall than the current system for some Americans, but not all. This plan would become more expensive as the income of the family increases, and so it would place a more significant burden on wealthier segments of society. Further, Democratic presidential hopeful John Delaney pointed out that Medicare-for-all would also take away the three choice options of healthcare currently provided to seniors – Medicare, Medicare plus, or a supplemental insurance plan – and force them into a "one size fits all" type of plan. Also, the government-sponsored Medicare and Medicaid programs cover only 80-90 percent of the healthcare costs with commercial, private supplemental insurance plans supplementing the remaining costs of healthcare. And if these commercial plans are taken away, many hospitals and healthcare providers will be drastically affected because they would not be paid adequately for their healthcare services (John Delaney, personal communication in HuckabeeOnTBN, Oct. 5, 2019).

As a practical matter, for any Medicare-for-all proposal to pass Congress, it must garner bipartisan support, a prospect that seems challenging and highly unlikely given the current political climate in the country. Moreover, recently, President Trump signed a new executive order that would strengthen the Medicare program for seniors by empowering them with more plan options, more access to new treatments and procedures, and would allow more consultation time with their providers, physicians, and other medical care providers. Such measures are meant to enhance and continue the Medicare program for all eligible seniors and to reduce the likelihood of Medicare-for-all, a proposal that many experts contend would bankrupt the system anyway and could ultimately lead to Medicare-for-none (The White House, Oct. 3, 2019).

Another payment option is a joint responsibility plan. Such an approach could be workable in conjunction with patient-centric services, wellness programs, and individual responsibility if all related stakeholders in the healthcare system collaborate effectively together. Further, this approach could be sustainable with the addition of employer-provided basic optimal cost healthcare for all/most, and with some form of supplemental insurance provided by federal or state healthcare funded/sponsored system to cover specialized or chronic long-term complications and specialty services needs (Doug Curran, MD, personal communication, Aug. 16, 2019, Sept. 6, 2019).

Payroll Tax (Premium) Measure

Perhaps, similar to social security, to receive healthcare benefits, one should be required to pay into the system. One means to accomplish this – at least for a significant portion of society – is via an enhanced payroll tax for healthcare that is paid by everyone and matched with an employer's contribution. To be eligible for basic coverage, one must generate at least a certain threshold level of premium (or payroll tax). Perhaps plan benefits and features could be enhanced as one's contribution increases – which would create an incentive to work additional hours.

A structure like this fixes the medical care cost component per hour for all employees since the costs of all medical services are spread across and applied to all payroll costs. Also, employers do not incur medical care costs only on behalf of those employees who work more than some eligibility threshold, but they would be incurred on all payroll hours. Such a structure would produce at least two benefits. First, it would increase the revenue generated to pay for medical care services by applying a medical care premium rate across a broad payroll base, and second, it would help to eliminate the employer incentive to limit employee hours, a practice that reduces the number of employees covered by employer-provided health insurance coverage. Also, if benefit features improved as one worked more hours, employees would have an incentive to increase their hours.

If approaches like this were in place and met the federal requirements for employers to provide coverage, there would be less incentive for employers to create so many part-time positions to keep employees below eligibility thresholds for medical benefits. The healthcare coverage benefits would be a byproduct of employment, and the basic cost would be the same rate per hour regardless of whether a person worked full or part-time.

Of course, the needs of those who are unable to work or are too young must also be addressed. The country would need a system to vet this segment of society for eligibility, and the cost of providing those benefits would need to be added to the program costs borne by all. But the basic goal of this approach is to motivate more individuals to get into the workforce to enhance their benefits and to eliminate the employer disincentive for creating employee positions not covered by medical insurance. This approach could address the healthcare funding needs of a significant percentage of the population. Of course, consideration must also be given to addressing medical contributions for independent contractor status workers as well.

Western countries are wealthy enough to discuss and even consider universal coverage plans. In fact, in many of the European countries, including Switzerland, Germany, and the UK, and France, universal health coverage is provided to all of their citizens. In most of the world, society as a whole is not in a position to offer such a medical safety net. However, if society as a whole wants health coverage, society must find a way to pay for it collectively – or individually when they use a service.

Patient-Centric/Consumer-Centric Focus

Regardless of which healthcare models are chosen, the patient/customer focus must be at the center of the system. According to Dr. Doug Curran, healthcare professionals must believe in and embrace a patient-centric focus in treating their patients. Dr. Curran recommends that there must be a collaborative partnership between physicians, healthcare providers, medical staff and personnel, and patients all working together for one's healthcare. Also, patients must take personal, pro-active responsibility for their own wellness through actively doing the right exercise program, eating healthy, maintaining proper weight, and controlling basics like blood sugar and blood pressure while at the same time cooperating with the physician's and medical professional's instructions and recommendations (Doug Curran, MD, personal communication, Aug. 16, 2019, Sept. 6, 2019).

When considered in the light of a patient-centric/customer-centric focus, most of the new, innovative models of healthcare are doing just that – keeping the patient/customer as the primary focus and tailoring creative healthcare programs to meet a person's specific needs in all or as many aspects as possible – cost, patient care, the basket of services, physician's access, attention and time spent with patients, and patient-physician communications. The focus of all healthcare services should be on a "basket of service" approach, which means that all healthcare must be customized to suit the specific needs of the patient at that particular time. And overall, the primary goal is to make healthcare affordable, provide improved services at lower costs, and continue to focus on optimal cost, sustainable healthcare!

Affordable Care Act (ACA) Related Issues

Because the ACA has been the law now for several years, it seems prudent and practical for the US to keep the good points of this healthcare program, and to eliminate/minimize any apparent weaknesses. Healthcare providers can work within the ACA structure. Some have been able to provide adequate healthcare at a considerably lower cost than elsewhere.

However, current health care costs are generally expensive, and they can vary widely. For example, some Texas entrepreneurs and small business owners spend around $1800/month for health insurance for a family of four (Doug Curran, MD, personal communication, Aug. 16, 2019, Sept. 6, 2019). Although that seems expensive, another business owner in Indiana pays about $4000/month for his family's health insurance, more than double the Texas amount! (Al Turnbeaugh, Ph.D., personal communication, Sept. 12, 2019). However, Dr. Curran points out that through some innovative and intentional cost-optimization measures, the Affordable Care Organization (ACO) group in Texas that he and 100 other primary care physicians work for have generated between $4 to 6 million per year cost savings and have helped save another 8% in insurance premium costs for their patients. They did so by working together and partnering with the insurance companies like United Healthcare, Aetna, and others, as well as focusing on proactive wellness programs and managing healthcare for patients to promote their well-being (Doug Curran, MD, personal communication, Aug. 16, 2019, Sept. 6, 2019).

Similarly, from his own recent personal experience as a patient after a successful kidney transplant procedure, Al Turnbeaugh (personal communication, Dec. 14, 2019) recommends that most people can take a proactive approach to their health and improved wellbeing through eating healthy, regular exercise, maintaining the proper weight, and regulating the control of blood sugar and blood pressure while cooperating with the physician's and medical professional's instructions and recommendations. By doing so, they may avoid or minimize expensive medical treatments, medicine and drugs, and other complications. Also, he suggests that more people must be educated about possibly serving as human donors to give "life" to others, who may need critical organs to increase their life span. Such efforts would cumulatively contribute toward overall lower healthcare costs and help promote healthy living with a higher quality of life.

Corporate Partnership Programs

Amazon, Berkshire Hathaway, and JP Morgan have been working on a corporate partnership healthcare program to offer competitive rates for healthcare plans to their three organizations' employees (Snider, 2018). Later on, they plan to provide these competitive plans of high-quality healthcare at optimal rates to the various employers and organizations in the rest of the country. Corporate partnership programs expect to benefit many people with their high-quality, affordable healthcare plans and excellent services offered at lower, optimal costs. Therefore, the current, dynamic healthcare environment demands some changes, new considerations, and exploring new, innovative approaches or models related to healthcare reform for the country.

SOLUTIONS AND RECOMMENDATIONS

The authors propose five innovative models to consider and choose from for the US population in the future. Figure 1 shows the innovative healthcare options model for the US population.

Hybrid Healthcare Plan Model

One of the innovative healthcare models may be referred to as the Hybrid Healthcare Plan option. Currently, the nation has primarily two major options for healthcare –

Figure 1. Innovative healthcare plans model for the US

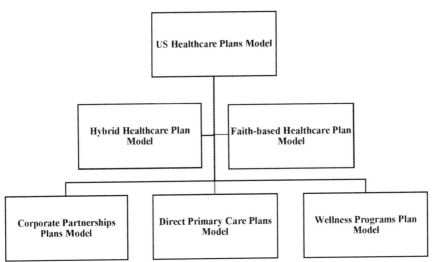

employer-sponsored private insurance healthcare plans, and the federally sponsored ACA public healthcare plan. The Republican lawmakers mostly seem in full support of the private insurance healthcare plan, and the Democratic lawmakers are primarily supportive of government-funded healthcare for all. However, neither partisan solution appears to be the most optimal, sustainable one for the country. Instead, a third option – the Hybrid Healthcare Plan option -- would merit serious consideration. The private insurance healthcare plans would continue to be used for the majority of the US population for most health-related services. However, for specialized care and expensive treatments, the government plan/s should subside these services costs. Government subsidy, provided through Medicare/Medicaid or some other related comprehensive healthcare program, is necessary as no family should be unnecessary burdened and often financially wrecked because of some life-threatening, critical and essential cancer treatments, transplants, and surgical procedures, which may require specialized care and treatments that are expensive. And concerning the healthcare premiums, co-pays, deductibles, etc., all these will continue to be paid by the individual but on a sliding scale related to one's income to be fair to all. (Huckabee, 2019). This Hybrid healthcare plan and other similar efforts would help provide an optimal cost, sustainable healthcare system for all people in the US.

Faith-Based Healthcare Plans Model

Faith-based healthcare plans are growing fast and increasingly becoming popular alternatives to consider, especially for people of faith in the US. According to the Alliance of Healthcare Sharing Ministries, which was founded in 2007, currently, about one million Americans depend on faith-based healthcare programs that allow the community of Christians to share their medical bills rather than use other private or public health insurers and programs (Hagar, 2017). Four such major organizations manage these faith-based healthcare programs – Christian Care Ministry (which offers the Medi-Share program), Liberty HealthShare, Samaritan Ministries, and Christian Healthcare Ministries.

For example, Chris and Jolie Jenkins, a young couple with a family of eight, use the faith-based healthcare sharing program as an affordable alternative to traditional health insurance plans. In 2016, the Jenkins' 7-year-old daughter suffered from a recurring infection. She required two doctor visits, three lab tests, and an ultrasound, and the ultrasound in itself cost around $1200, or an emergency visit for a family with kid/s at 2 am for fever or cold cost around $1000! (Hagar, 2017). Incidentally, Chris Jenkins knows this information firsthand as he worked as an emergency medicine physician at the local hospital; and though he could have chosen his employer-provided healthcare plan, he found out that his family's share for such coverage would be expensive. Instead, the family had opted for a healthcare sharing ministry plan in place of the traditional insurance, and the cost of treatment for their child was $500 with no copay to be concerned about (Hagar, 2017). So, for many Americans, these types of healthcare options are more cost-effective and beneficial to them, and also they give them a feeling and sense of community spirit of helping one another with healthcare services and costs as and when needed by a family. Further, the ACA model allows religious small and large nonprofit organizations to share the healthcare cost between their members as an alternative under the ACA mandatory insurance programs.

An essential principle for the faith-based healthcare programs is "shared money, shared beliefs." Members, who agree to follow Christian, Biblical values-based standards and rules, are allowed to contribute a monthly amount to the pool or "share box." When a billable-medical incident occurs, the member initially pays for it out-of-pocket, often with cash for the lower "self-pay" fee that many healthcare providers offer, and then submits it to the health share community for reimbursement (Hagar, 2017). Other health share organizations like Christian Care Ministries ask members to use in-network providers like traditional insurance programs. And the physicians, hospitals, or clinics send their bills directly to the organization, which negotiates discounted rates and then pays on behalf of the member-patient. Payments are made from the health share pool of money generated from the monthly contributions, averaging about $400 a month/couple and $529/month for a family, according to Liberty HealthShare ministry, to the healthcare service providers of the member/s. Or sometimes, the members' expenses are presented to other members in the pool, who may voluntarily send financial help directly to the member who submitted the claim (Zamosky, 2018). According to one of the health share ministries, Medi-Share, its members have helped one another pay more than $1 billion in healthcare costs since its founding in 1993, and it has about 220,000 members subscribing to the ministry programs currently (Hagar, 2017). From another health share organization, Dale Ellis, chief executive of Liberty HealthShare, says, "It's such a different paradigm, it's really relational, it's our money going every month to another person who needs it" (Hagar, 2019, p.5). It is all a matter of attitude that differentiates the share members from insurance premium-paying personnel. And as a result of the emphasis on community and relationships, an entitlement attitude between the insurer and the insured is minimized and replaced with an attitude of truly caring for one other's health and helping one another in a true Christian spirit.

Corporate Partnership Plans Model

Corporate partnership plans, such as the collaboration between Amazon, JP Morgan Chase, and Berkshire Hathaway, are increasingly becoming popular as the nation grapples with healthcare reform. The principal goals of all the new innovative models are to lower the cost of healthcare and increase the high-quality delivery of healthcare services. The timing for the need for such programs now is exact and perfect as healthcare spending constituted about 18% of the US economy in 2016, and it is continuously increasing higher, and totaling nearly $10,348 per person in the US in 2018 (Bomey, 2018).

Recently, Amazon, JP Morgan Chase, and Berkshire Hathaway have set up a new non-profit called Haven with a website (https://havenhealthcare.com/) to manage all of their 1.2 million employees' healthcare needs. This trend of corporate healthcare programs that Amazon has started offering is similar to the Apple AC Wellness Clinic, which the company had launched for its employees in early 2018. Also, Amazon is experimenting with a new healthcare program by launching its Amazon Care website to offer virtual primary care for its Seattle-based employees (Comstock, 2019). This offering includes a telemedicine app, online chat with a nurse, medication delivery, and app-enabled house calls to the employee's office or home. Amazon does not employ at this time any doctors; instead, the company is contracting with a local clinic called Oasis Medical Group (Comstock, 2019) to provide the primary care services, and it does not include emergency care services.

These corporate partnership programs would have several dramatic effects on healthcare. They show the need for innovation and creativity in healthcare options for consumers. Amazon's CEO Jeff Bezos has revolutionized the enormous multi-billion dollar retail industry by using some disruptive innovative type strategies based on the strategic concept of "disruptive innovation" pioneered by Harvard Business School professor Christensen (Christensen, 1997). Several longtime and nationally renowned competitors that could not compete well or adapt to new trends in online buying, and influenced mainly by Amazon's strategies, are struggling to survive in this industry while Amazon is flourishing. These giant corporate leaders are similarly trying to impact healthcare too! They plan to do something grand in healthcare through bold thinking and innovative strategies.

Also, with their tremendous reputations of success and impact preceding them, several corporate leaders are gaining momentum in healthcare innovations. The Health Transformation Alliance, formed in 2015 by American Express, Macy's, Verizon, and Caterpillar, is partnering with other corporate leaders, including JP Morgan Chase and Berkshire's subsidiary, BNSF Railway (Bomey, 2018). One of the most significant factors to drive their innovative strategies related to healthcare is the non-profit motive. Similar to the giant conglomerate healthcare provider Kaiser Permanente, which includes several successful and increasingly growing for-profit and non-profit organizations in several locations in the US, Mr. Bezos and Mr. Buffet too have set up Haven as a non-profit organization. The two successful leaders clearly understand the significance of the long-term implications rather than a short-term focus on quarterly earnings, especially for solving problems in healthcare; this would be a distinctive competency and unique selling point for Haven. They would promote themselves as being more socially responsible seeking an "enlightened" self-interest in the long run rather than looking at short-term outcomes of self-interest and immediate profits, which many of their competitors in the industry, such as the leading for-profit insurance companies, pharmaceutical companies, and many healthcare providers are doing.

Further, the new partnerships would aim to achieve their goals of lower costs and high-quality healthcare by reducing the bureaucracies of healthcare. They would consider cutting some jobs or reducing the rate of job growth – the healthcare industry in 2016 employed 12.4 million people, according to the Bureau of Labor Statistics, which is eight times more than the total workforce of Walmart worldwide (Bomey, 2018). And similar to the technological innovation that Amazon used effectively to bring about massive changes in the retail industry, the Haven group could use automation to change the healthcare industry too. Data analysis innovations, together with hi-tech integration, automated healthcare tests, lab work, and food preparation activities, may be enhanced through automation and the use of artificial intelligence, which could lead to substantial savings for the corporate partnership companies.

Another key implication is the increased use of telemedicine in healthcare. Just as remote online banking has grown over the years, and online shopping has almost become the norm today for many products and many younger people, telemedicine may also increase in use and demand in healthcare (Bomey, 2018). With expanded telemedicine, healthcare providers may share physicians and nurse practitioners, and other medical personnel, thereby helping reduce costs. Also, some changes in the drug pricing and distribution channels, especially related to pharmacy benefit managers (PMBs) such as Express Scripts and CVS Health Caremark, could potentially lower the costs. By offering online pharmacy and cutting out the middleman again, Amazon, through Haven, could deliver its products and services at discounted prices without compromising the quality in healthcare.

Also, due to its vast experience in successfully changing consumer buying behavior over the years, which was considered almost impossible to do, Amazon may be able to repeat changing patient behavior, too. Using various kinds of technology and apps, Haven can send its patients reminders to take their medicine regularly, eat more healthy, get healthcare services promptly when needed, and take better care of their health overall. Companies immensely benefit when they can get their employees to live healthier lives. "We know that healthier workers not only cost less but are also more productive," said Jean Abraham, a healthcare administrator, and professor at the University of Minnesota (Bomey, 2018). Finally, by reshaping the payment methods to healthcare providers, Haven can lower its costs. It would tie the payment to the quality of healthcare provided in the future rather than the number of services provided as currently structured, referred to as fee-for-value. The three corporate giants, with all their resources, brainpower, firepower, and influence, can make such an innovative trend happen.

In describing another new trend and innovation in healthcare, the increasing use of Artificial Intelligence (AI), leading cardiologist Dr. Eric Topol contended that technology companies like Apple, Google, Microsoft, and Amazon are becoming more involved in healthcare through the use of AI models to benefit physicians and medical professionals. As he puts it, "As machines get smarter and take on suitable tasks, humans might actually find it easier to be more humane" (Farr, 2019, p. 1). AI technology models would help with the busy work that physicians and medical professionals do like inputting medical records, data analysis, "deep learning" from people's data and lifestyles using algorithms, etc. which may lead to higher patient-based quality services and patient satisfaction. Therefore, corporate partnership programs may very well be ready to revolutionize the healthcare industry as they did in the retail sector and be planning to achieve the significant outcomes of lower cost, higher quality healthcare, and sustainability in healthcare.

Direct Primary Care Programs Model

Prior to the use of insurance to pay for healthcare, patients paid their physicians directly for their services. Today, the new direct primary care model is increasingly used in healthcare and is going back to this direct patient-physician relationship, including personalized care and attention, a more significant impact on patients' health, direct patient payment for services, etc. Many physicians realized that they were not spending much time with their patients as they got bogged down with insurance paperwork and data entry. And they were not enjoying practicing medicine in the traditional family medicine practice or finding it meaningful, according to Dr. Hsieh of Granger, Indiana. "I felt very strongly that we were not delivering the kind of care that could be the best for the patient, and I explored other ways I could continue to practice the way I wanted (Gallegos, 2019, p. 1). Another direct primary care provider, PeakMed in Colorado, provides unlimited access to individuals and families to their personal physician for a flat fee; patients can text or call their physician at any time and as often as they wish. Jon Hernandez, PeakMed's CEO, says that "by changing the economics of healthcare today and improving quality and access to care, we can overhaul the experience and redefine both health and care" (Betz, 2018, p. 2).

In an American Academy of Family Physicians (AAFP) 2018 survey, direct primary care physicians described how they had structured their "new" practices. They said that 80% of them charge a fee directly to the patient, and most opt-out of insurance and do not bill any third party; 56% are more than 15 years post-residency; 72% of practices have been operating less than three years; 54% of the practices started from scratch, and 34% converted from an existing practice; 57% of practices have employer-based contracts; 58% of the practices supplement their income through other practice opportunities; 345 patients is the average panel size, and 596 is the average target panel size; and importantly 91% of physicians would promote the model to others (Gallegos, 2019). Direct primary care is growing fast as more physicians are moving toward adopting the new model. In 2009, only 100 practices were involved with direct primary care, but today in 2019, around 1000 practices in 48 states are caring for more than 300,000 patients, according to Jay Keese, the executive director of the Direct Primary Care Coalition (Gallegos, 2019).

Some of the advantages of the direct primary care model include better health outcomes resulting from more access to physicians; lower, transparent costs based on a flat fee; higher quality care from a synergistic relationship between physician and direct primary care practice and the patients; and healthcare available access irrespective of age, pre-existing conditions, insurance coverage or nature of the health condition and illness (Betz, 2018).

However, direct primary care has some limitations too. The direct care contracts do not usually cover the specialist's treatment or hospital stays; patients with Medicare, Medicaid or ACA plans may have limited funds to pay for the primary care related services; and for practices offering exclusively direct primary cost, the revenue potential may be restricted to patients who receive their care (Betz, 2018). Also, it takes time and preparation, marketing, and restructuring to manage a successful direct primary care practice, primarily if a physician, used to a panel size of 2500, is looking to fill in 600-800 patients. Over six years, Dr. Rob Lamberts switched by leaving his traditional practice to the new direct care model providing care for his 800 patients. He charges them $35 to $70 a month depending on age and offers a family fee of $150-175 for up to five family members. The services that he provides include extended physician access, office visits, discounted in-house lab charges, discounted medications dispensed from his office, and with substantially less paperwork. But Dr. Lamberts says that his quality of life is much better than before, and so is his quality of patient care (Gallegos, 2019). Similarly, family physician Dr. Brian Forest, founder of Apex Healthcare Direct in Apex, North Carolina, when asked to rate his job satisfaction on a scale of 1-10, said, "I'd have to call it a 20. Practicing medicine this way, which puts the focus on the care of the patient and providing the best quality of care you can, is just simply fantastic" (Carlson, 2015, p. 22).

Direct primary care practices need to choose from the direct-to-consumer route or direct-to-employers option to provide services. The first targets patients as members, and the other contracts with employers for services to their employees. Some practices choose both options. Ultimately, the physician's reputation for providing high-quality care and service to patients is critical for a successful direct primary care practice, and patients should know about you, the physician, according to Dr. Hsieh (Gallegos, 2019). It is a shift in healthcare from fragmented care to connected ecosystems, all transitioning seamlessly (Davis & Gourdji, 2019). The practice must have staff that helps run the logistics of the primary care practice, run everything smoothly through patient education and advocacy, and assist patients in navigating specialist visits, medication, payment, and other related services. "It's a different mindset," says Dr. Lambert. "You suddenly are focused on keeping patients away from the office rather than having a full office....keeping people well rather than benefitting from people getting sick. That's a challenge to lose the mindset and to suddenly celebrate if you have a day that's not very busy or your office is empty. That's a good thing." (Gallegos, 2019, p. 13).

Wellness Programs Model

Similar to the several innovative alternative programs, wellness programs are also gaining momentum in healthcare. As part of a Centers for Medicare & Medicaid Services (CMS) pilot program, ten states in the US would be offering health-based wellness programs. The ten states may use incentives such as lower premiums for those residents that do achieve their health outcomes. However, for those state residents whose medical conditions prevent them from participating, states must offer some alternative programs. Also, the states are required to ensure that wellness programs will not lead to coverage loss for the participants or increase the cost for the federal program (HealthMarkets, 2019).

Another type of direct primary care/wellness program referred to as the concierge medicine model is gaining popularity recently. Some differences between the two types are the cost, billing to insurance, per patient panel, physician-patient "face time," and radiology, labs, routine procedures, etc. The direct primary care model monthly subscription/member fee is $40-$100, whereas, for the concierge medicine model, it ranges from $100 to $30,000 (Carlson, 2015). For the direct primary care model, there is no billing to insurance, 600-1500 is the patient panel size, and up to 80 to 90 percent cash discounts or catastrophic insurance will cover lab tests and other related costs. For the concierge medicine, some practices bill to insurance, and some practices do not, 100 to 800 is the patient panel size, and lab tests, etc. are often billed to insurance (Carlson, 2015).

Concierge medicine appeal is flourishing with about 5000 physicians who are practicing concierge medicine currently, and this number is expected to increase in the future – for example, Florida-based MDVIP was pioneered in the year 2000 and has grown to a network of more than 800 physicians (Lincoff, 2015). In this type of practice, concierge doctors focus on preventive care more than traditional physicians do. "If you keep the patient out of the hospital or the ER, it saves patients a lot of money. The people that buy into this model are really trying to buy into a personalized engagement model focused on prevention," said Bret Jorgensen, CEO of MDVIP (Lincoff, 2015, p. 6.).

Several innovations in direct primary care have been pioneered at the Academic Innovations Collaborative of the Harvard Medical School Center for Primary Care. And some of the leading direct primary care practices include Iora Health, MedLion, Paladina Health, Qliance, and White Glove Health, which are also among the largest direct primary care services organizations in the country. Dr. Russell Phillips, the director of the Harvard Medical School Center for Primary Care, says, "Iora's been very successful in recruiting some of our top residents. Direct primary care is a creative and innovative approach that we can all learn from.... I'm supportive of trying to find new ways of doing primary care better" (Carlson, 2015, p. 23). Also, Jason Hwang, chief medical officer of PolkaDoc, says, "If I were a graduating resident looking for a job, I think these direct primary care opportunities would be very attractive to me" (Carlson, 2015, p. 23). Further, several scholars and experts in healthcare concur that direct primary care will be the standard way primary care will be practiced in the coming years. Direct primary care is here to stay, now, and in the future.

In all these five "new" innovative models discussed, by practicing some servant leadership principles (Selladurai and Carraher, 2014), healthcare leaders and executives can help reform and transform their organizational personnel and staff, including physicians, nurses, and all medical-related members throughout their organizations. They can enhance the healthcare organizations and ensure positive patient experiences through implementing more of a patient/consumer-centric focused organizational climate. Top executives at healthcare organizations can achieve patient-consumer centricity by helping define it and by modeling their patient-centered behaviors (Davis & Gourdji, 2019). Commitment to patient-centricity needs more action than mere words. David Feinberg, CEO of Geisinger Health System, a regional health system in Pennsylvania, showed commitment to patient care and brought a new meaning to the concept of patient-centricity. He introduced a "satisfaction guaranteed or money-back" refund policy called ProvenExperience implemented through an app, which patients used to provide instant feedback on their healthcare experiences. In the first year, Geisinger had to refund nearly $500,000 to its patients. Despite implementing this refund, the Geisinger Health System sincerely valued what its patients think of its services. "We put our trust in you, the patient, because you've put your trust in us," said Dr. Alistair Erskine, CIO of Geisinger (Davis & Gourdji, 2019, p. 12).

With a clear focus on patient/consumer-centricity, healthcare organizations can achieve the critical outcomes of improved patient satisfaction, lower healthcare costs, enhanced quality and delivery of healthcare services, and overall sustainability, just as Amazon has done in the online industry. Amazon did so in revolutionizing the online buying behavior by providing total consumer-centric experiences to its customers. Interestingly, this type of customer-focus is best valued and exemplified by Amazon CEO Jeff Bezos, who continually reminds his organization that the empty chair in all their meetings is a reserved seat that always represents their customers! (Koetsier, 2018). This customer-centric mission and vision that are driving the entire organization may very well be continued at the new healthcare partnerships like Amazon Haven, Amazon Care, and others with the high likelihood of similar outcomes, including improved patient satisfaction, lower healthcare costs, enhanced quality and delivery of healthcare services, and overall sustainability.

FUTURE DIRECTIONS

Future research studies must continue to explore more innovative and creative healthcare options to offer participants in the US in the future relevant to the changes in technology, healthcare, and demand for the kinds of needed services prevalent at that time. Research must be directed toward testing the five innovative healthcare options discussed in this chapter for their effectiveness in terms of being cost-effective, affordable for all, high-quality, patient-centered, and sustainable in the long run. Also, research must explore how these patient/consumer-centric models would need to be continuously improved in terms of satisfying relevant and critical outcomes. Further, research must continue to explore, if and as necessary, whether healthcare would continue to be a private, employer-sponsored program, or federal government-sponsored program, or state government-sponsored, or some combination of these.

CONCLUSION

In this chapter, the authors have proposed and presented five innovative models of healthcare as alternative options to traditional healthcare options and programs for the US population. These "new" healthcare models provide alternatives that address significant outcomes such as cost containment or lower costs of healthcare, more optimal delivery of benefits and services, higher employee satisfaction, improved patient-provider relations, and optimal sustainability.

REFERENCES

Betz, E. (2018). Advantages and limitations of the direct primary care model. *MGMA STAT*. Retrieved from https://www.mgma.com/ data/data-stories/ advantages-and-limitations- of-the-direct-primary-c

Bomey, N. (2018, Feb. 25). How Amazon, JPMorgan, Berkshire could transform American healthcare. *USA Today (Online)*. Retrieved from https://www.usatoday. com/ story/money/ 2018/02/25/ amazon-jpmorgan- berkshire-health-care/ 350625002

Carlson, R. (2015, March 1). Direct primary care practice model drops insurance and gains providers and consumers. *Physician Leadership Journal*. Retrieved from https://www.thefreelibrary.com/ Direct+primary+care+ practice+model+drops+ insurance+and+gains... -a0409422676

CBS. (2019). *Carol's second act*. Retrieved from https://www.cbs.com/ shows/ carols-second act/about/

Centers for Medicare & Medicaid Services. (2018). *National Health Accounts Historical: NHE Tables*. Retrieved from https://www.cms.gov/ research-statistics-data- and-systems/statistics

Christensen, C. (1997). *Disruptive Innovation*. Retrieved from https://www. christenseninstitute.org/ disruptive-innovations/

Christensen, C. (2018). *Christensen Institute: Healthcare*. Retrieved from https:// www.christenseninstitute.org/ results/?_sft_topics= healthcare

Comstock, J. (2019, September 24). *Amazon launches Amazon Care, a telemedicine-driven care offering for Seattle employees*. Retrieved from https://www. mobihealthnews.com/ news/nortamerica/ amazon-launches-amazon-

Davis, S., & Gourdji, J. (2019). *Making the healthcare shift: The transformation to consumer-centricity*. New York: Morgan James Publishing.

Everett, B. (2019, July 15). Republicans ready to dive off a cliff on Obamacare. *Politico*. Retrieved from https://a.msn.com/ r/2/AAEj9o3?m= en-us&referrerID=InAppShare

Farr, C. (2019, March 14). Everything we know about Haven, the Amazon joint venture to revamp healthcare. *Health Tech Matters*. Retrieved from https://www.cnbc.com/ 2019/03/13/ what-is-haven-amazon- jpmorgan-berkshire- revamp-health-care.html

Farr, C. (2019, March 13). Cardiologist Eric Topol explains how artificial intelligence can make doctors more humane. *Health Tech Matters*. Retrieved from https://www.cnbc.com/2019/03/13/eric-topol-interview-with-christina-farr-on-ai-and-doctors.html

Folland, S., Goodman, A. C., & Stano, M. (2013). *The economics of health and health care* (7th ed.). Boston: Pearson.

Gallegos, A. (2019). Direct primary care: What makes a practice successful? *Family Practice News*, *49*(7), 1–23.

Gottlieb, J., & Shephard, M. (2018, September 6). How large a burden are administrative costs in healthcare? *Econofact*. Retrieved from https://econofact.org/how-large-a-burden-are-administrative-costs-in-health-care

Hagar, S. (2017, Feb. 5). Health share ministries offer alternatives to ACA. *TCA Regional News*.

HealthMarkets. (2019, October 1). *Healthcare Reform News Updates. CMS announces 10-state pilot wellness program for ACA marketplace*. Retrieved from https://www.healthmarkets.com/resources/health-insurance/trumpcare-news-updates/

Himmelstein, D. (2014, Sept. 8). A Comparison of hospital administrative costs in eight nations: US costs exceed other nations by far. *The Commonwealth Fund*. Retrieved from https://www.commonwealthfund.org/publications/journal-article/2014/sep/comparison-hospital-administrative-costs-eight-nations-us

Huckabee, M. (2019, August 17). *Free healthcare for everyone! Bad idea!* Retrieved from https://www.youtube.com/watch?v=4IacUBgGz7w

Huckabee, M. (2019, October 5). *Is John K. Delaney too moderate for the democratic elections? Find out!* Retrieved from https://www.facebook.com/HuckabeeOnTBN/videos/2485494795013107/

Kessler, G. (2019, September 24). Biden's bungled attack on medicare-for-all. *The Washington Post*. Retrieved from https://www.washingtonpost.com/politics/2019/09/24/bidens-bungled-attack-medicare-for-all/

Koetsier, J. (2018, April 5). *Why every Amazon meeting has at least one empty chair?* Retrieved from https://www.inc.com/john-koetsier/why-every-amazon-meeting-has-at-least-one-empty-chair.html

Lincoff, N. (2015, June 30). *The future of healthcare could be in concierge medicine*. Retrieved from https://www.healthline.com/health-news/the-future-of-healthcare-could-be-in-concierge-medicine-063015

Lundy, J. (2018, June 5). Sharing health costs with faith: Ministries offer coverage, savings as an alternative to traditional insurance. *TCA Regional News.*

Mello, M., Chandra, A., Gawande, A., & Studdert, D. (2010). National costs of the medical liability system. *Health Affairs.* Retrieved from https://www.healthaffairs. org/ doi/10.1377/hlthaff.2009.0807

Next, A. (2014). *The freedom and empowerment plan: The prescription for conservative consumer-focused health reform.* Alexandria, VA: America Next.

Selladurai, R., & Carraher, S. (2014). Lead like the greatest leader! Case Study. In R. Selladurai & S. Carraher (Eds.), *Servant leadership: Research and Practice* (pp. 350–355). Hershey, PA: IGI Global. doi:10.4018/978-1-4666-5840-0.ch026

Snider, M. (2018, January 30). Amazon, Berkshire Hathaway, JPMorgan Chase to tackle employee healthcare costs, delivery. *USA Today (Online).* Retrieved from https://www.usatoday.com/ story/money/ americasmarkets/2018/01/30/ amazon-berkshire-hathaway- jpmorgan- chase-tackle-employee-health-care-costs-delivery/1077866001/

Stack, S. J. (2016). Health Care Reform in the United States: Past, Present, and Future Challenges. *World Medical Journal, 62*(4), 153–157.

The White House. (2019, October 3). *President Donald J. Trump's healthcare agenda puts seniors and American patients first.* Retrieved from https://www. whitehouse.gov/ briefings-statements/ president-donald-j-trumps- healthcare-agenda-puts-seniors-american- patients-first/?utm_source= ods&utm_medium= email&utm_campaign= 1600d

Twachtman, G. (2019, May). CMS creates Primary Care First for small, solo practices. *Family Practice , 49*(5), 1–4.

Zamosky, L. (2018, December 18). *Healthcare sharing ministries: A leap of faith?* Retrieved from https://www.healthinsurance.org/ other-coverage/healthcare-sharing-ministries-a-leap-of-faith/

ADDITIONAL READING

Alix, E., Bryant, J., Sanson-Fisher, R., Fradgley, E., Proietto, A., & Roos, I. (2018). Consumer input into health care: Time for a new active and comprehensive model of consumer involvement. *Health Expectations, 21*(4), 707–713. doi:10.1111/ hex.12665 PMID:29512248

American Academy of Family Physicians. (2014). *Direct primary care: An alternative to the fee-for-service framework.* Retrieved from https://www.aafp.org/dam/AAFP/documents/ practice_management/ payment/DirectPrimaryCare.pdf

Carlasare, L. (2018, August). Defining the place of direct primary care in a value-based care system. *Wisconsin Medical Journal, 117*(3), 106–110. PMID:30193018

Chase, D. (2013, July 10). Direct primary care regulatory trends. *Forbes.* Retrieved from https://www.forbes.com/ sites/davechase/2013/07/10/ direct-primary-care-regulatory-trends/

Cheney, C. (2016). Acquisition and assimilation: Capella healthcare's model. *HealthLeaders, 19*(2), 14–15.

Doherty, R. (2015). Assessing the patient care implications of "concierge" and other direct patient contracting practices: A policy position paper from the American college of physicians. *Annals of Internal Medicine, 163*(12), 949–952. doi:10.7326/M15-0366 PMID:26551655

Huff, C. (2015, January). New practice model evolves: 'direct care.' *ACP Internist.* Retrieved from https://www.acpinternist.org/archives/2015/01/practice.htm

Medley, J. (2017). *Direct primary care: An alternative to fee-for-service.* Retrieved from https://www.firstprimarycare.com/ direct-primary-care-an-alternative-to-fee-for-service/

Von Drehle, D. (2014, December 22). Medicine is about to get personal. *Time.* Retrieved from https://time.com/3643841/medicine-gets-personal/

KEY TERMS AND DEFINITIONS

Corporate Partnership Plans Model: Companies that partner together in pooling their resources to offer innovative healthcare plan/s that would benefit all the companies' employees.

Direct Primary Care Plans Model: The physician and healthcare provider/s interact directly with their patients, in terms of more direct contact, time spent, services provided, direct payment agreements, etc.

Enlightened Self-Interest: Pursuit of profit or self-interest with social responsibility perspectives to be sustainable in the long term.

Faith-Based Plans Model: Healthcare plans that are related to Christian faith and values in this context.

Hybrid Plans Model: A blending or combination of two or more alternative plans into one plan.

Innovative Alternative Model: New healthcare-related change/s to the existing system, which involves implementing or putting into action an alternative strategy, plan, or program that may be measured in terms of effectiveness.

Patient/Customer-Centricity: The healthcare provider/organization emphasizes a total focus on the patient and is customer-centered.

Stakeholders: All of the individuals and groups that have some "stake" or interest in the organization.

Chapter 3

Shifting Toward Consumer-Centricity:
Insights and Lessons From Emerging Transformations

Jeff Gourdji
Prophet, USA

Scott M. Davis
Prophet, USA

ABSTRACT

In the face of government reform and competitive disruption, healthcare organizations are in need of consumer-centric transformation: transformation that will help them win when consumers shop for a doctor, plan, or medicine and engage them in their care to form a partnership that will improve outcomes and lower costs. The authors interviewed 70 senior executives at leading provider systems, health plans, and pharmaceutical manufacturers to understand their transformation agenda. Interviews asked such question as What initiatives and changes are underway? Where have they had success? What will come next? Where have they struggled?" And, most importantly, What can others learn from them? Davis and Gourdji uncovered five shifts and share practical advice and examples of what these leaders are doing to set them in motion.

DOI: 10.4018/978-1-7998-2949-2.ch003

THE ERA OF THE E-CONSUMER

Change has been on the horizon for many years for healthcare organizations, both in how they do business and in how they engage consumers. In the past, experts discussed the need for healthcare organizations to drive preference and selection–how organizations convince consumers that they are the best hospital, plan or medication. But the healthcare landscape has changed drastically from this time; conversations have shifted focus to driving engagement, relationships and loyalty—much like other consumer businesses. Today's healthcare world belongs to the "e-consumer."

The e-consumer is not a technology term. The genesis is the "e-patient," a concept coined in the 1990s by the late Dr. Tom Ferguson, M.D., an American physician who advocated for participatory medicine and the increasing role of patients in managing their own healthcare. E-patients, he says, are **empowered, engaged, equipped and enabled**. E-patients are not just patients who engage for purposes of self-diagnosis. These individuals also engage in their own health management, partnering closely with organizations in order to find the solutions that work best for them.

The e-patient, however, is a concept limited to direct interactions with healthcare organizations. It is important that patients are engaged when they are ill; but their behavior outside the clinic, hospital or doctor's office has significant implications and cannot be disregarded. That's why the concept has been expanded. Similar to the e-patient, the e-consumer is **empowered, engaged, equipped and enabled**, but for the e-consumer, moments of health are just as important as moments of sickness. Serving e-consumers means giving them tools that see them through recovery and beyond and designing services that cure and empower them.

The Growing Population of E-Consumers

Today, only the beginning of consumer centricity in healthcare is emerging and while there is still a long way to go to achieve full consumer centricity, traditional healthcare organizations are taking smalls steps while contemplating bigger moves that others can learn from.

Many healthcare organizations are at a disadvantage when it comes to consumer centricity, because they were not built to meet the expectations of consumers today. Providers historically have taken a paternalistic approach to care, in which the doctor always knows best. Payers were built to serve employers and manage costs. And pharmaceutical companies have driven their business through providers, not patients. The challenges are several:

A Limited View of the Health Journey

Across the healthcare spectrum, organizations have historically focused on a specific part of the health journey. Healthcare providers are structurally designed to serve patients who are sick and need treatment, not consumers who are managing their health. Providers, payers, and pharmaceutical companies all focus on patients at the point of care, not across the health journey.

Learning the Wrong Lessons

Healthcare organizations sometimes follow the steps of tech companies by latching onto trends without considering how those trends will perform in healthcare or if they are even relevant. They invest in programs like apps or updated websites, which serve only as Band-Aids for a larger problem and sometimes even make it worse. In the pharmaceutical industry alone, 26 percent of the more than 700 apps created are used only once—and nearly three-quarters of them are abandoned by the 10th use.[1]

Hesitation to Adopt New Technology

Healthcare is a highly regulated industry and patient lives are at stake; so, when it comes to embracing and adopting new technologies, there is substantial hesitation and resistance. "Change is hard when it comes to considering the technological infrastructure that enables great leaps forward. Health systems and insurers are behind on implementing new technologies because they fear—rightly so—some of the security risks that come with cloud-based capabilities. But instead of considering

Figure 1. Holistic view of the healthcare journey

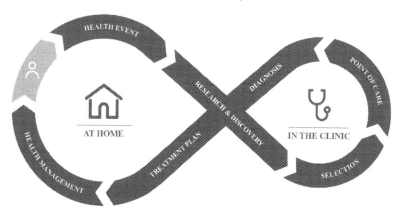

ways to contain or protect against these risks, some folks just make it a blanket rule not to use them," says Sterling Lanier, CEO of Tonic Health, a data collection and payments platform (S. Lanier, personal communication, May 5, 2017).

Cumbersome Legacy Systems

Many traditional healthcare organizations are hindered by their legacy technology systems that were designed for a different era. Integrating new data into old systems is cumbersome, resulting in an inability to share and access information in a consumer-centered way. Moreover, when it comes to collaboration with different players in the healthcare ecosystem, fragmentation is a challenge. There is no easy way for life-science companies to communicate with care teams and no easy way for providers care teams to help resolve conflicts with payers.

A Future of Uncertainty

On top of the structural barriers that organizations grapple with during transformation, they are also at the mercy of ever-changing healthcare policies that can disrupt or entirely uproot current structures as have not been seen in the United States where healthcare is highly politicized. "We have to be thoughtful of how we move because there is this general fear that all of the sudden these changes could be obsolete," says Mark Modesto, Chief Marketing Officer of Chicago's Northwestern Medicine (M. Modesto, personal communication, June 6, 2017).

What this Research Tells Us

To understand what the healthcare industry is currently doing and can to do to reshape itself, the authors conducted in-depth interviews with more than 70 organizations around the globe and surveyed almost 250 executives at leading healthcare enterprises, including large hospital systems; payers; and pharmaceutical, medical device and digital health companies in the United States, Asia and Europe. These organizations include some of the most prominent names in healthcare, including Mayo Clinic, Intermountain Health, Aetna and Pfizer. The authors set out to understand what these organizations are currently doing to be consumer-centric, where they would like to be in the future, and what challenges they face in getting to their ideal state. From the interviews, five shifts that organizations can make now to become more consumer-centric were identified.

Figure 2. A summary of the five shifts to consumer-centricity

	THE FIRST SHIFT From Tactical Fixes to a Holistic Experience Strategy	*Healthcare organizations often start enhancing consumer experiences in one-off initiatives (i.e., reducing waiting-room times). However, by executing on a holistic experience that ladders up to a unifying strategy, they can move their organization to the next level of consumer centricity.*
	THE SECOND SHIFT From Fragmented Care to Connected Ecosystems	*Although payers, providers and pharma companies are finding new ways to work together, the healthcare journey remains fragmented for most consumers, causing frustration and inefficiency. But, when healthcare organizations operate in a connected, integrated ecosystem, rather than as a standalone entity, they can better engage consumers and solve the pain points that are preventing long-term health.*
	THE THIRD SHIFT From Population-Centric to Person-Centered	*Healthcare organizations often focus on creating products, services and experiences for groups of similar consumers, such as those who have the same condition or those who fall into the same demographic. To be truly consumer-centric, it is critical for healthcare organizations to create products, services and experiences for consumers based on their individual needs.*
	THE FOURTH SHIFT From Incremental Improvements to Pervasive Innovation	*Healthcare organizations often settle for small, time-consuming improvements to established systems and processes that were never designed with the consumer in mind. To put the consumer at the center, organizations must reimagine their approach to innovation to truly reinvent the consumer experience. They can consistently adopt both an innovative and a minimally viable product mindset, using a portfolio of approaches to spark wholesale, enterprise-wide change.*
	THE FIFTH SHIFT From Insights as a Department to a Culture of Consumer Obsession	*Establishing insights as a function is critical to gathering intelligence, but it's not enough. Healthcare organizations can go further by creating a culture of consumer obsession, where everyone in the organization always keeps the consumer front and center.*

THE FIRST SHIFT: FROM TACTICAL FIXES TO A HOLISTIC EXPERIENCE STRATEGY

At Novant Health, consumer experience is approached holistically. It is built into every strategic element we have. –Carl Armato, CEO, Novant Health (C. Armato, personal communication, July 17, 2018)

The healthcare industry, for the most part, fails to deliver cohesive experiences. A burdensome healthcare journey can lead to higher costs and lower health outcomes. To increase connections throughout the journey, organizations can develop a holistic experience strategy to guide the design of experiences under a unifying definition of what consumer centricity means for their organization.

Despite the importance of consumer experience (CX), many organizations continue to focus on one-off initiatives like reductions in nighttime noise, better dining options and more efficient parking instead of creating a cohesive journey aligned with a broad strategy. "You have to think about your customers, whoever they may be, more holistically and less transactionally," says Dennis Murphy, CEO of Indiana University Health (D. Murphy, personal communication, June 6, 2017). "When people come to our healthcare system, they aren't touching us just once. How well it's connected and how seamless it is drives satisfaction and engagement as important as any individual experience." The problem of creating fragmented experiences is likely driven by the fact that healthcare organizations often measure success through touchpoint feedback. 71 percent of the organizations surveyed report relying on experience-satisfaction scores (e.g., appointment satisfaction) or touchpoint metrics (e.g., waiting-room time) to evaluate how well an organization is delivering. While this type of measurement works for touchpoint optimization, it leads to addressing consumer pain points in a disjointed manner.

Organizations need to define what consumer centricity means for them and allow that to inform a holistic experience strategy, clarifying goals and tactics to successfully activate it.

Here are ways for organizations to get started:

- Define consumer centricity for the organization in a way that is consistent with the business model and organizational strategy.
- Codify the definition of consumer centricity so it can be socialized and activated across the business.
- Develop a roadmap of initiatives that will deliver a consumer-centric experience and identify bold moves that will jump-start momentum.
- Build a strong organizational engine with the appropriate structure and expertise to deliver the holistic experience.

Synchronize Consumer Centricity and the Business Model

While many healthcare organizations have woven consumer centricity into written missions or visions, leaders tell us that translating consumer centricity into a living, organizational strategy is challenging—fully realizing that a consumer-centric strategy requires significant changes to overall mindsets, organizational structure, employee incentives and investment priorities.

Lesson from Intermountain Healthcare: Go Ahead, Break Your Business Model

"We recognized that traditional modes of healthcare, where we wait until people are ill just to treat them in our facilities, were not serving our patients or our customers in the way that we need to serve them," says Dan Liljenquist, Senior Vice President and Chief Strategy Officer at Intermountain (D. Liljenquist, personal communication, March 3, 2018).

Changes within the industry pushed Intermountain to re-evaluate whether its current mission, of being "a model healthcare system," could lead to success. After deliberation and debate, the organization decided to change its mission to help people "live the healthiest lives." The problem, though, was that the system was designed to carry out the previous mission, not the new one. The system had a traditional hospital- and facility-based care model and even owned its payer network and medical group in order to drive additional volume to its own hospitals. The two strategies clashed: One aimed to keep hospitals full and efficient, and the other aimed to keep people out of the hospitals.

In 2017, to address the conflicting models, Intermountain restructured into two areas. One consists of specialists, primarily oriented around the hospitals; this area was focused on getting the lowest cost per case and determining how to get the best value on care given at its facilities. The system also split its medical group in half, creating a community-based care group aimed at per-member and per-month cost reduction. The focus for this second area became engagement outside the facilities, medication adherence and identification of health problems before they become critical. This restructuring ensures that the community-based care group is fully engaged, both economically and clinically, in keeping people well and out of facilities.

Learn from Piedmont Healthcare: What's Your Manifesto?

To succeed in a highly competitive environment, Piedmont knew it needed to reimagine the consumer experience both to increase consideration and selection among consumers and to unify the organization around a common brand experience. The result of this effort was the "Piedmont Way," a manifesto guiding all aspects of the patient experience. The system wrote a statement about the organization's mission "The Piedmont Way". Piedmont's five experience principles support this mission: Lead with Human, Connect the Journey, Anticipate Needs, Create Uplifting Moments and Enrich with Technology.

Jump-Start with Bold Moves

To truly deliver on consumer centricity, organizations need to make bold and deliberate moves that galvanize the organization to act.

Learn from Geisinger Health: Put Money on the Line

When David Feinberg, M.D., became CEO of Geisinger Health System, he shifted the organization's focus to the consumer experience. Within his first year, he told *Becker's Hospital Review* that his ultimate goal was "eliminating the waiting room and everything it represents. A waiting room means we're provider-centered—it means the doctor is the most important person and everyone is on their time."[2]

Figure 3. Piedmont Healthcare experience principle

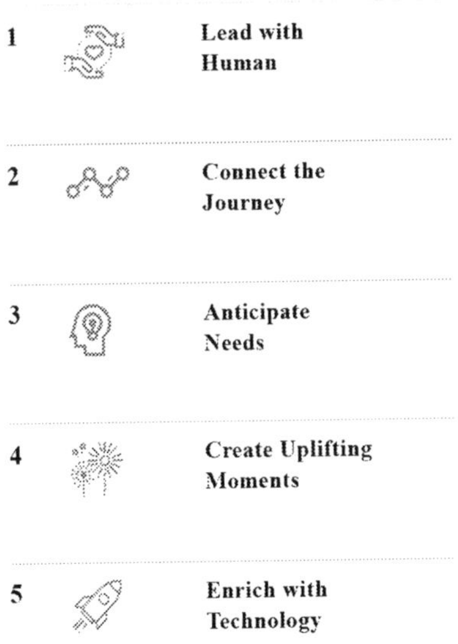

1		**Lead with Human**
2		**Connect the Journey**
3		**Anticipate Needs**
4		**Create Uplifting Moments**
5		**Enrich with Technology**

"Geisinger set an aggressive goal of achieving a Net Promoter Score (NPS) in the top 10 percent of all brands, which would require it to move from its current score of 24 to nearly 50. "Everyone talks about putting the patient first, and that's great—but to make it actually happen, we needed to take a big step that would force us to change," says, says Alistair Erskine, M.D., who was Geisinger's Chief Informatics Officer at the time of our discussion (A. Erskine, personal communication, May 11, 2017). To accomplish that, Geisinger announced ProvenExperience, a refund program with a special app that allowed patients to easily provide feedback on their experiences and receive refunds on their copays for poor experiences. Within a year of launching the program, Geisinger had refunded less than $500,000 to patients. ProvenExperience galvanized the organization to operate with the consumer at the center of everything it does and to demonstrate to patients that the hospital system trusts and values feedback. "The point is not so much the money part. It's about signaling that 'Look, we put our trust in you, the patient, because you've put your trust in us,'" Dr. Erskine says.

Seek Digital Dominance

Piedmont Healthcare launched several initiatives—from virtual visits and online scheduling to physician ratings and reviews—in order to propel the organization forward. "If you don't put a stake in the ground and tell everyone, 'This is what our consumer requires of us, so we're going to go after it and succeed,' it can be very difficult to get people on board," says Matt Gove, who was then Piedmonts' Chief Consumer Officer (M. Gove, personal communication, August 8, 2017).

Intermountain Healthcare is also using a bold approach, laying out deliberate steps to be "the first digitally-enabled, consumer-centric, integrated delivery system." CEO Marc Harrison, M.D. explains (M. Harrison, personal communication, September 6, 2017). "We're taking cues from Amazon, financial technology companies, Starbucks and the like. We are going to inject that holistically into a real digital transformation of an integrated health system to truly understand and serve people the way they want to be served."

Build the Right Team

Of course, these efforts are only as strong as the team behind them. CX leaders are most effective when they have a blended background in healthcare, strategy or consumer-centric industries. Three CX leader archetypes emerged in our research:

- **The Invested Healer**. Leaders with a background in medicine or clinical care, they have hands-on experience working with patients, deeply understand the clinical experience and have a personal interest in improving the overall patient experience.
- **The Best-Practice Strategist**. These leaders come from industries like consulting, where they have worked with organizations in many sectors to solve a range of business challenges similar to those in healthcare.
- **The Lifelong Consumerist**. Experts from consumer-centric industries, such as packaged goods, bring a consumer-first mindset.

Establish the Right Organizational Structure

And no matter where CX sits in the organization chart, they need strong, clear connections to the CEO and also need to be well respected and supported. There are three ways in which CX teams can be successful:

CX Lives Under Marketing: At Aetna, CX is part of the Marketing Department. This works at Aetna, because marketing is seen as essential to strategic decisions. Marketing can deliver quick wins to build credibility, or the organization can invest in the marketing team through a strategic hire.

A Separate CX Team: Piedmont Healthcare has a centralized CX team comprised of cross-service line players within the Physician Enterprise Group. This elevates the importance of CX within the organization. Katie Logan, VP of Customer Experience at Piedmont, says that having her team sit within the Physician Enterprise Group is important, since executing much of the consumer-centric strategy requires the support and cooperation of physicians and their operations (K. Logan, personal communication, February 28, 2018). "We are laying the foundation for some of these pieces and how we will execute and implement them," she says. "We want to deploy [CX] across the entire organization with some level of consistency; and by starting at the top of the funnel, we can work our way through the customer journey."

A Decentralized Team: Biotechnology company Amgen has a dedicated patient engagement team focused on consistently incorporating the voice of the patient throughout the value chain. "The real change that we believe the organization needs, is to be decentralized," says Jessica Nora, Amgen's Executive Director of Patient Engagement Strategy, "so we have a group of patient centricity leaders, which are high potential executive directors and directors, sponsored by their vice presidents." (J. Nora, personal communication, June 29, 2017). These dedicated leads sit across the organization to ensure the patient voice is being elevated and represented across functions and regions. They are responsible for developing a patient centricity network within their functions and making progress against specific goals.

THE SECOND SHIFT: FROM FRAGMENTED CARE TO CONNECTED ECOSYSTEMS

I cannot be responsible for population health if I am waiting for those three hours a year when I interact with a patient. I have to consider how to extend my influence and show up differently.—John Haney, Area Vice President Southeast, Johnson & Johnson (former VP, Healthcare Strategic Marketing) (J. Haney, personal communication, June 27, 2017)

Healthcare journeys are frustrating and fragmented, making engagement and health outcomes difficult to improve. "The system is so fragmented," says Jeffrey Dachis, CEO of One Drop, "it is a burden on patients and is incredibly disempowering." (J. Dachis, personal communication, May 31, 2017) Consumers are responsible for managing connections between their many providers, their health plan and their pharmacy. Even more damaging, treatment plans fail to consider the many factors that influence a consumer's health, leading to suboptimal outcomes. To do better, healthcare organizations focus on developing solutions that package discrete parts of the journey in a single offering. In the Second Shift, how organizations can move from fragmented care to connected ecosystems is explored.

Challenge for Healthcare: Connecting the Broken Pieces

A connected healthcare journey seems unimaginable, because healthcare organizations still struggle to reduce fragmentation within their own organizations let alone handle service gaps in the broader industry.

Fragmentation hinders the development of solutions both inside organizations and in their outside collaborations. Providers like Kaiser Permanente, Intermountain Healthcare or Geisinger Health System that have built integrated delivery networks from the ground up are an obvious exception, as they started with a strong cultural foundation that encourages both integration and coordination with the consumer at the center. If healthcare organizations want to engage patients in a way that reduces costs and improves outcomes, those organizations need to go beyond their traditional responsibilities, create a solution-oriented mindset and serve consumers differently.

Organizations need to move away from simply addressing a single pain point or developing a new product or service touchpoint and, instead, start moving toward offering fully integrated solutions. Connecting the factors of an ecosystem is no easy task, and the majority of healthcare organizations are just starting the process. This shift is more challenging for payers than for other players, and 68 percent of payers report that they are only in the beginning stages.

Figure 4. Overview of the healthcare ecosystem

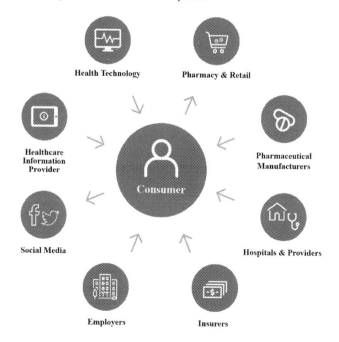

"Plus Product" Solutions Engage Customers

To make this transition, a model is proposed that was shared by Jean-Michel Cossery, former VP of Oncology North America at Eli Lilly and Co. That model outlines three types of offers that an organization can make to consumers. The first is *Product,* a stand-alone drug, service or plan. The primary objective of this *Product* offering is to push the product, which consumers then learn to use on their own. The second is a *Product Plus*, which means the single drug, service or plan is enhanced with "wraparound" services such as educational materials, patient-support programs or digital tools, such as an app. The primary objective of *Product Plus* is still to push the product; but at this stage, and at the most basic level, the organization assists the consumer in using the product. The third offering, called a *Plus Product,* takes a comprehensive solution-oriented approach to serving the patient—layering on elements, as needed, to create an ecosystem and drive the desired outcome. The primary objective of the *Plus Product* is to engage the consumers, guide them through the journey and build a relationship with them.

Getting to *Plus Product* requires:

- Building a thorough, deep understanding of consumer pain points.
- Understanding other players within the healthcare ecosystem that can help address the pain points and develop a holistic solution.
- Aligning with a willingness to collaborate across business silos. The components of a *Plus Product* often fall outside the walls of a single organization, requiring coordination and partnership.

Learn from Mount Sinai: Identify Where Consumers Get Stuck

In 2015, New York's Mount Sinai Health System partnered with the 32BJ Health Fund, which provides benefits to members of the U.S.'s largest union of property service workers, to co-design a bundled Total Joint Replacement (TJR) package with

Figure 5. Developing plus product solutions

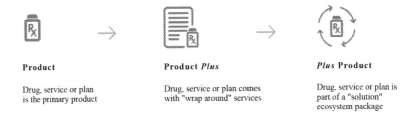

Product	Product *Plus*	*Plus* Product
Drug, service or plan is the primary product	Drug, service or plan comes with "wrap around" services	Drug, service or plan is part of a "solution" ecosystem package

amenities that address common challenges that patients face. The two organizations understood that given the complexity of the operation and its burden on patients, they needed to connect the ecosystem with a *Plus Product* solution.

The Health Fund understood that TJR surgeries can be challenging for its members: coordinating resources for a successful surgery and recovery can be difficult. To uncover specific challenges related to TJR, 32BJ conducted comprehensive focus groups with its members. The research revealed that members lacked important information and navigation assistance to ensure a healthy recovery. As a result, many patients incorrectly believed that they would need to recover in a skilled nursing facility.

Consumer-First Solutions

The *Plus Product* solution that the hospital and the Health Fund created was designed specifically to meet the needs of the Fund's members. The final bundle program for TJR includes additional services that address the key challenges identified in the research. The hospital system provides a care guide to work, one-on-one, with patients from the day they schedule surgery through their recovery. The care guides act as advocates and help members understand how to take care of themselves during their recovery period. To help members during their recovery, the Fund waives copays on the first 10 physical therapy visits within the first 50 days after discharge. The final component of the TJR surgery bundled package, known as a reference price, pushes patients to go to settings that are at or under the reference price of joint replacement surgery in the Mount Sinai program. "When we looked at this procedure, we saw where the gaps were; and we believe it's our responsibility to fill those for the patient, using the entire ecosystem at hand," says Lucas Pauls, Plan Sponsor Channel Lead, who helped manage the partnership (L. Pauls, personal communication, August 8, 2017).

Leveraging Strengths

Given the various components of the *Plus Product* solution, the Fund and Mount Sinai leveraged their unique strengths to share the investment and logistics of the solution. Combining their expertise led to an efficient and successful program that addresses TJR in its entirety, not just the operation itself.

Lower Costs, Happier Patients

Within the first year of the program, Mount Sinai, 32BJ and patients experienced improved outcomes and lower costs. Patients reported high satisfaction with their

Figure 6. Mount Sinai Health Systems' plus product solution: total joint replacement

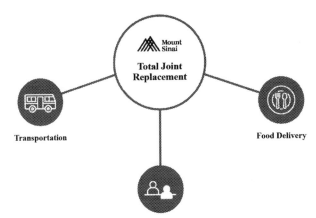

experience, and the number of skilled nursing facility discharges dropped by 12 percentage points. In addition to improved health outcomes, the reference price on the TJR surgeries led to a four-fold increase in the volume of TJR surgeries at Mount Sinai. Because members sought out more reasonably priced hospitals, the program led to nearly $13,000 in savings per operation switched to Mount Sinai. By considering the broader care journey and speaking directly with patients about their needs, organizations can create added value that produces win-win situations. At Mount Sinai, care became far more than just the procedure; rather, it was about the many additional factors shaping recovery.

Learn from Geisinger Health: Write an Rx for Food, Not Medication

Pennsylvania's Geisinger Health System is all too familiar with the costs associated with diabetes and took on the challenge of tackling this public health issue. Geisinger Health understood that the biggest challenge for improving and sustaining health among diabetic patients was not something that could be solved with medication alone; rather, it required a change in behavior. Geisinger Health identified that consumers who struggle the most with behavioral change are low-income, food-insecure consumers. Those people have limited access to, and are unable to afford, nutritious, fresh foods that help slow or reverse the progression of the disease. To tackle this challenge, Geisinger Health designed the Fresh Food Farmacy.

This "pharmacy" looks less like a traditional pharmacy and more like a grocery store. The shelves are stocked with healthy staples like whole-grain pasta and beans; refrigerators hold fresh produce, low-fat dairy, meats and fish. This pharmacy is not just for grocery shopping; it also serves as an educational lab, where participants learn from registered dietitians how to prepare recipes and adopt eating habits that lead to a healthy lifestyle. After their visit, participants go home with a "prescription" of five days' worth of free, fresh food. The Fresh Food Farmacy program targets low-income patients, so providing free food solves the financial burden.

Adding Value, Increasing Health

Since its launch, the Fresh Food Farmacy has proven to be beneficial for both consumers and the health system. The Fresh Food Farmacy program costs Geisinger nearly $1,000 per participant. The outcomes, however, far outweigh the upfront costs. Geisinger Health evaluates the success of the program by patients' A1C levels, which measure the amount of glucose in the blood. Through research and analysis, Geisinger Health determined that the program saves $8,000 for every one-point decrease in a patient's A1C levels. Within the first year, many of the participants in the program saw a three-point decline in their A1C levels, resulting in savings of nearly $24,000.[3]

Craft Packages That Connect Healthcare Players

Pharma companies like Germany-based global pharmaceutical company Boehringer Ingelheim (BI) are leveraging partnerships with digital companies to offer value-added services to consumers. BI partnered with Propeller Health, a digital health company involved in chronic obstructive pulmonary disease (COPD) care management. Propeller Health makes a chip that attaches to BI's RESPIMAT® inhaler and tracks a patient's adherence data. That allows the physician to monitor adherence and, if necessary, get in touch with the patient before he or she becomes ill. The data also creates a comprehensive view of the patient's progress so that individuals can view their own condition management. By notifying care teams when adherence is low and giving patients a snapshot of their progress, the BI RESPIMAT makes patients aware of their condition before it becomes critical.

As healthcare organizations around the globe continue to be under pressure to deliver value over volume, this type of solution—which allows physicians to remotely identify problems before they become emergencies—will be even more beneficial. "We are now a far stronger enabler of [physicians'] business when their incentives shift to value," says Paul Fonteyne, CEO of BI USA. "We feel much more patient-focused, because we know we developed the medications to avoid costly events that no patients would desire for themselves." (P. Fonteyne, personal communication, June 14, 2017) By engaging people in this way—giving them ownership of their own data and helping them communicate with physicians—BI proactively manages the challenges facing patients with COPD instead of being entirely reactive.

THE THIRD SHIFT: FROM POPULATION-CENTRIC TO PERSON-CENTERED

People define value differently. For someone like myself, who is healthy and busy, high-value care is all about convenience and access. And that's very different from someone who has two different chronic diseases and moves in and out of homelessness.– Niyum Gandhi, EVP and Chief Population Health Officer, Mount Sinai Health System (N. Gandhi, personal communication, July 6, 2017)

From communications that don't resonate to engagement plans that don't fit the consumer's lifestyle, organizations continue to make healthcare—which is inherently a personal experience—something that feels impersonal and disconnected.

In the Third Shift, healthcare organizations learn to leverage their understanding of what's relevant to *groups* of consumers in order to tailor experiences that suit the needs and preferences of *individual* consumers. Seeing each consumers as a 'person," and not part of a population, is core to this shift.

The Challenge for Healthcare: Seeing Past Population-Based Myopia

Healthcare organizations have access to enormous amounts of data that hold the potential to create personalized experiences across the non-clinical aspects of care, such as appointment scheduling, billing or treatment plan adherence. Despite having a wealth of data, the healthcare industry has yet to unleash its potential. When healthcare leaders were surveyed about personalized experiences, more than half reported that they fail to use data to customize communication channels and content. "You think about all the other things that go on," says Sheri Dodd, Vice President and General Manager of Medtronic Care Management Services, a service business within Medtronic, plc, a medical device company, "like making sure questions are relevant to the patient's condition, reading and comprehension skills. Relatability matters in patient engagement," (S. Dodd, personal communication, August 23, 2017)

Gaining a more nuanced understanding of consumers requires two stages: First, healthcare organizations can use insights from groups of similar consumers (sometimes called personas) to create products, services, experiences and communications. Second, using insights from the selected personas, organizations can build on that foundation and incorporate an individual's data to personalize the product or service. "There is a huge opportunity to understand more about patients and what is happening in their lives and use that understanding to benefit the patient through better medicines and services," says Frank Cunningham, Vice President, Managed Healthcare Services, Eli Lilly and Company (F. Cunningham, personal communication, July 20, 2017).

How to Make the Shift: Use Insights to Inform Products And Services

One path to increasing personalization is leveraging consumer insights that go well beyond a demographic understanding. Engaging consumers in their health requires a behavioral change that demographics alone can't drive. Instead of looking at the market as a heterogeneous group of people, a segmentation analysis identifies personas that represent groups of people with common characteristics.

Learn from Novant Health: New Personas Reveal Better Prospects

In 2013, Novant Health, a North Carolina-based hospital system, announced a strategic plan to formally unify all programs, services and facilities under a single operating unit. After several mergers, acquisitions and partnerships, the four-state integrated health system expanded to include 13 hospitals, 500 outpatient clinics, 1,300 physicians, nine million customers and $4 billion in revenue. The challenge was to unify the system, which previously operated under 350 different brand names, and to gain relevance. To do this well, Novant Health had to gain a deeper understanding of the groups within the populations so it could design mechanisms to engage consumers in relevant ways. "We had to agree that the right way forward was to compare ourselves to iconic brands outside of healthcare—not to aspire to be them but, rather, to be inspired by them—and connecting with individual consumers in ways that meet their unique needs," said David Duvall, then the Novant Health Senior Vice President, Chief Marketing and Communications (D. Duvall, personal communication, March 1, 2018).

Part of getting to a single, unified system involved creating services that resonate with Novant Health's different populations of consumers. To do that, Duvall's team conducted rigorous research to derive a segmentation solution that was both strategic and achievable. The research examined thousands of patients, potential patients and caregivers on multiple levels, from price sensitivity and smartphone usage to time spent on the internet and social media engagement. The research uncovered six key personas:

Novant Health identified the first two segments as a primary focus and used cross-functional teams to design products and services to meet the needs of each group.

Figure 7. Novant Health's consumer segmentation

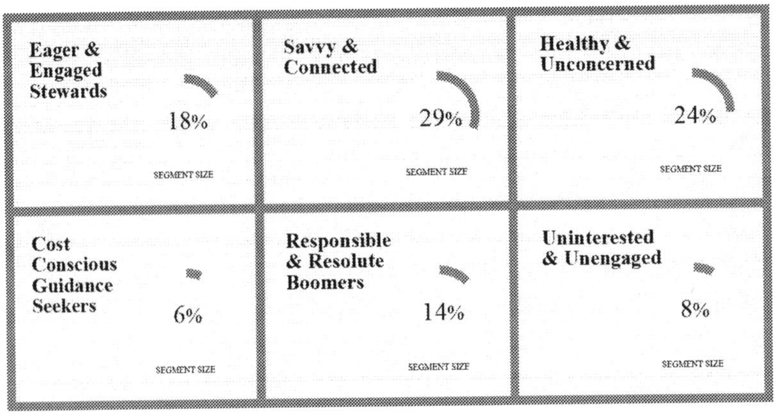

Eager & Engaged Stewards 18% SEGMENT SIZE	Savvy & Connected 29% SEGMENT SIZE	Healthy & Unconcerned 24% SEGMENT SIZE
Cost Conscious Guidance Seekers 6% SEGMENT SIZE	Responsible & Resolute Boomers 14% SEGMENT SIZE	Uninterested & Unengaged 8% SEGMENT SIZE

Segmentation enabled the system to identify common needs that resonate most with target segments. Because Novant Health needs to serve all consumers, however, the organization identified the top needs in all segments, such as cost clarity, access and digital integration. Those insights led to the development of services such as *Your Healthcare Costs*, an online feature that helps consumers understand complex healthcare finance information. Insights from the segmentation also led to the development of *Care Connections*, a 24-hour virtual care hub with services such as nurse triage, online scheduling, wellness coaching, discharge follow-ups, medication management and psychosocial consults. The insights catalyzed the hospital system's digital transformation, leading to the development of products such as *HoldMyPlace* for urgent-care reservations, *Open Schedule* for viewing physician availability and online scheduling through *MyChart*.

Mine People's Data for More Relevance

Creating services and offerings based on insights from different segments allows for more relevant engagement with consumers. Organizations don't have to stop there, though. They can take it a step further and create personalized experiences using the data collected on individual consumers. The challenge in healthcare is capturing and identifying the right data to drive more personal offerings.

Delivering on Your Data Promises: Use Data for Good

Organizations need a Consumer Data Value Exchange (CDVE): a mechanism for determining what consumers will receive in return for sharing personal data. Developing an effective CDVE requires a few key steps: The organization theorizes

Figure 8. Consumer data value exchange (CDVE) model

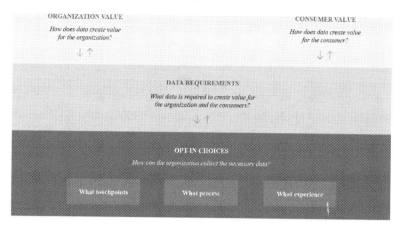

how data can add value for both the consumer *and* the business, what touchpoints in the journey are appropriate for data collection and what the process (e.g. opt-in) for data collection will look like. Then, the organization codifies it in a specific, motivating value-exchange proposition that will resonate with consumers. Finally, the organization deploys the value exchange proposition.

The CDVE strategy is not common in healthcare, but some organizations are attempting it. PatientsLikeMe, slated to become part of United Health Group, Inc, as of July 2019, is a network that allows patients living with chronic conditions to track and share their experiences and improve outcomes. PatientsLikeMe aggregates data submitted by patients and sells it to companies creating new drugs, devices, equipment, insurance plans and medical services. By selling data, PatientsLikeMe helps companies accelerate the development of new solutions for patients. The organization's CDVE, called "Data for Good," is the foundation of PatientsLikeMe's business model. As the company explains, "Your data has a heartbeat that gives life to medical research. Donate your data for you, for others, for good."

THE FOURTH SHIFT: FROM INCREMENTAL IMPROVEMENTS TO PERVASIVE INNOVATION

On both the competitive side and the consumer expectation side, we are seeing that the definition of consumer centricity keeps getting elevated. We have to continue to innovate and push ourselves to maintain both consumer relevance and a competitive edge. – Indiana University Health Chief Executive Officer Dennis Murphy (D. Murphy, personal communication, June 26, 2017)

The healthcare industry is anything but stagnant, though it is risk-averse. That cautiousness continues to widen the gap between consumer expectations and what healthcare organizations can deliver. And it dramatically impacts their ability to influence consumer behavior outside the clinic.

To adapt to the changes that consumers demand, healthcare organizations need to make the Fourth Shift: moving from incremental improvements to relentless and pervasive innovation. This shift explores how organizations can spark innovation and maintain it over time, making it an integral part of the way in which the organization runs its business and serves consumers.

The Challenge for Healthcare: Make Fresh Thinking Less Frightening

Clinical innovation demands incredible precision and caution and requires multiple rounds of testing and analysis until the final product has been perfected and approved by appropriate governing bodies. While long processes are warranted in clinical research, they stifle healthcare experience and engagement innovation, which need not be scrutinized in the same way. This risk aversion isn't surprising, given the amount of regulation within the healthcare industry. Organizations have good reason to be risk-averse, as they seek to avoid litigation, HIPAA violations and privacy breaches.

Solving Healthcare's Idea Shortage

If healthcare organizations want to keep up with the competition and improve engagement, they need to radically transform innovation practices that run through the organization. Healthcare organizations can spark innovation in a few different ways:

- Mirror the strategy of startups and apply the Minimal Viable Product (MVP) concept to innovation.
- Form an internal startup or incubator program to unite the most innovative minds in the company for brainstorming and designing new ideas.
- Outsource innovation to external organizations.

Applying the MVP Approach

One technique they can use is from the startup industry. Minimal Viable Product (MVP) is a trial-and-error approach by which an organization releases an idea as version 1.0 and then continues to make updates and improvements until the product becomes final. The MVP approach accelerates the innovation process by securing the minimum amount of resources required to prove impact and gather evangelists, who will then help improve and expand the product.

"We want to focus on what we call 'low-resolution' solutions before we spend millions of dollars on the 'high-resolution' solution. Let's put our focus into building the right thing for consumers rather than wasting time on perfection," says Robin Glasco, Chief Innovation Officer at Blue Cross Blue Shield of Massachusetts until September 2018 (R. Glasco, personal communication, March 6, 2018).

Learn from Advocate: Same-Day Mammograms Ignite Bigger Changes

One of the Midwest's largest health systems, Advocate Health Care (Advocate Aurora Health since April 2018) used an MVP approach to begin its journey to same-day appointment scheduling. As Advocate worked to deepen its relationship with consumers, the organization found that convenience and access were two areas where the system could improve. The ideal solution would be online, same-day self-scheduling so that consumers could have more freedom to decide when they receive healthcare. Structurally, this would be a big ask of the system's IT department and physicians, *and* it would require a massive cultural change. So Advocate started small, leveraging an MVP approach and mindset.

The process began with a project called "Call Today, Be Seen Today," which allowed same-day scheduling for mammograms. The organization realized that consumers did not just want educational materials about breast cancer; they also wanted greater access to care. If Advocate could expand access, Advocate would also expand business. "We realized this consumerism goes far beyond an advertising campaign," says Advocate's Chief Marketing and Digital Officer, Kelly Jo Golson (K. J. Golson, personal communication, June 1, 2017). By focusing on mammography, Advocate could control the number of changes necessary to implement the new program, quickly measure results and make real-time updates before investing in an entire restructuring. Advocate experienced double-digit growth after "Call Today, Be Seen Today" was activated, as the new program doubled the number of same-day appointments made and tripled the number of new appointments made. More importantly, the program increased engagement in the breast cancer awareness campaign, which both benefits consumers' long-term health and drives mammogram business to the system.

After the success of "Call Today, Be Seen Today," Advocate rolled out the 2.0 version of the initiative, which included same-day results.

Figure 9. The MVP approach in action at Advocate Aurora Health Care

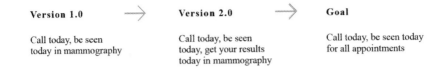

Create an Internal Startup

One way to overcome the risk aversion that plagues healthcare is to separate innovation efforts from the core business.

The challenge of risk aversion is particularly acute in the pharmaceutical industry. The regulatory nature of pharma not only stifles experience innovation but also fails to attract entrepreneurial minds with risk-taking attitudes. To solve that, some pharma companies are creating a separate, internal function with a completely different culture that inspires innovative thinking. German pharmaceutical company Boehringer Ingelheim, for example, formed a digital innovation lab called BI X. The team operates like a startup, working closely with all three business units of the company: human pharma, animal health and biopharmaceuticals. BI X is a space for collaboration among specialists in data science, agile software development and user-experience design.

In addition to being physically separate from the parent pharmaceutical company, the digital innovation lab has its own recruitment process to attract innovative talent. By operating internally, BI still benefits from the proprietary innovation that comes out of the lab. The BI X Lab launched in summer of 2017, and the organization invested 10 million euros in the lab within the first year.

Learn from BCBSMA: Finding its Soul in Human-Centered Design

In the survey, progress on the shift to pervasive innovation, is slight. In fact, only 14 percent of providers and 15 percent of pharma companies believe they have made the Fourth Shift, while not a single payer reported having done so. Some payers are fighting that resistance to innovation by using both separate internal functions and external thought partnerships to propel innovative efforts.

When Robin Glasco started at Blue Cross Blue Shield of Massachusetts as Chief Innovation Officer, a lot of innovative activity was happening in the competitive landscape, and BCBSMA wanted to increase its focus on weaving the discipline of innovation into the fabric of the organization. "We define innovation not as a thing but as a continuous state of reimagining what is possible—with the mission of transforming how we deliver health care. Our house in the future won't operate like our house in the past," says CEO Andrew Dreyfus (A. Dreyfus, personal communication, March 20, 2018). "Everything—from the plumbing and the wiring to the design and the fact that it's even like a house with four walls, a roof and windows—will change."

Glasco formed the internal innovation function, which hosts training and boot camps throughout the year to teach those involved in the organization how to carry innovation into other departments. Glasco and her team walk attendees through the multiple stages of innovation (e.g. empathy, problem definition, ideation, prototyping) and explore the necessary mindsets (e.g. action orientation and radical collaboration). The boot camp is impactful because BCBSMA associates are joined by external participants such as students, professors, physicians and CEOs and are exposed to new ways of thinking about and applying innovation. "We don't define innovation as a noun or a verb. We define it as a mindset of continuously reimagining what is possible. It requires us to embrace a bias toward action, collaboration with different minds, and a culture of prototyping. That's innovation – it's more than a two-day boot camp," Glasco says (R. Glasco, personal communication, March 6, 2018).

THE FIFTH SHIFT: FROM INSIGHTS AS A DEPARTMENT TO A CULTURE OF CONSUMER OBSESSION

Maturing our organization in its consumer centricity is about listening to our members and acknowledging what they are saying with action. It's about integrating their voice into ours. —Doug Cottings, Staff Vice President, Market Strategy & Insights, Anthem (D. Cottings, personal communication, September 8, 2017)

In the first four shifts, the importance of developing an experience strategy, connecting ecosystems, personalizing experiences and driving pervasive innovation was discussed. Making these shifts hinges on knowing what the consumer needs and wants and incorporating that into strategic and tactical decision-making to ultimately drive consumer preference and engagement. "At the end of the day, it is a competitive marketplace and everybody has choice. If we want to be their choice, we have to understand our customers deeply – where they are today; what tensions they face; and, how best to deliver solutions and experiences that relieve those tensions in the most relevant way," says Veronica Chase, Vice President of Marketing at Eli Lilly and Co (V. Chase, personal communication, July 11, 2017). In the Fifth Shift, how organizations can build an Insights Operating System (IOS), a system whose function is to help organizations get to the right insights, drive the right decisions at the right time and win with the right consumers, is addressed.

The Challenge for Healthcare: Insights are Trapped in the Wrong Places

Healthcare organizations were designed to meet a basic human need—and the extent to which they engaged consumers in meeting that need has had little impact on their success. Now that healthcare organizations are responsible for lowering costs and driving consumer engagement and satisfaction, it is imperative that they understand consumers in a different way.

Insights for All: Build Your New IOS

To become insight-driven, organizations must be able to surface relevant consumer knowledge that will influence decision-making. The combination of knowledge and action forms the new IOS, an organizational structure that is equal parts consumer insight processes and outcome-oriented decisions.

The center of the IOS is where relevant knowledge is uncovered and where a team with the right capabilities and processes sits. Once the insights team has developed the capability to identify the right knowledge, the next step is to equip the organization to act. Action requires mechanisms and processes for sharing information and for making consumer insights foundational for all decision-making. Both parts of the IOS are critical to its success.

The First Layer of IOS: Surface the Right Data

Identifying consumer insights requires the work of an experienced team that understands how data becomes an insight and how an insight turns into action. This is the first part of the IOS.

A strong insights team, say from a CPG company like Procter & Gamble, understands the process and effort required to uncover deep and meaningful insights from raw data. Once in the appropriate context, the data point becomes information that can be organized and structured for strategic usage. That information becomes knowledge when it is given meaning and implications, at which point it becomes a business learning. Knowledge becomes insight when it solves a problem and can be integrated and actionable.

Four different insight team archetypes have been observed: The Data Reactor, The 360 Reporter, The Business Strategist and The Culture Catalyst.

- **The Data Reactor.** These teams operate at a basic level, conducting reactive project fulfillment research. They have limited connection to senior leaders. Their focus is on hindsight and tactical research and they have little involvement with functions beyond marketing. These teams react but never anticipate. They report but rarely implement.
- **The 360 Reporter.** These teams conduct both strategic and tactical research, integrating multiple sources of data to mine insights on individual behavior with a perspective on potential drivers of future behavior. This team represents the consumer to senior executives, sharing interesting trends and insights from the research but have a limited role in strategic decision-making.
- **The Business Strategist.** These teams also present the voice of the consumer to senior executives, but their role is more advanced. They are present during planning and decision-making. The knowledge of the team spans across the entire organization, and these teams are sought out enablers for tackling big strategic challenges.
- **The Culture Catalyst.** These strategic insights teams have extensive involvement and responsibility across functions and a direct line of sight into the executive suite. These teams are part of the strategic planning process and help set the agenda on which initiatives are highest priority. The work of these teams and their profile are integral to driving both three- to five-year strategic plans and world-class consumer experiences.

Organizations that want to build a consumer-obsessed culture should aim to be Business Strategists or Culture Catalysts; however, most live as Data Reactors or 360 Reporters. When healthcare organizations are surveyed about the role of their current market research/insights team, only 12 percent responded that their insights team was able to catalyze culture change.

Figure 10. Insight operation system (IOS) maturity levels

BASIC			*ADVANCED*
The Data Reactor	**The 360 Reporter**	**The Business Strategist**	**The Culture Catalyst**
These teams operate at a basic level, conducting reactive project fulfillment research. They have limited connection to senior leaders.	*This approach is slightly more advanced, and teams conduct both strategic and tactical research, integrating multiple sources of data to mine insights on individual behavior with a*	*In this model, teams also present the voice of the consumer to senior executives, but their role is more advanced and they are present during planning and decision-making.*	*This strategic insights team has extensive involvement and responsibility across functions and a direct line of sight into the executive suite. Their knowledge base helps drive the organization*
Their focus is on hindsight and tactical research and they have little involvement with functions beyond marketing. With a team like this, a healthcare organization cannot be consumer-obsessed and will struggle to engage consumers in new ways. These teams react, never anticipate, but rarely implement.	*perspective on potential drivers of future behavior.* *This team represents the consumer to senior executives to share interesting trends and insights from the research, but this team has a limited role in strategic decision making. They focus more on storytelling and less on behavior changing.*	*The knowledge of this team spans across the entire organization and they are sought out enablers for tackling big strategic challenges.*	*forward by focusing on both insight and foresight.* *They are a part of strategic planning and help to set the agenda on what initiatives are highest priority. Their work and profile are integral to driving both three-to-five-year strategic plans and world-class consumer experiences.*

The Journey to Becoming a Culture Catalyst

Processes Needed to Support Insight Development

In addition to acquiring talent with relevant capabilities for uncovering insights, organizations need to ensure that their teams have processes in place that support proactive insight development and not just reactive data collection.

Learn from Aetna: Consolidating Insights and Marketing Magnifies Value

When David Edelman joined Aetna, he understood that insights would be critical to decision-making and effectively change member and enterprise behavior. Uncovering insights would require strengthening the organization's enterprise intelligence. At the time of his arrival, the marketing, branding and insights teams operated separately from each other, working in silos. Post-consolidation, Edelman evaluated the talent on his team to ensure they were up for the task and were aligned with the jobs they needed to accomplish.

Edelman also created Insight Ambassadors to work with other functions throughout the organization and collaborate on recommendations. Insight Ambassadors, which come from marketing, partner with business unit leads to talk about the implications of consumer insights on the business and align them with strategic goals. "This team's role is to be senior advisors—as well as designers and executers of programs—and strategic counselors to the business, drawing on the insights. They need to take that work to the business unit and help [the business unit] understand how to use it," Edelman says (D. Edelman, personal communication, April 25, 2017). Today, Aetna's marketing, brand and insight functions are fully integrated and operating at a high level.

Learn from Lilly: Rewrite the Job Description

Given the new demands of healthcare insights teams, some organizations have found that the talent they previously had for what would have been sufficient for a Data Reactor was no longer sufficient for the needs of the business. Dave Moore, Senior Director of Global Insights and Analytics at Lilly until late 2017, says that as Lilly began making concerted efforts to become more consumer-centric, it had to adjust its approach to recruiting and training insight talent (D. Moore, personal communication, February 14, 2018). The company began to hire talent with skills in data synthesis, integrating data from multiple sources and with a high IQ for data-informed storytelling. Lilly also rotates people in and out of the insights function to ground them in the business, allowing them to eventually bring their consumer-focused lens to other functions. Acquiring talent with a more strategic lens has helped Lilly's insights team move from 360 Reporter to Business Strategist.

The Second Layer of IOS: Turn Insights into Action

Even if an organization uncovers groundbreaking insights, those insights are helpful only if the rest of the organization can act on them. Anthem's Doug Cottings explains that action is the next frontier for his team, which began as a pure Data Reactor and has evolved into a 360 Reporter. Since Cottings joined Anthem, the team has gained a deeper understanding of the member experience and has established a Voice of Consumer (VOC) platform to host a wide variety of data—from demographic and claims data to data about what hold music the member hears or how long the member was actually on hold. The team, however, has yet to unlock its full strategic potential. "We can play a more consultative role, but that will require democratizing the VOC so everyone has access to it," says Cottings (D. Cottings, personal communication, September 8, 2017).

This is where the second part of the IOS comes into play. All too often, research is conducted or data is gathered but never used—not because it wasn't insightful, but because the data didn't make it into the hands of people who could use it at the right time. Three ways to disseminate insights have been observed: self-service mechanisms, targeted communications and formal or informal cross-functional partnerships.

Self-Service Mechanisms

To ensure that insights are available cross-functionally, organizations can establish dashboards and portals that are regularly updated with relevant data and analysis. Lilly, for example, has a knowledge-management hub that houses the research conducted over the past 12 years. The hub contains key summaries, visuals and lessons for every business or therapeutic area. The hub gives other functions an essence of what the organization knows about consumers now and how this knowledge has evolved over time.

Targeted Communications

Having an ongoing database of insights is good, but organizations should also establish processes to call out key insights. Those communications become an opportunity to spell out implications for business goals and highlight key changes in the market. On a quarterly basis, Lilly issues a newsletter full of research and insight updates, which is a direct way for the team to communicate its most recent findings and highlight key insights.

Perhaps even more powerful than a newsletter or a town hall are Lilly's immersive insights sessions. Lilly believes the best way to bring insights to life is through employees who have an appreciation for the consumers they serve and the challenges they face in dealing with and managing their conditions. Lilly inspires this appreciation by holding live workshops in which insights are brought to life through immersive experiences. Employees meet patients who are invited in to talk about their condition.

Cross-Functional Partnership

At organizations like Novant Health, where the data and analytics capability is still in the building process, cross-functional teams consult the insights team to learn exactly how insights might be used. The process began when Mathias Krebs, Senior Director, Insights & Analytics, would approach teams to learn about the challenges they faced and solve those issues using insights. Over time, Krebs and his team built a reputation for both understanding the problems and then delivering and incorporating the insights that would help most (M. Krebs, personal communication, March 9, 2018). While the process is largely informal, it has allowed for close partnerships—with insights used in the most effective ways. "The demand for insights has grown organically," says Krebs. "It is informal at the moment, but teams come to us because they understand the value of the knowledge we hold and the ways we can help them."

When Stacey Geffken, Director of Product Development and Market Research, joined Geisinger Health Plan, the market research function was firmly a Data Reactor. The team primarily evaluated the organization's performance in the market and occasionally conducted focus groups. "Essentially, the team started as a small group of people just debating what they thought the consumer wanted," says Geffken (S. Geffken, personal communication, March 30, 2018). Chris Fanning, Chief Marketing Officer, brought on Geffken to improve that function because Fanning believes that consumer insights need to be integral to the way the organization develops products and experiences. "Consumer centricity cannot be viewed simply as a marketing piece. It has to be tied to all strategic goals," says Fanning (C. Fanning, personal communication, May 1, 2017).

Change started first by bringing consumers into Geisinger offices to share, first-hand, what their experience with the Geisinger Plan looked like. From there, Geffken and her team established a baseline of consumer understanding by routinely collecting structured feedback about the experience, implementing NPS, conducting an annual key driver study and developing touchpoint surveys to build out a voice of the customer platform. The team has greatly improved the efficiency of solving consumer pain points and has given member experience teams greater insight into how they can better serve members.

CONCLUSION: THE PATH TO TRANSFORMATION

Research has uncovered a few different paths that organizations a can take to jump-start their efforts—recognizing, of course, that change may emanate from anywhere in the organization.

Executive Led: Top Down Transformation

C-Suite executives are in a unique position to accelerate the journey to consumer centricity. With an initial focus on the First Shift, they can uniquely jump-start the journey by defining what it should look like at their organization and by role-modeling consumer-obsessed behaviors. As previously noted, Dr. David Feinberg shifted Geisinger Health's direction toward consumer centricity when he joined the organization. "He made a clear case for focusing on the patient experience as a primary target and for focusing overall on a brand that we have called 'Caring' that represented how we set up a healthcare ecosystem in which you step into a hospital and don't even realize you're in the hospital," says Alistair Erskine (A. Erskine, personal communication, May 11, 2017).

Research shows that the strongest changes begin at the very top of the organization and travel down. That requires executives to articulate their vision in ways that are accessible to employees and to model behaviors that support consumer obsession. Novant Health CEO Carl Armato did that when he orchestrated the creation of the People's Credo, which outlines the ways employees should treat each other, and the Standards of Service, which outlines the ways employees should treat consumers. Setting a standard for both the consumer and the employee experience led to what Armato calls "the human experience" (C. Armato, personal communication, July 18, 2017).

Beyond the large-scale, more official moves, executives should be cognizant of their position as role models and demonstrate ways to weave consumer centricity into the organization. Indiana University Health's CEO Dennis Murphy sends handwritten notes and certificates to employees receiving awards for consumer-centric behaviors to demonstrate, in a very personal way, leadership's recognition of and appreciation for the work. Murphy also makes rounds on hospital floors to talk with patients who have the fewest visitors. "I make sure those people get a chance to talk to somebody. I go into the patient's room, get them water and help them feel personally supported. It sets an example that you don't fully appreciate until you leave the floor and somebody tells you that the staff was blown away that you talked with that specific patient," says Murphy (D. Murphy, personal communication, June 26, 2017). Executives may have the highest positions in the organization; but when it comes to making the biggest impression on culture, they are often most impactful at the ground level.

Marketing Led: Bringing Functional Change

As the function typically responsible for knowing consumers best, marketing often plays a key role in transformation. Some marketing leaders have a seat next to the executive leaders and can take the approach outlined for executive leaders. That is what happened for Matt Gove, Chief Consumer Officer at Piedmont Healthcare. Working closely with CEO Kevin Brown, Gove drove alignment regarding what consumer centricity would look like at the health system, developed a roadmap of moves and then implemented appropriate programs such as same-day scheduling and physician ratings and reviews. Many marketing leaders, however, do not have the influence to spark wide-scale change. Those who are still strengthening their teams and building organizational authority need to take another approach and focus their initial efforts on insights.

Focusing on the Fifth Shift will help leaders establish a stronger insights capability and uncover the insights that will lead to action. Aetna's Dave Edelman bolstered the enterprise intelligence function by consolidating marketing, branding and insights under his leadership. "Our early quick wins came in the form of helping our sales teams take greater advantage of digital channels and bring the power of smarter analytics into their go-to-market strategies. That led to some immediate wins and established our credibility," says Edelman (D. Edelman, personal communication, April 25, 2017).

Once marketing leaders have developed the organizational foundation for consumer insight development, they can move to the Third Shift to apply those insights for greater consumer personalization and even greater impact. Marketing can also play a key role in establishing any external partnerships that may enhance the organization's ability to create personalized experiences. As insights begin to flow through the organization to inform key decisions, marketing begins to influence innovation efforts.

Marketing is typically viewed as the team that understands the consumer best; so making inroads in the Third and Fifth Shift should be the focus. Those leaders should consistently use the consumer's voice to win over leadership.

Building a Movement from the Ground Up

Leaders across other functions—such as operations, customer service, digital or IT—may not have the influence of executive leadership or marketing, but they can play a critical role in igniting change. They may not have the power to mandate the creation of an insights team or a segmentation analysis, but they can identify consumer pain points in their purview and work closely with the research team to determine what insights are currently available.

If other business leaders work from the ground up and gain advocates along the way, they, too, can ignite change by diligently connecting everything they do back to the consumer and ensuring that their efforts ladder up to the greater strategy.

THE FUTURE OF CONSUMER CENTRICITY

For any of the five shifts to take hold, time, investment and patience is required regardless of whether the move is a wholesale transformation or a step toward change in an on-going journey. But as the organization moves forward, it will begin to see results. Beyond improved business outcomes, organizations will enjoy the impact that consumer centricity can have on the patients they serve. Consumer centricity is the solution that will allow healthcare businesses to grow, the consumers they care for to thrive and the communities they live in to flourish.

NOTE

This chapter has been condensed from *Making the Healthcare Shift: The Transformation to Consumer-Centricity*, with permission (Morgan James 2019)

REFERENCES

Aubrey, A. (2017, May 8). *Fresh Food By Prescription: This Health Care Firm Is Trimming Costs - And Waistlines.* Retrieved from https://www.npr.org/sections/thesalt/2017/05/08/526952657/fresh-food-by-prescription-this-health-care-firm-is-trimming-costs-and-waistline

Becker's Hospital Review. (2015, December 7). *The corner office: Dr. David Feinberg on raising the patient experience to a whole new level*. Retrieved from https://www.beckershospitalreview.com/hospital-management-administration/the-corner-office-dr-david-feinberg-on-raising-the-patient-experience-to-a-whole-new-level.html

Gourdji, J., & Davis, S. (2019). *Making the Healthcare Shift: The Transformation to Consumer-Centricity*. New York: Morgan James.

King, D. A. (2018, February). *Using technology to drive behavioural change in healthcare*. Retrieved from https://www.warc.com/content/article/bestprac/using_technology_to_drive_behavioural_change_in_healthcare/120037?utm_source=DailyNews&utm_medium=email&

ADDITIONAL READING

Elton, J., & O'Riordan, A. (2016). *Healthcare disrupted: next generation business models and strategies*. Hoboken, NJ: Wiley.

Emanuel, E. J. (2015). *Reinventing American health care: how the Affordable Care Act will improve our terribly complex, blatantly unjust, outrageously expensive, grossly inefficient, error prone system*. New York, NY: PublicAffairs.

Glorikian, H. (2017). *MoneyBall Medicine: Thriving in the New Data-Driven Healthcare Market*. Boca Raton, Florida: CRC Press. doi:10.1201/b21953

Gourdji, J., & Davis, S. (2019). *Making the Healthcare Shift: The Transformation to Consumer-Centricity*. New York: Morgan James.

Neuwirth, Z. (2019). *Reframing Healthcare: A Roadmap For Creating Disruptive Change*. Charleston, SC: Advantage Media Group.

Rosenthal, E. (2018). *An American sickness: how healthcare became big business and how you can take it back*. New York: Penguin Books.

KEY TERMS AND DEFINITIONS

Best-Practice Strategist: These leaders come from industries like consulting, where they have worked with organizations in many sectors to solve a range of business challenges similar to those in healthcare.

Consumer Data Value Exchange (CDVE): A mechanism for determining what consumers will receive in return for sharing personal data.

Consumerism: The protection or promotion of the interests of consumers.

E-Consumer: Empowered, engaged, equipped, and enabled healthcare consumers.

Insights Operating System (IOS): A system whose function is to help organizations get to the right insights, drive the right decisions at the right time and win with the right consumers.

Invested Healer: Leaders with a background in medicine or clinical care, they have hands-on experience working with patients, deeply understand the clinical experience and have a personal interest in improving the overall patient experience.

Lifelong Consumerist: Experts from consumer-centric industries, such as packaged goods, bring a consumer-first mindset.

Plus **Product:** A comprehensive solution-oriented approach to serving the patient, layering on elements, as needed, to create an ecosystem and drive the desired outcome.

ENDNOTES

[1] https://www.warc.com/content/article/bestprac/using_technology_to_drive_behavioural_change_in_healthcare/120037?utm_source=DailyNews&utm_medium=email&

[2] https://www.beckershospitalreview.com/hospital-management-administration/the-corner-office-dr-david-feinberg-on-raising-the-patient-experience-to-a-whole-new-level.html

[3] https://www.npr.org/sections/thesalt/2017/05/08/526952657/fresh-food-by-prescription-this-health-care-firm-is-trimming-costs-and-waistline

Section 2

Chapter 4
Effective Teamwork and Healthcare Delivery Outcomes

Adam Greer
Ascension St. John Medical Center, USA

Roshini Isabell Selladurai
In His Image Family Medicine Residency, Ascension St. John Medical Center, USA

Andrea L. Pfeifle
Indiana University, USA

Raj Selladurai
Indiana University Northwest, USA

Charles J. Hobson
Indiana University Northwest, USA

ABSTRACT

The chapter focuses on high-performing people and effective teamwork in healthcare at accountable care organizations (ACOs). Studies have found that patients are more satisfied when they engage with providers who understand and express their 'soft-skill' competencies. The model presented will illustrate how teamwork training and innovative care, Leader-less Group Discussions, interprofessional education and communication, and leadership/top management support have been found to positively impact effective teamwork, which in turn would synergistically impact the quadruple aim of patient experience, quality of patient care, lower cost, and provider satisfaction. Patient satisfaction is closely linked to provider related outcomes such as employee performance, job satisfaction, and reducing costs.

DOI: 10.4018/978-1-7998-2949-2.ch004

INTRODUCTION

Teamwork is critical to effective patient care, high quality, and reducing costs. This chapter will focus on the role of teamwork in healthcare with a special emphasis on the emerging vehicle of the Accountable Care Organization delivering the care. The chapter will first look at some background information on the significance of teamwork within the healthcare arena. Then the authors will move on to discuss an analysis of the impact of effective teamwork on the quadruple aim, followed by a case study of the Ascension St. John Healthcare System ACO in Tulsa, OK. Next, the chapter will look at solutions to identified problems and challenges that a greater emphasis on teamwork could potentially address. Finally, the study will look at areas of future research to fill in gaps on how teamwork can be most effectively utilized to improve patient outcomes, quality of patient care, provider satisfaction, and reduce costs.

BACKGROUND

Studies have shown that effective teamwork and communication are crucial elements for quality healthcare in terms of safe and reliable delivery of healthcare services (Leonard & Frankel, 2011). In other industries such as business, aviation, and nuclear power/energy, research over the last several decades has proven that effective teamwork is a significant factor for safe and effective performance. Contained within the voluminous literature on teamwork are seven major models identifying essential team-related behaviors/competencies. Beginning chronologically in 1950, these include: Bales (1950), Stevens and Campion (1994), Cannon-Bowers, Tannenbaum, Salas, and Volpe (1995), Chen, Donahue and Klimoski (2004), Baker, Horvarth, Campion, Offerman, and Salas (2005), Salas, Sims, and Burke (2005), and Hobson, Strupeck, Griffin, Szostek, Selladurai, and Rominger (2013). All of these studies the surging interest in the vital role that teamwork plays in healthcare delivery was manifestly evident in a recent special issue of the American Psychologist entitled: The Science of Teamwork (May-June 2018). In the section on teamwork in applied organizational settings, three of the seven ((43%) articles focused on the healthcare industry: overall healthcare (Rosen, DiazGranados, Dietz, Benishek, Thompson, Pronovost, & Weaver), primary care (Fiscella & McDaniel), and intensive care (Ervin, Kahn, Cohen, & Weingart). Clearly, enhancing teamwork is at the forefront of efforts to improve the effectiveness and efficiency of healthcare delivery systems.

ANALYSIS

In Figure 1 and the discussion that follows, the authors focus on a conceptual model of effective teamwork and its synergistic impact on the Quadruple Aim of patient experiences, quality of patient care, lower costs, and provider satisfaction.

The model proposes that the effective teamwork factors of teamwork training and innovative patient care, leader-less group discussion, interprofessional education and communication, and leadership/top management support would help enhance effective teamwork, which in turn would impact positively the four critical outcomes of the Quadruple Aim, namely patient experiences, quality of patient care, lower costs, and provider satisfaction.

Teamwork Training and Innovative Patient Care

Rosen et al. (2018) reviewed published research on the use of teams in healthcare from 2000 to 2017. Among their major conclusions was the well-documented relationship between effective teamwork and important patient, staff, and organizational outcomes. Successful teamwork resulted in safer, higher quality, and more cost-efficient patient

Figure 1. Effective teamwork and impact on the quadruple aim

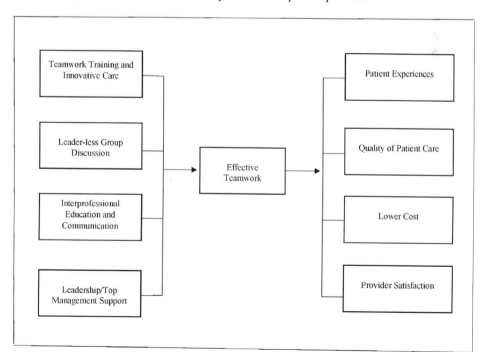

care. Fiscella and McDaniel (2018) cogently argued that the traditional, MD-centric model of primary care needs to be replaced with a more team-focused model. They concluded that successful implementation and utilization of teamwork was linked to improvements in all significant outcomes, including safety, care quality, cost, and patient satisfaction. Ervin et al. (2018) examined teamwork within intensive care units. They found that the use of teamwork within interprofessional models of patient care led to decreases in both morbidity and mortality.

The positive role of effective teamwork to improve healthcare delivery outcomes is significant and necessary for today's healthcare organizations competing in a dynamic patient-centered environment. In a recent healthcare-related study, about 25 to 30 percent of hospitalized patients have reported that they experienced an unfavorable or adverse event, and much of it was avoidable (Classen, Resar, Griffin, et al., 2011) if more effective teamwork had been implemented by the caretakers at the facility. Further, Davis and Gourdji (2019) have emphasized the need for healthcare organizations to become more patient- or consumer-centric cultures. Just as in the case of Amazon, which has revolutionized online shopping/buying consumer behavior with a consumer-centric culture and philosophy, in healthcare too, the consumer always must come first. It is imperative that the healthcare system organizations must be structured with the customers at the central focus of everything throughout the organization. This is a large but needed shift in thinking from the previous system being organized around providers. Both these experts have emphasized that the whole healthcare system and its various partnering organizations should move from being fragmented care to more of a connected ecosystem (Davis & Gourdji, 2019). Organizations that allow for greater fluidity of patient information will help reduce costs through the elimination of unnecessary testing and increase quality by allowing providers across specialties and levels of care to access patient medical history more readily.

Leonard and Frankel (2011) also have recommended this cultural shift in healthcare, and for the highly skilled, trained, and competent individual healthcare professionals to learn how to collaboratively work together as a team to provide high-quality, safe, patient care. They believe that effective teamwork in healthcare must require teaching, training, and the practice of specific teamwork-based techniques, tools, competencies, and behaviors to all healthcare stakeholders, including leadership support for teamwork, understanding, and adapting to the safety culture of the work environment. Both senior leadership and clinical leaders must support and promote teamwork for it to be effectively implemented. Also, both the leadership levels must ensure a safety culture in which teamwork is encouraged and able to flourish in the healthcare organization. Everyone in the organization must be treated with respect and be free to express his/her voice if and when they notice problems with patient care to create a sustainable high-reliability organization that makes patient safety a top priority. Also, the safety culture-enhanced teamwork priority was supported by a recent two-year study of 180 work teams where Google found five attributes that characterize effective teams. These included dependability, structure and clarity, meaning and significance, impact, and the most significant one, namely psychological safety --free expression of one's opinions in a setting created where employees can feel safe in letting their guards down (Schneider, 2019). Similarly, in a Michigan Keystone ICU project, the goal of reducing infections was found to be more attainable among those who felt comfortable speaking up and expressing their opinions than those who did not in this clinical study (Leonard & Frankel, 2011).

Effective teamwork in healthcare would emphasize behaviors such as structured communication, which includes frequently used briefings to get the team members together focused on goals and tasks at hand. High-performing teams routinely would use briefings to build team spirit, commonality in purpose, goals, and tasks, and to ensure the whole team is on the same page. Also, such cohesive teams would understand the context of the work environment and know exactly the information, resources, and the personnel that they need to work together effectively. With awareness of the "bigger picture," the effective team can offer more proactive solutions rather than reactive responses to events. Several studies have shown that teamwork briefings reduce delays and optimize the use of resources with little or no waste (Leonard & Frankel, 2011). Another case study also showed the significant benefits of briefings for the teams in that the use of frequent perioperative surgical briefings resulted in a 31% reduction in intraoperative delays (Mukherjee & Sexton, 2008).

The focus on training in building effective teamwork is crucial in healthcare organizations; it must be interdisciplinary, system-wide, and interactive with all physicians taking active roles in the teambuilding training processes. When the physician's involvement in the training processes is high, it results in more effective training for all. And when all the medical team members learn and practice together, the teamwork is enhanced through higher procedural knowledge ("I know how to do this as we have done it before") and cohesive social agreement ("I know how to use these tools as we have agreed how we will use them"). High-quality patient care is a result of effective teamwork in practice system-wide. This is best illustrated by Kaiser Permanente that provided perinatal safety in the system across 36 hospitals using multidisciplinary teamwork training; teaching clinical processes and reliability in multidisciplinary settings (for example, fetal heart rate interpretations), and practicing emergency scenario building on their clinical units such as shoulder dystocia or prolonged fetal bradycardia (Leonard and Frankel, 2011). The use of practical simulation, when done regularly and systematically, helps provide the delivery of safer patient care. Studies have shown positive effects of the use of simulation in various procedures in obstetrics (Draycott, 2008), and a 60% decrease in adverse events and claims (Pettker et al., 2009).

Further, effective teamwork in surgery in the Veterans Administration health system has also shown positive outcomes. These included a 18% decrease in mortality rates, lower nursing turnover, fewer interruptions from nurses leaving to get supplies during surgery, higher perceptions of improved teamwork and collaboration, and avoiding 100+ adverse events that were estimated to have saved the system $12 million (Neily, Mills, et al., 2010). Also, studies have shown the positive effects of knowledge integration on patient-centric teamwork, and on team performance with patient-centered teamwork serving as a mediating variable affecting the effects of knowledge integration on team performance (Korner et al., 2016).

In addition to teamwork training, David Feinberg, CEO of Geisinger Health System, a regional health system in Pennsylvania, showed commitment to innovative patient care and brought a new meaning to the concepts of patient-centricity, patient experiences, and feedback, and the quality of patient care. He introduced a "satisfaction guaranteed or money-back" refund policy called ProvenExperience implemented through an app, which patients used to provide instant feedback on their experiences as patients. In the first year, Geisinger had to refund nearly $500,000 to its patients. Despite implementing this refund, the Geisinger Health System sincerely valued what its patients think of its services. "We put our trust in you, the patient, because you've put your trust in us," said Dr. Alistair Erskine, CIO of Geisinger (Davis & Gourdji, 2019, p. 12).

Leaderless Group Discussion (LGD)

The authors believe that there are major opportunities to improve the performance of teams in healthcare by more widely adopting the "leaderless group discussion" (LGD) to assess and develop teamwork skills at the individual level. The LGD is a type of work-sample evaluation in which a small group (5-7) engages in a problem-solving simulation for 20 to 60 minutes, and no formal leader is appointed (Gatewood, Field, & Barrick, 2016). Trained raters observe and assess individual group member performance using various teamwork rubrics. This can be done while the group is interacting, or better, by videotaping the interaction and then reviewing the tape.

The validity of a work sample test is based upon the extent to which its content reflects significant job-related tasks or activities. Given the documented importance of team-based problem solving in many healthcare occupations (Ervin, Kahn, Cohen, & Weingart, 2018; Fiscella & McDaniel, 2018; Rosen, Diaz Granados, Dietz, Benishek, Thompson, Promovost, & Weaver, 2018), the LGD offers an invaluable, content valid approach to measuring individual performance.

Contained within the voluminous literature on teamwork are seven major models identifying essential team-related behaviors/competencies. Beginning chronologically in 1950, these include: Bales (1950), Stevens and Campion (1994), Cannon-Bowers,

Tannenbaum, Salas, and Volpe (1995), Chen, Donahue, and Klimoski (2004), Baker, Horvarth, Campion, Offerman, and Salas (2005), Salas, Sims, and Burke (2005), and Hobson, Strupeck, Griffin, Szostek, Selladurai, and Rominger (2013). Hobson, Szostek, Griffin, Lusk, and Rydecki (2017) reviewed this body of research and formulated an integrative meta-model, consisting of critical behaviors that were common across the seven. This meta-model is organized into two well-known, widely documented categories: task and social. For the task category, there is one primary competency (task completion), composed of 10 specific behaviors, including both positive and negative ones. The social category consists of three primary competencies, with the number of specific behaviors in parentheses: communication (11 items), member relations (8 items), and disagreement management (12 items). The full meta-model is provided below.

META-MODEL

Task Category

Task Completion Competency

1) Positive Behaviors
    a. Agrees with a team member
    b. Answers teammate's question
    c. Builds on another's idea/piggy-backs on the idea (beyond mere agreement)
    d. Takes notes on team discussion
    e. Seeks clarification by asking questions/paraphrasing another's input
    f. Keeps the team focused and "on-track"
    g. Keeps track of time
    h. Helps the team establish goals/plans
    i. Provides team-based feedback/praise/reinforcement
    j. Expresses own opinion that adds value to the discussion
2) Negative Behaviors
    a. Brings up a topic that is unrelated to team discussion
    b. Dominates discussion by failing to allow others to talk
    c. Distracts team with inappropriate humor, repetitive/nervous behavior, and/or by being overly pessimistic, negative, dramatic, or by complaining excessively

Social Category

1. Communication Competency

1) Positive Behaviors
   a. Speaks in a clear/understandable manner
   b. Displays open body language (sitting upright, slight lean forward, oriented toward team, arms/legs/hands not crossed)
   c. Maintains appropriate eye contact with teammates while speaking
   d. Maintains appropriate eye contact when listening to teammates
   e. Uses non-verbal comprehenders while listening (uh-huh, head nods, etc.)
2) Negative Behaviors
   a. Speaks in an unclear/not understandable manner
   b. Speaks in a verbose, rambling manner
   c. Appears distracted, disinterested, pre-occupied
   d. Allows note taking to interrupt active listening
   e. Displays closed, defensive body language (slouching, leaning back, oriented away from the team, crossed arms/legs/hands)
   f. Avoids eye contact

2. Member Relations Competency

1) Positive Behaviors
   a. Recognizes and praises team members' contribution
   b. Insures input and participation of all team members/invites quiet teammates to participate
   c. Expresses empathy toward team members
   d. Uses appropriate humor to reduce anxiety and stress
   e. Calls teammates by first name
2) Negative Behaviors
   a. Interrupts speaker
   b. Engages in a side conversation while teammate is talking
   c. Disregards a teammate's input

3. Disagreement Management Competency

1) Positive Behaviors
   a. Plays devil advocate
   b. Uses critical analysis, rather than emotions, to evaluate ideas/actions
   c. Constructively disagrees with teammate ideas

    d.   Employs an integrative (win-win) approach to disagreement resolution

    e.   Expresses willingness to compromise

    f.   Mediates disagreement among teammates

    g.   Accepts feedback from teammates without defensiveness or "shutting down"

    h.   Asks teammates about agreement concerning proposed team decisions

2)   Negative Behaviors

    a.   Gives personalized, derogatory criticism to teammates

    b.   Responds defensively/aggressively to feedback from teammates

    c.   Refuses to compromise; insists that his/her idea is the only correct one

    d.   Withdraws from interaction after feedback from teammates

Hobson et al. recommended a 5-point scoring format (0-4), based upon the frequency of occurrence of each behavior. Procedures for calculating an overall score were also provided.

The use of the LGD to measure individual teamwork skills became popular in business and industry when the managerial assessment center was introduced by AT&T in 1956 (Bray, Campbell, and Grant, 1979). Subsequently, it has been widely utilized to screen candidates for hiring/promotion and as a platform for performance coaching (Arthur and Day, 2011; Gatewood et al., 2016; Thornton Rupp, 2006).

Within higher education, several studies have been conducted in which the LGD was successfully utilized to assess and improve teamwork skills in undergraduates (Chen, Donahue, & Klimoski, 2004; Hobson, Strupeck, Griffin, Szostek, Selladurai, & Rominger, 2013) and MBA students (Costigan & Donahue, 2009; Hobson, Strupeck, Griffin, Szostek & Rominger, 2014). Innovative universities are also employing the LGD as an evaluation tool in screening student applicants, including a prominent, highly rated MBA program and two Midwestern Physician Assistant programs.

In summary, the LGD offers a proven, content-valid, behaviorally-based methodology to assess individual teamwork skills. Given the vital and growing importance of teamwork in the provision of patient services, healthcare institutions could utilize the LGD in two major ways: (1) as a screening tool in making a hiring and/or promotion decisions to insure candidates demonstrate high levels of teamwork and competence and (2) as a framework for assessing and developing teamwork skills of current employees. Similarly, schools preparing students for healthcare professions could also use the LGD to screen applicants and as a vehicle to assess and enhance student teamwork skill levels. The authors have found that in both business and educational settings, employing the LGD for skill measurement and development is best accomplished by videotaping group interaction and using the tapes to foster self-awareness and motivation to improve.

Leveraging Interprofessional Education

Communication and teamwork are essential for providing quality health care and achieving the Quadruple Aim (Bodenheimer & Sinsky, 2014), and several resources and tools exist to support the integration of these skills into practice within and across settings. Increasingly, these resources and tools are being utilized to inform and improve team performance in the health care setting. Yet much of the health care workforce has not been trained to work or think interprofessionally. Instead, they have been isolated from other team members for the vast majority of their education and hence, unskilled with essential interprofessional collaborative practice competencies, unaware of the various roles and responsibilities of other team members, and lacking experience collaborating to improve health and health care outcomes.

Preparing graduates as team-ready to join the clinical workforce must include training in and experience applying core competencies for interprofessional practice: Roles/Responsibilities, Values/Ethics for Interprofessional Practice, Roles/Responsibilities, Interprofessional Communication, and Teams and Teamwork (IPEC, 2011; IPEC, 2016; HPAC, 2019); as well as cultural humility and cultural competency, education about vulnerable populations, and systems-based quality improvement focused on eliminating health care disparities (Casey, Chisholm-Burns, Passiment et al, 2019). Accreditors and academic training programs at the graduate and undergraduate level are increasingly incorporating interprofessional education, where health professions students, residents, and fellows learn about, from, and with each other with the intention of improving care and care outcomes (IPEC, 2011; WHO, 2010; Zorek & Raehl 2012). However, these new skills and values taught at this level are easily lost when new clinicians enter the workforce to work in organizations using traditional approaches to delivering care that is siloed and hierarchical in nature (IOM, 2015; Josiah Macy, Jr. Foundation, 2013).

To affect a long term, sustainable change in health care delivery that supports effective teamwork and achieves the Quadruple Aim, interprofessional education must be effectively supported by a new and different clinical learning environment where teamwork and innovative care delivery models are embraced at the macro, meso, and micro-levels. While newly evolving, characteristics of this new clinical learning environment must include teamwork and also likely include patient-centeredness, a continuum of learning, reliable communications, shared accountability, and evidence-based practice centered on interprofessional care (Weiss et al., 2019).

Leadership/Top Management Support

For effective teamwork to be implemented in healthcare organizations, top management leadership and support are crucial. Interestingly, Mayo Clinic CEO

John Noseworthy has emphasized their primary goal this way: "Every step we take, every tactical strategy decision we make, is based on what is in the best interest of the patient –and that is the only interest to be considered. At Mayo Clinic, we put patients first. That is the foundation of our culture" (Davis & Gourdji, 2019, p. 97). And with collaborative, close-knit teamwork permeating among all of the healthcare providers, including physicians, staff, medical personnel, and administrators, they can provide a patient-centered culture in their organizations, and subsequently, patients would be able to receive the high-quality care they deserve and expect.

Further, Berry and Beckham (2014) have discussed team-based care and how Mayo Clinic presented a cancer patient Don with access to high-quality, efficient patient care, which is the main goal for accountable care organizations (ACOs). He had been given a prognosis of "immediate surgery" as the best option though he would have lost his ability to speak. Don sought a second opinion at Mayo, and Mayo's three cancer specialists met with him and recommended radiation and chemotherapy but not surgery. After three months of treatment at Mayo, Don is cancer-free! He received high-quality patient care rendered in an integrated, teamwork-based system that leveraged and synthesized experience, information, and technology. Mayo Clinic's success stems from its commitment to two fundamental values, which are significant strengths: The patient's needs come first, and emphasis on integrated, team-based medicine (Berry & Seltman, 2008). These values/ strengths contributed to Mayo's high performance on critical quality outcomes such as readmissions, complications, resource use, survival rates, and affordability, which is commendable and worthy to emulate (Consumer Reports, 2013). Patient feedback on Mayo's patient care is very positive, and more than 90% of them share favorable opinions and feedback with others (Berry & Seltman, 2008). Teamwork was more than encouraged; it was demanded at Mayo. Also, Mayo emphasized the sharing of knowledge, integration of all services centered on the patient, and a fixed salary for physicians to ensure they have no incentive to provide higher or lower patient care; these are all synthesized to provide care that is customized to the needs of the patient (Clapesattle, 1941). Mayo has many strengths, including long-term sustainability as a healthcare organization for over 150 years, a worldwide continually glowing reputation, and its practice of some servant leadership principles such as exemplary, sacrificial leadership, strong value for people and productivity, and deep concern for relationships and results (Selladurai & Carraher, 2014). Above all, its strong commitment to patient care and organizational teamwork have helped Mayo to serve as an excellent healthcare model for other healthcare systems to emulate.

To further illustrate the value of effective teamwork and its impact on the critical outcomes, the author/s performed a case study of an ACO in Tulsa, Oklahoma. This ACO allows analysis and encourages the use of specific skills, which foster efficient high-performing teams and have an impact on the four quadruple aims -- patient experiences, quality of patient care, lower costs, and provider satisfaction.

Case Study

Introduction

Healthcare reform has become a topic of much debate since the Affordable Care Act (ACA) was signed into law in 2010. One way that change has been implemented in the United States is through Accountable Care Organizations (ACO's). With an emphasis on the quadruple aim (previously known as the triple aim) of patient experience, population health, reducing costs, and most recently added improved provider satisfaction, ACO's have incorporated a heavy emphasis on building effective teams in order to meet the ever-increasing need for quality healthcare while at the same time reducing costs. Having multiple team members working at the top of their license from physicians, administrators, nurse practitioners, registered nurses, medical assistants, front staff, and many others involved in the healthcare of a patient population requires excellent communication between all parties involved.

Since ACO's incorporate a large number of people and organizations, teamwork is critical to accomplishing the four above stated goals. As part of this research, one of the authors performed a case study interviewing two leaders in the Ascension St. John Health System ACO in Tulsa, OK. Ann Paul is the ACO President and Chief Strategy Officer, while Troy Cupps is the Director of Value-Based Programs and ACO Operations. According to A. Paul (personal communication, July 11, 2019) and T. Cupps (personal communication, July 8, 2019), the Ascension St. John ACO is made up of greater than 20 organizations and affiliates that partner together to make referrals easier to process, help with flow of information between organizations, improve patient quality, and reduce costs.

Teamwork Across the Spectrum of Care

When looking at quality improvement, one of the most important aspects is to have a quality improvement program with an annual plan. This program is multifaceted and requires a great deal of communication and teamwork among the people on all levels within the organization. The theory of diffusion of innovation is a bell-shaped curve that group people into several categories of innovators, early adopters, early majority, late majority, and laggards. Laggards will usually the last to accept innovation, while innovators are so far ahead of the curve that the majority would not follow, and so early adopters are critical to have on boards and committees when formulating a plan because people will be willing to support them. The majority of people are either in the early or late majority. Using the diffusion of innovation theory, one can create a team framework rather than a "top-down" framework to structure the organization. Not only do the people creating the plan need to work together well to make it most effective, but the vision needs to be adequately presented to the providers, managers, employees, etc. The model used to communicate this vision, goals, and objectives is a multimodal communication approach, which requires multiple methods of communication. Ascension St. John has incorporated strategies of email, podcasts, and weekly meetings to communicate these goals and objectives.

One of the most important aspects of cost savings within the ACO is preventing hospitalizations by providing excellent outpatient care, especially the timeframe within 30 days of being discharged from the hospital. Care managers have been hired within the Ascension St. John clinics to help bridge this gap between discharge from the hospital and follow up with primary care physicians, which has substantially decreased hospital readmission rates. Having care managers both in the hospital and the clinics make communication across the continuum of care both between providers and to the patient more fluid and effective. Also, having the same EMR for the different levels of care, including urgent care, hospital, and clinics, helps increase quality by making information about what happened to the patient available to all potential providers in real-time, which also helps eliminate duplicate testing thus reducing costs.

Multiple levels of the health system have to work together as well. Separate organizations within the same ACO also work together to make patient information flow more freely between organizations with different Electronic Medical Records (EMR's). For example, Harvard Family Physicians has contracted with Ascension St. John to supply care to patients as part of the larger network. Tulsa Bone & Joint is a local independent orthopedic surgeon group that has also contracted with Ascension St. John to be the primary source of orthopedic care to patients within the ACO, thus creating a system to allow the flow of information to occur more readily than with other orthopedic providers. Ascension St. John has also contracted with QuikTrip (a local gasoline supplier) to coordinate medical care to their employees in an attempt to reduce costs by increasing efficiency and increase quality. If there is an issue with a QuikTrip employee being able to access care to a specialty, the ACO office attempts to help these employees access healthcare or resolve any medical access issue that they are attempting to resolve previously on their own. These formal contractual relationships have quality improvement goals that have financial incentives tied to them. Early on in forming these relationships, Ascension St. John initially focused largely on improving quality of care prior to the financial focus on shared savings provided by Centers for Medicare and Medicaid Services (CMS) (Medicare Shared Savings Program, 2019). Having these organizations all sharing financial incentives allows for greater cooperation between the organizations to help meet the quality measures and requirements for each organization to receive its share of the incentive. These contractual relationships also make warm handoffs for patient healthcare easier, allowing for smoother transitions between providers and increased patient satisfaction. A significant goal is to have every service that is required by all patients across the entire continuum of care within the same system, but this is very rare, and Kaiser is the system that comes the closest at this point.

Attributes of Top Performing Teams

One of the most significant pitfalls that potentially distract from effective teamwork is complacency diminishing creativity. The early life of any organization requires a great deal of creativity and vision.

However, as the structure begins diffusing into the organization and initiatives are built out at a deeper level, the system transitions away from vision to maintenance stages. This transition can lead to a lack of new ideas being created, a lack of innovation in meeting new goals. Another pitfall is not to allow staff members to be recognized for their accomplishments or successes. Ensuring that each member feels valued and is attributed to the work they perform helps maintain a positive culture.

On the other hand, the longer a team works together without a turnover, the more efficiently they can perform because more time can be spent innovating and doing rather than training new hires when team members leave. As long as the team member fits well into the culture of the team, retention of top talent is a key element of effective teamwork. The Ascension St. John Healthcare System has five (5) ACO staff employees that have been working in the office for several years with minimal turnover, so this has helped tremendously in defining roles and maximizing teamwork efficiency. Fortunately, each of the employees was carefully selected as a high performing individual who makes the team function at a high level. Making expectations known up front is critical to be able to recruit high-functioning matches between potential employees and organizations. Exposing new employees to all the resources available helps reduce employee turnover. This has to be specific to the new role/employee combination and empowers one to do his/her job with maximum efficiency. A positive attitude when facing failure is also helpful when working as a team. Since many programs and ideas end up not succeeding, being able to take what is learned and move on to the next project quickly is extremely important.

Technology advances such as email and Skype have become an integral aspect of communication among the team internally and when helping diffuse information throughout the organization. Since organizations cannot allow outside employees to access their own EMR's, MyHealth was created as a website that allows for patient data to be accessed across healthcare systems by uploading data to the website for providers to access. Making this data available without having a separate log on is the next step in increasing the availability of information without the hindrance of accessing a different website.

The primary measure of outcomes is defined by CMS within an ACO. Currently, there are 23 quality measure benchmarks that are used when providing financial incentives to ACO's. These measures are a combination of reporting and performance based on the measure specifications and the year of phasing in the quality measures. The benchmarks are listed below:

CAHPS: Getting Timely Care, Appointments, and Information
- CAHPS: How Well Your Providers Communicate
- CAHPS: Patients' Rating of Provider
- CAHPS: Access to Specialists
- CAHPS: Health Promotion and Education
- CAHPS: Shared Decision Making
- CAHPS: Health Status/Functional Status
- CAHPS: Stewardship of Patient Resources
- CAHPS: Courteous and Helpful Office Staff
- CAHPS: Care Coordination
- Risk-Standardized, All Condition Readmission
- All-Cause Unplanned Admissions for Patients with Multiple Chronic Conditions
- Ambulatory Sensitive Condition Acute Composite (AHRQ Prevention Quality Indicator (PQI))
- Falls: Screening for Future Fall Risk
- Preventive Care and Screening: Influenza Immunization
- Preventive Care and Screening: Tobacco Use: Screening and Cessation Intervention
- Preventive Care and Screening: Screening for Clinical Depression and Follow-up Plan
- Colorectal Cancer Screening
- Breast Cancer Screening
- Statin Therapy for the Prevention and Treatment of Cardiovascular Disease
- Depression Remission at Twelve Months
- Diabetes Mellitus: Hemoglobin A1c Poor Control
- Hypertension (HTN): Controlling High Blood Pressure

SOLUTIONS AND RECOMMENDATIONS

Many potential solutions can be utilized from the above analysis on teamwork. The healthcare sector can learn a great deal from the already extensive research on teamwork within the business arena, as this has proven to be effective in increasing employee satisfaction, improving efficiency, and increasing quality. Implementing what business research has already acquired in the healthcare sector can be done through screening applicants for essential characteristics for members of high functioning teams in the hiring process. Part of the interview could include incorporating the applicant on an already established high functioning team. For current employees, the Leaderless Group Discussion method described above can be used to evaluate members of already established teams, and feedback is given to help increase their impact. These could even be built into currently established performance reviews.

There are many ways that policy could potentially influence the incorporation of effective teamwork into healthcare in the future. The research that currently exists regarding teamwork in healthcare is already strong in showing increased efficiency and patient satisfaction but could be strengthened by being more focused on patient-oriented outcomes. This would require lobbying congress for more funding to NIH for research. Professional organizations such as the AMA (American Medical Association), AAP (American Academy of Physicians), ACP (American College of Physicians), ABMS (American Board of Medical Specialties), and other such organizations could provide professional development opportunities that promote the importance of teamwork. Allowing physicians currently in practice to obtain CME in this important area could greatly benefit the teams where said physicians are already serving. A valuable current resource is the AAPL (American Association for Physician Leadership) for physician targeted education on teamwork. Another strategy could be to incorporate the role of teamwork within current accreditation standards and in the education process through medical schools and residency programs. Allowing students and residents to participate in interdisciplinary teams early will help them function more effectively throughout their professional careers.

FUTURE DIRECTIONS

Looking forward, there are several different directions that are being explored in healthcare reform that could positively impact the integration of teamwork into healthcare delivery to improve care outcomes. Reimbursement for providers is one area that is quickly evolving. Many different models are being proposed and utilized, and which may be tested, such as capitation, value-based models such as pay for performance, CMS shared savings, etc. Many organizations are using a mixed model for reimbursement of providers, including RVU's, quality metrics, and patient-panel. One area of potential improvement could be incorporating cost savings into provider reimbursement, perhaps allowing the providers involved to earn potential bonuses that come from the shared savings based on their ability to reduce costs.

Having the entire complement of the medical staff involved in meeting quality metrics and rapid cycle improvement events or interventions will be important going forward. The Ascension St. John system currently uses medical assistants to call patients who are due for colonoscopies and mammograms in order to make sure that patients are up-to-date on their colon and breast cancer screenings, so enabling staff to help coordinate specific areas of care will help increase overall quality by increasing the early detection of potentially curable common diseases. Care managers are also critical to the process of creating a fluid continuum of care across the spectrum of acuity of medical care. Calling patients after a visit to the emergency room or hospitalization to ensure that medications are correct, a follow-up appointment with PCP has been scheduled, appropriate referrals placed, and additional needs met is extremely helpful in preventing readmission (reducing costs) and increasing quality of care. To accompany these improvements, it will be necessary for organizations to emphasize prevention and to incentivize innovation to develop, implement, and continuously improve and reward new practice models demonstrating Quadruple Aim outcomes and return-on-investment when team care is integrated into care delivery. Also, the conceptual model of effective teamwork and impact on the Quadruple Aim discussed in the chapter may be tested empirically in healthcare organization/s to measure the effectiveness of the use of teamwork, its results analyzed, and findings reported/used for further discussion and potential replication in other healthcare organizational settings to benefit all the stakeholders.

Additionally, new and expanded academic-practice partnerships will be needed to augment and support these improvements in healthcare delivery. More and better integration of residents, fellows, health professions and public health learners into interprofessional teams as they emerge in the workforce (i.e., interprofessional education) will leverage change and serve to differently prepare the future healthcare workforce to provide safer, more productive, more efficient, more responsive care and improve outcomes.

CONCLUSION

Teamwork will be critical for healthcare reform to be successful going forward. Many studies have already shown that effective teamwork is critical in achieving the goals of the quadruple aim, but more research is needed to show correlation with patient outcomes and opportunities made available through medical organizations for further training. Incorporating interprofessional training into higher medical education would be beneficial in creating a teamwork atmosphere that would ideally help create a culture of interdependent care. Using tools such as Leaderless Discussion Groups can facilitate more effective teamwork among already established teams and can be used in the hiring process or with performance reviews. Reimbursement reform that is more focused on quality rather than productivity and emerging vehicles of care, such as ACO's will become more important as the demand for reducing costs and increasing patient satisfaction becomes more heavily emphasized. Although there is a great deal of uncertainty in the future of healthcare reform, effective teamwork has been and will continue to be critical for the delivery of low cost, quality care that ensures both patient and provider satisfaction.

REFERENCES

Arthur, W., & Day, E. A. (2011). Assessment centers. In S. Zedock (Ed.), APA Handbook of Industrial and Organizational Psychology (vol. 2). Washington, DC: American Psychological Association. doi:10.1037/12170-007

Baker, D. P., Horvath, L., Campion, M. A., Offermann, L., & Salas, E. (2005). The ALL Teamwork Framework. In T. S. Murray, Y. Clermont, & M. Binkley (Eds.), *International Adult Literacy Survey, Measuring Adult Literacy and Life Skills: New Frameworks for Assessment*. Ottawa: Ministry of Industry.

Bales, R. F. (1950). A set of categories for the analysis of small group interaction. *American Sociological Review, 15*(2), 257–263. doi:10.2307/2086790

Bartrom, S., & Stanton, T. (2011). High performance work systems: The gap between policy and practice in healthcare reform. *Journal of Health Organization and Management, 25*(3), 281–297. doi:10.1108/14777261111143536 PMID:21845983

Berry, L., & Beckham, D. (2014). Team-based care at Mayo Clinic: A Model for ACOs. *Journal of Healthcare Management, 59*(1), 9–13. doi:10.1097/00115514-201401000-00003 PMID:24611420

Berry, L., & Seltman, K. (2008). *Management lessons from Mayo Clinic*. New York, NY: McGraw Hill.

Bodenheimer, T., & Sinsky, C. (2014). From triple to quadruple aim: Care of the patient requires care of the provider. *Annals of Family Medicine, 12*(8), 573–576. doi:10.1370/afm.1713 PMID:25384822

Bray, D. W., Campbell, R. J., & Grant, D. L. (1979). *Formative years in business: A long-term AT&T study of managerial lives.* R.E. Krieger Publishing Co.

Cannon-Bowers, J. A., Tannenbaum, S. I., Salas, E., & Volpe, C. E. (1995). Defining competencies and establishing team training requirements. In R. Guzzo & E. Salas (Eds.), *Team effectiveness and decision making in organizations* (pp. 333–380). San Francisco: Jossey Bass.

Casey, B. R., Chisholm-Burns, M., Passiment, M., Wagner, R., & Riordan, L. (n.d.). *Weiss KB for the NCICLE Quality Improvement: Focus on Health Care Disparities Work Group.* The role of the clinical learning environment in preparing new clinicians to engage in quality improvement efforts to eliminate health care disparities. Retrieved from http://ncicle.org

Centers for Medicare and Medicaid. (2019). *Medicare shared savings program.* Retrieved from https://www.cms.gov/Medicare/Medicare-Fee-for-Service-Payment/sharedsavingsprogram/index.html

Chen, G., Donahue, L. M., & Klimoski, R. J. (2004). Training undergraduates to work in organizational teams. *Academy of Management Learning & Education, 3*(1), 27–40. doi:10.5465/amle.2004.12436817

Clapesattle, H. (1941). *The doctors Mayo.* Minneapolis, MN: University of Minnesota Press.

Classen, D. C., Resar, R., Griffin, F., Federico, F., Frankel, T., Kimmel, N., ... James, B. C. (2011). "Global trigger tool" shows that adverse events in hospitals may be ten times greater than previously measured. *Health Affairs, 30*(4), 581–589. doi:10.1377/hlthaff.2011.0190 PMID:21471476

Consumer Reports. (2013, May). *Safety still lags in ILS hospitals.* Retrieved from http://www.consumerreports.org/cro/magazine/2013/05/safety-still-lags-in-u-s-hospiitals/index.htm

Costigan, R. D., & Donahue, L. (2009). Developing the great eight competencies with leaderless group discussion. *Journal of Management Education, 33*(5), 596–616. doi:10.1177/1052562908318328

Davis, S. M, & Gourdji, J. (n.d.). *Making the Healthcare Shift: The Transformation to Consumer-Centricity.* New York, NY: James Morgan Publishing.

Draycott, T., Sibanda, T., & Owen, L. (2009). Does training in obstetric emergencies improve neonatal outcome? *BJOG, 112*, 177–182. PMID:16411995

Ervin, J. N., Kahn, J. M., Cohen, T. R., & Weingart, L. R. (2018). Teamwork in the intensive care unit. *The American Psychologist, 73*(4), 468–477. doi:10.1037/amp0000247 PMID:29792461

Fiscella, K., & McDaniel, S. H. (2018). The complexity, diversity, and science of primary care teams. *The American Psychologist, 73*(4), 451–467. doi:10.1037/amp0000244 PMID:29792460

Gatewood, R. D., Feild, H. S., & Barrick, M. R. (2016). *Human Resource Selection* (8th ed.). Boston: Cengage Learning.

Health Professions Accreditors Collaborative. (2019). *Guidance on developing quality interprofessional education for the health professions*. Chicago, IL: Health Professions Accreditors Collaborative.

Hobson, C. J., Strupeck, D., Griffin, A., Szostek, J., & Rominger, A. S. (2014). Teaching MBA students teamwork and team leadership skills: An empirical evaluation of a classroom educational program. *American Journal of Business Education, 7*(3), 191–212. doi:10.19030/ajbe.v7i3.8629

Hobson, C. J., Strupeck, D., Griffin, A., Szostek, J., Selladurai, R., & Rominger, A. (2013). Facilitating and documenting behavioral improvements in business student teamwork skills. *Business Education Innovation Journal, 5*(1), 83–95.

Institute of Medicine. (2015). *Measuring the impact of interprofessional education on collaborative practice and patient outcomes*. Washington, DC: National Academies Press.

Interprofessional Education Collaborative Expert Panel. (2011). *Core competencies for interprofessional collaborative practice: Report of an expert panel*. Washington, DC: Interprofessional Education Collaborative.

Jost, T. J., & Pollock, H. (2016). Making healthcare truly affordable after healthcare reform. *The Journal of Law, Medicine & Ethics, 44*(4), 546–554. doi:10.1177/1073110516684785 PMID:28661251

Korner, M., Lippenberger, C., Becker, S., Reichler, L., Müller, C., Zimmermann, L., ... Baumeister, H. (2016). Knowledge integration, teamwork, and performance in healthcare. *Journal of Health Organization and Management, 30*(2), 227–243. doi:10.1108/JHOM-12-2014-0217 PMID:27052623

Leonard, M., & Frankel, A. (2011). Role of effective teamwork and communication in delivering safe, high-quality care. *The Mount Sinai Journal of Medicine, New York, 78*(6), 820–826. doi:10.1002/msj.20295 PMID:22069205

Macy, J., Jr. Foundation. (2013). Transforming patient care: Aligning interprofessional education with clinical practice redesign. New York, NY: Author.

Mukherjee, N., & Sexton, J. (2008). Impact of preoperative briefings on operating room delays. *Archives of Surgery, 143*(11), 1068–1072. doi:10.1001/archsurg.143.11.1068 PMID:19015465

Neily, J., Mills, P., & Young-Xu, Y. (2010). Impact of a comprehensive patient safety strategy on obstetric adverse events. *Journal of the American Medical Association, 304*, 1693–1700. doi:10.1001/jama.2010.1506 PMID:20959579

Pettker, C., Thung, S., & Norwit. (2009). Impact of a comprehensive patient safety strategy on obstetric adverse events. *American Journal of Obstetrics Gynecology, 200*, 492e1-492e8.

Rosen, M. A., DiazGranados, D., Dietz, A. S., Benishek, L. E., Thompson, D., Pronovost, P. J., & Weaver, S. J. (2018). Teamwork in healthcare: Key discoveries enabling safer, high-quality care. *The American Psychologist, 73*(4), 433–450. doi:10.1037/amp0000298 PMID:29792459

Salas, E., Sims, D. E., & Burke, C. S. (2005). Is there a "Big Five" in teamwork? *Small Group Research, 36*(5), 555–599. doi:10.1177/1046496405277134

Schneider, M. (2017, July 19). *Google spent 2 years studying 180 teams. The most successful ones shared these 5 traits.* Retrieved from https://www.inc.com/michael-schneider/google-thought-they-knew-how-to-create-the-perfect.html

Selladurai, R., & Carraher, S. (2014). Lead like the greatest leader! Case Study. In R. Selladurai & S. Carraher (Eds.), *Servant leadership: Research and Practice* (pp. 350–355). Hershey, PA: IGI Global. doi:10.4018/978-1-4666-5840-0.ch026

Stevens, M. J., & Campion, M. A. (1994). The knowledge, skill, and ability requirements for teamwork: Implications for human resource management. *Journal of Management, 20*(2), 503–530. doi:10.1177/014920639402000210

Thornton, G. C. III, & Rupp, D. E. (2006). *Assessment centers and human resource management.* Mahwah, NJ: Lawrence Erlbaum. doi:10.4324/9781410617170

Weiss, K. B., Passiment, M., & Riodan, L. (n.d.). Wagner R for the National Collaborative for Improving the Clinical Learning Environment IP-CLE Report Work Group. *Achieving the Optimal Interprofessional Clinical Learning Environment: Proceedings From an NCICLE Symposium.* Retrieved from http://ncicle.org

World Health Organization. (2019). *Framework for action on interprofessional education and collaborative practice*. Geneva, Switzerland: World Health Organization.

Zorek, J., & Raehl, C. (2012). Interprofessional education accreditation standards in the USA: A comparative analysis. *Journal of Interprofessional Care, 27*(2), 123–130. doi:10.3109/13561820.2012.718295 PMID:22950791

ADDITIONAL READING

Abu-Rish, E., Kim, S., Choe, L., Varpio, L., Malik, E., White, A. A., ... Zierler, B. (2012). Current trends in interprofessional education of health sciences students: A literature review. *Journal of Interprofessional Care, 26*(6), 444–451. doi:10.310 9/13561820.2012.715604 PMID:22924872

Brandt, B., Lutfiyya, M. N., King, J. A., & Chioreso, C. (2014). A scoping review of interprofessional collaborative practice and education using the lens of the Triple Aim. *Journal of Interprofessional Care, 28*(5), 393–399. doi:10.3109/13561820.2 014.906391 PMID:24702046

Cox, M., Cuff, P., Brandt, B. F., Reeves, S., & Zierler, B. (2016). Measuring the impact of interprofessional education on collaborative practice and patient outcomes. *Journal of Interprofessional Care, 30*(1), 1–3. doi:10.3109/13561820.2015.11110 52 PMID:26833103

Frenk, J., Chen, L., Bhutta, Z. A., Cohen, J., Crisp, N., Evans, T., ... Zurayk, H. (2010). Health professionals for a new century: Transforming education to strengthen health systems in an interdependent world. *Lancet, 376*(9756), 1923–1958. doi:10.1016/ S0140-6736(10)61854-5 PMID:21112623

Institute of Medicine. (2015). *Measuring the impact of interprofessional education on collaborative practice and patient outcomes*. Washington, DC: National Academies Press.

Josiah Macy Jr. Foundation (2013). Transforming patient care: Aligning interprofessional education with clinical practice redesign. In M. Cox & M. Naylor (Eds.), Transforming Patient Care: Aligning Interprofessional Education with Clinical Practice Redesign. Atlanta.

National Academy of Medicine. (2017). *The role of accreditation in achieving the Quadruple Aim for health*. Washington, DC: National Academies Press.

Reeves, S., Fletcher, S., Barr, H., Birch, I., Boet, S., Davies, N., & Kitto, S. (2016). A BEME systematic review of the effects of interprofessional education: BEME Guide No. 39. *Medical Teacher*, *38*(7), 656–668. doi:10.3109/0142159X.2016.1173663 PMID:27146438

Reeves, S., Perrier, L., Goldman, J., Freeth, D., & Zwarenstein, M. (2013). Interprofessional education: Effects on professional practice and healthcare outcomes (update). *Cochrane Database of Systematic Reviews*, 3. PMID:23543515

Vlasses, P., & Zorek, J. A. (2016). Interprofessional education accreditation standards across US health professions. National Center for Interprofessional Practice and Education, Inaugural Learning Together at the Nexus: National Center Summit on the Future of IPE, Minneapolis, MN, August 22 & 23, 2016.

KEY TERMS AND DEFINITIONS

Accountable Care Organizations (ACOs): Healthcare organization that is partially reimbursed based on increased quality and decreased cost of care provided to patients assigned to it.

Effective Teamwork: Two or more people working together synergistically to accomplish more than the sum of individuals alone.

Interprofessional Education: Occasions when members or students of two or more professions learn about, with and from each other, to improve collaboration and the quality of care and services (Center for the Advancement of Interprofessional Education, 2019).

Leaderless Discussion Group: The LGD is a type of work-sample evaluation in which a small group (5-7) engages in a problem-solving simulation for 20 to 60 minutes, and no formal leader is appointed (Gatewood, Field, & Barrick, 2016).

Quadruple Aim: Patient care that encompasses four overarching goals of enhancing the patient experience, improving population health, reducing costs, and provider satisfaction.

Chapter 5

The Economics of Health:
An Overview of the American Healthcare System

Sean Michael Haas
The University of Texas at Dallas, USA

Sanjana Janumpally
The University of Texas at Dallas, USA

Brendan Lamar Kouns
The University of Texas at Dallas, USA

ABSTRACT

The American healthcare system is vast and complex. An overview of the United States' healthcare system provides a view into the interrelated dynamics between three categories of factors: consumers, intermediaries, and providers. Consumers demand health inputs in order to produce health status that allows them to live productive lives. Intermediaries, such as insurance companies and government programs, reduce the direct cost of healthcare for consumers. Providers, such as hospitals and physicians, amongst others, have historically exhibited a degree of monopolistic power in the healthcare market. The modern trend towards managed care organizations, firms that vertically integrate multiple aspects of the healthcare market, aims to reduce costs imposed by such providers.

DOI: 10.4018/978-1-7998-2949-2.ch005

INTRODUCTION

Why does the United States spend so much money on healthcare? This is a popular question in modern socioeconomic discourse, as the United States spends more on healthcare than any other country in the world by a large margin (OECD 2019). This disparity attracts a lot of attention from researchers looking to design reform measures. However, this leads to additional questions, such as; how does the market for healthcare function in the United States? And, is it efficient in allocating resources? In order to answer these questions, the various facets of the American healthcare system must be examined in detail in order to untangle their interdependence and highlight inefficiencies.

Healthcare is a fundamentally essential factor in modern societies. The individual incentive to prolong one's life and alleviate discomfort means that healthcare is universally demanded by consumers. Even healthy individuals will likely face medical adversity at some point that requires professional treatment. Moreover, the extension of life expectancy across the population through advances in healthcare has led to increased economic output over time. Economically, the healthcare industry makes up a large portion of both capital and labor in the United States. Due to the importance of healthcare in modern society, the system faces a high degree of public scrutiny and criticism. Such criticism is warranted as the United States' healthcare system contains many inefficiencies that are uncovered through an economic examination; from disproportionate spending and cost increases, to problems in information transmission and distorted market dynamics.

An overview of the United States' healthcare system provides a view into the inter-related dynamics between three categories of factors: consumers, intermediaries and providers. Consumers demand health inputs in order to produce health status that allows them to live productive lives. Intermediaries, such as insurance companies and government programs, reduce the direct cost of healthcare for consumers. Providers, such as hospitals and physicians, have historically exhibited a degree of monopolistic power in the healthcare market. The modern trend towards managed care organizations, firms that vertically integrate multiple aspects of the healthcare market, aims to reduce costs imposed by such providers.

Consumers

The first category of components involved in the American healthcare system are consumers. This category looks at the demand side of the healthcare market by including consumption behavior, the prices paid by consumers, and the demand of healthcare products and services in the market.

In a basic sense, the demand side of the healthcare market is made up of consumers who purchase health inputs seeking utility gain through improved health status. The term "health inputs" refers broadly to healthcare products and services that are purchased by consumers. The term "health status" refers to an individual's overall quality and quantity of life. Health status is captured by four indicators including life expectancy, avoidable mortality, chronic disease morbidity, and self-rated health (OECD 2019). However, consumer demand for health inputs in the market is not this simple. Theoretically, a perfectly competitive market should allow for the efficient allocation of resources that maximizes societal well-being (OpenStax 2016). This theoretical situation is indicated by the presence of both productive and allocative efficiency, meaning that products are produced at the minimum average cost for producers and the prices paid by consumers are equal to the marginal cost of production. Thus, the benefit derived by consumers purchasing the products is equal to the societal cost of allocating the resources towards producing those products.

While such theoretical perfect competition may lead to the maximization of societal well-being, real-world markets rarely mimic the theoretical textbook examples. In the United States healthcare markets, there are several fundamental characteristics that impede such optimal resource allocation. Healthcare markets are inherently beset by imperfect and asymmetric information, as well as exhibiting vast product differentiation (Gaynor and Vogt 2000). Product differentiation refers to goods that are fundamentally different from the goods offered by other firms in the market, whereas imperfect and asymmetric information refer to inequalities of information between parties in a transaction (OpenStax 2016). Encapsulating product differentiation, most health inputs purchased by consumers are specialized to fit an individual diagnosis made by a medical professional and are thus inherently heterogeneous and non-transferable (Gaynor and Vogt 2000). This means that consumers are unable to trade their health inputs among each-other on a secondary market, and instead must interact with the primary producer, leading to an imbalance in market power between producers and consumers.

Both characteristics of product differentiation and information asymmetries lead to the imbalance in market power between producers and consumers, resulting in monopolistic competition in healthcare markets (Folland et. al. 2013). Monopolistic competition describes a market where there are multiple firms competing against one another, but their products are differentiated to allow for greater producer power. The result is an intermediate market between perfect competition and pure monopoly, as producers can set prices and quantities, but their demand curve still exhibits a degree of elasticity. Monopolistically competitive firms are not productively or allocatively efficient, and consumer prices are higher than under perfect competition (OpenStax CNX 2016).

Demand in healthcare markets differs from demand exhibited by many other types of consumer products, as healthcare may be considered both a luxury good as well as a reputation good (Grossman 1972, Hagist and Kotlikoff 2005, Satterthwaite 1981). The demand curve for healthcare is highly elastic, exhibiting an income elasticity greater than one (Hagist and Kotlikoff 2005). This means that health inputs are perceived by consumers to be luxury goods, and that changes in consumer income have a dramatic impact on demand. Similarly, as a reputation good, consumers rely on information from social networks to select healthcare providers (Folland et. al. 2013).

Despite the primary effect of changes in relative costs that cause consumer demand for health inputs to behave like a luxury good, there are differences in the intrinsic qualities of both human health and health inputs themselves. Health inputs are not directly desired by consumers; but rather consumers seek the health status that comes from utilizing health inputs (Folland et. al. 2013, Grossman 1972). In this regard, health inputs can be viewed as a productive good that produces health status as an output, and this output allows individuals to work productively when they otherwise would not be able to (Folland et. al. 2013). However, due to diminishing marginal returns, additional health inputs have a decreasing marginal impact on output. This means that consumers' health status improves as they consume additional health inputs, however the rate of change becomes reduced over time. Moreover, consumers take an active role in improving their health status by not only purchasing these health inputs passively, but also allocating their own time to utilizing those inputs (Grossman 1972). However, the improved health status gained by purchasing and utilizing health inputs does not have a pre-determined time span of efficacy. A consumer who purchases health inputs is unable to know with certainty how long their health status will improve, or if it will improve at all, due to the vast differences in individual diagnoses and underlying health status between individuals. Despite this variability in the time span of efficacy, health inputs can be viewed as an investment good that produces improved future health status as an output (Folland et. al. 2013, Grossman 1972). This improved future health status allows individuals to exhibit an increase their working capability, earn additional income and improve their quality of life. As an investment good, increased consumption of health inputs should produce dramatic increases in future economic output for society.

Over the last century in the United States, there has been a dramatic increase in both the consumption of health inputs and the increased efficacy of those inputs. This increase in healthcare consumption has led to a vast increase in public health status, as shown by changes in mortality and life expectancy. In the first half of the 20th century, life expectancy rose from 47 years in 1900 to 63 years in 1940 (Cutler and Miller 2004). Much of this decrease in mortality can be attributed to reductions in infectious disease exhibited as a result of clean water technologies

(Cutler and Miller 2004). In the latter half of the 20th century, mortality rates in the United States decreased further, as newborn life expectancy increased by 6.97 years from 1960 to 2000, driven by improvements in infant care and cardiovascular disease treatment (Folland et. al. 2013, Cutler, Rosen and Vijan 2006). However, these improvements in life expectancy exhibited by the United States over the last century have occurred alongside large increases in healthcare spending (Cutler et. al. 2006). The next section looks at the growth in healthcare spending in the United States to analyze the societal costs and benefits of this trend.

Healthcare Costs & Spending

The healthcare sector is a large and ever-growing portion of the United States economy, as shown through data on National Health Expenditures (NHE). The National Health Expenditure Accounts measure annual spending in the United States on healthcare goods, services, public health activities, government administration, insurance costs and healthcare investment (Center for Medicare and Medicaid Services 2018).

As shown in Table 1, the absolute increase in NHE has been substantial in the last several decades. Rising from $27.2 billion in 1960 to $3,492.1 billion in 2017 (Centers for Medicare and Medicaid Services 2018). These increases occurred alongside vast population growth, as the US population grew from 186 million in 1960 to 325 million in 2017 (Centers for Medicare and Medicaid Services 2018). However, the increase in NHE is disproportionately larger than the growth in the US population. Viewing changes in NHE as a percentage of US Gross Domestic Product provides a view on the increasing role of healthcare in the overall economy. In 1960 national healthcare expenditures as a percentage of US GDP amounted to only 5.0%, however this metric has grown over the following years, rising to 8.9% in 1980, 13.4% in 2000, before reaching 17.9% in 2017 (Centers for Medicare and Medicaid Services 2018, Folland et. al. 2013, Werling et. al. 2014). Looking at changes in NHE on a per-capita basis provides a more granular view of consumer spending on healthcare. Over this time period NHE per capita rose from $147 in 1960 to $8,086 in 2009, growing by a multiple of 55 (Folland el. al 2013). Adjusting for inflation through the Consumer Price Index, real NHE per capita in 2009 was 7.6 times higher than real NHE per capita in 1960. This illustrates the dramatic increase in both healthcare spending and healthcare prices, which have occurred even when the economy has exhibited brief periods of deflation such as in 2009 (Folland et. a. 2013). The increase in NHE has outpaced inflation in the United States over this time period and is expected to continue to outpace economic growth rates in the near future (OECD 2019).

Table 1. National Health Expenditures and Other Data (1960 – 2017)

Table 1 National Health Expenditures and Other Data (1960 - 2017)								
Expenditure Amount	**1960**	**1970**	**1980**	**1990**	**2000**	**2010**	**2017**
National Health Expenditures (Amount in Billions)	$ 27.2	$ 74.6	$ 255.3	$ 721.4	$ 1,369.2	$ 2,598.6	$ 3,492.1
Gross Domestic Product (Amount in Billions)	$ 542.4	$ 1,073.3	$ 2,857.3	$ 5,963.1	$ 10,252.3	$ 14,992.1	$ 19,485.4
U.S. Population (Millions)	186	210	230	254	282	309	325
National Health Expenditures (Annual Percent Change)		13.1	15.3	11.9	7.2	4.1	3.9
U.S. Population (Annual Percent Change)		1.2	1.0	1.2	1.0	0.8	0.7
Gross Domestic Product (Annual Percent Change)		5.5	8.8	5.7	6.5	3.8	4.2
National Health Expenditures (Per Capita Amount)	146	355	1,108	2,843	4,855	8,411	10,739
National Health Expenditures as a Percent of Gross Domestic Product (Percent)	5.0	6.9	8.9	12.1	13.4	17.3	17.9

Source: Centers for Medicare and Medicaid Services (2018)

Healthcare spending in the United States has risen precipitously over the last several decades, but how does this compare with other advanced economies? Utilizing data from the OECD can provide a reference point to compare healthcare spending over time. The Organization for Economic Co-Operation and Development includes 36 member countries that are considered developed economies with high levels of income. The United States exhibits a much larger amount of healthcare spending compared to the OECD average. In 2018 average healthcare spending per capita was around $4,000 adjusted for purchasing power across OECD member countries, whereas the United States healthcare spending per capita was around $10,000 (OECD 2019). This increase in spending compared to other advanced economies has not coincided with improved health outcomes, as the United States exhibits a lower life expectancy than the average for OECD countries (OECD 2019, Papanicolas et. al. 2018). In recent years the United States has continued to spend a disproportionately large proportion of GDP on healthcare relative to other advanced economies. As a percentage of GDP, healthcare spending in the United States is around 16.9% relative to the OECD average of 8.8% (OECD 2019). Moreover, this disparity in healthcare spending between the United States and OECD member countries has persisted over several decades and is indicative of the longer-term trend in increasing healthcare expenditures.

While annual healthcare spending per capita in the United States has increased from $146 in 1960 to over $10,000 in 2017, such metrics do not accurately show the shift in payment sources within the American economy. Most healthcare expenditures are paid by governments, as indicated by the change in real government healthcare spending, which rose by a factor of 6.9 from 1970 and 2002 (Cutler et. al. 2006, Hagist and Kotlikoff 2005). Possible explanations for these increases include that consumers may be purchasing a larger quantity of health services, the quality of the services purchased may be increasing, or the inflation rate of healthcare costs may be greater than the overall inflation rate exhibited by the United States (Folland et. al. 2013). While some hypothesize that changing demographics are a source of increased healthcare expenditures, Hagist and Kotlikoff 2005 find that benefit levels, care received by individuals at any given age, has risen at a faster rate than the increase in healthcare expenditures, meaning that the age composition of the population is not directly responsible for the increased costs of healthcare.

The dramatic increase in healthcare spending in the United States, both in isolation and in relation to other OECD countries, has produced massive economic benefit on aggregate through decreasing mortality rates across the adult population. From 1960 to 2000, increased spending on healthcare led to higher lifetime costs of $19,900 per year of additional life expectancy, though this cost is dramatically higher for the elderly population aged 65 and older, where the average cost per additional life year reached $84,700 (Cutler et. al. 2006). However, improving life expectancy has significant economic value to society that can be measured through several theoretical frameworks. In the United States, the statistical value of human life for prime-aged workers averages around $7 million (Viscusi and Aldy 2003). On aggregate, the increases in life expectancy in the United States from 1900 to 2000 have been found to be worth over $1.2 million per person, adding around $3.2 trillion per year to national wealth (Murphy and Topel 2006).

Economic Analysis of Healthcare Costs

Every society has limited resources. Economic analysis allows societies to efficiently allocate scarce resources in order to maximize aggregate outcomes. Regarding healthcare, the objective of this analysis is to determine whether the benefits of healthcare expenditures are worth the cost. This cost can be viewed as both an opportunity cost as well as a financial cost. There is an opportunity cost of allocating resources towards healthcare rather than utilizing those resources elsewhere in the economy. This opportunity cost must be considered alongside the direct financial cost to consumers (Olsen et. al. 1999).

While large amounts of healthcare spending are indicative of allocating greater amounts of societal resources towards healthcare, additional resources do not directly translate into improved health outcomes for individuals (OECD 2019). Analyzing both the financial and opportunity costs of healthcare spending can illustrate some of the variation in healthcare spending between countries. This analysis is performed through three primary methods; cost-effectiveness analysis, cost-utility analysis, and cost-benefit analysis (Olsen et. al. 1999). Cost-effectiveness analysis (CEA) examines individual benefit in terms of the specific health inputs consumed, meaning that this analysis does not translate across various diagnoses (Olsen et. al. 1999). Cost-utility analysis (CUA) aims to provide a transferable analysis of health outcomes that can be used across multiple diagnoses. CUA is typically measured in terms of quality-adjusted-life-years, which can be used to compare the efficacy of various health inputs across multiple individuals (Olsen et. al. 1999). These analyses are augmented by cost-benefit analysis (CBA), which expresses outcomes in monetary units in order to compare the financial costs of healthcare to a monetary benefit received by consumers (Folland et. al. 2013, Olsen et. al. 1999).

The significant variability of healthcare costs across different types of medical diagnoses further complicates the analysis of healthcare expenditures. Individual health status often varies between greatly between consumers, and similar health inputs may not produce identical outcomes. This leads to vast variation in the financial cost of saving one year of human life, as found by utilizing CEA. Medical interventions ranged in cost per life-year saved from less than $0 to over $1,000,000 (Tengs et. al. 1995). Often the cost of this additional life-year is unknown and only estimated until after treatment is deemed successful. Some treatments were found to save more resources than they consumed, such as childhood immunizations; whereas other treatments consumed a larger proportion of resources than they saved, such as intensive cardiovascular care (Tengs et. al. 1995). Large variations in cost were also present between different areas of society, such as interventions as a result of transportation accidents compared to occupational incidents. (Tengs et. al. 1995).

The existing literature shows that the dramatic increases in healthcare spending for both individuals and governments in the United States over the last several decades have been largely beneficial to society (Cutler et. al. 2006). While more resources have been allocated to the healthcare economy, in recent decades reductions in mortality and extensions in life expectancy have yielded significant economic value (Cutler et. al. 2006, Viscusi and Aldy 2003). The next section examines the presence of uncertainty in healthcare markets that lead to market inefficiencies.

The Presence of Uncertainty

The United States healthcare markets have large amounts of uncertainty that distort market dynamics and lead to inefficiencies. Uncertainty is present in the problems of imperfect and asymmetric information, as well as product uncertainty. Individual consumers cannot accurately predict their future health status without error, described as imperfect information. In many cases, low-probability events such as motor-vehicle accidents lead to an unexpected change in health status that requires immediate healthcare treatment. This leads to significant uncertainty and irregularity on the demand side of healthcare markets, as consumers seek many health inputs reactively rather than proactively (Arrow 1963, Folland et. al. 2013). Moreover, consumers often have less knowledge about health inputs and their own health status than producers, which is described as asymmetric information. Consumers are often not only purchasing health inputs from producers, they are also seeking information and advice. This information asymmetry means that consumers may not change healthcare providers due to inferior outcomes, meaning that inefficient providers may stay in business rather than failing (Newhouse 2002). Finally, product uncertainty is present in the notion that consumers cannot accurately predict the efficacy of all healthcare treatments, which leads to an additional source of uncertainty on the demand side of healthcare consumption. However, product uncertainty is present on the supply side of the market as well, as healthcare providers cannot guarantee the efficacy of many treatments and services (Arrow 1963, Folland et. al. 2013).

The presence of vast product differentiation, combined with these sources of uncertainty, leads to an imbalance of market power between healthcare producers and consumers. This imbalance manifests as monopolistic competition in the healthcare market, where producers have power over both pricing and the quantity of production and market forces do not efficiently allocate resources in the healthcare economy. Such market failures then lead to the creation of non-market institutions that aim to correct these failures, such as the government programs of Medicare and Medicaid (Arrow 1963, Saveoff 2004). These institutions are intermediaries that stand between producers and consumers, which will be examined in the next section.

Intermediaries

The second category of factors involved in the United States Healthcare system are the intermediaries that operate between consumers and providers in the market. These intermediaries include payment systems such as various forms of insurance, as well as the non-market institutions of Medicare and Medicaid.

Healthcare in the United States differs from many other countries in source of payment due to the presence of insurance (Folland et. al. 2013, Hagist and Kotlikoff 2005). Most American consumers do not pay directly for healthcare products and services. Many consumers purchase health insurance in one form or another, that requires them to pay regular premiums in exchange for avoiding the direct cost of healthcare services. Though most Americans receive insurance through employment, and insurance benefits have been associated with higher wages for employees (Folland et. al. 2013). Moreover, the United States government does not guarantee health insurance coverage for all individuals within the population, but rather provides for most healthcare costs for disadvantaged groups, such as the poor and elderly, through the programs of Medicare and Medicaid (Hagist and Kotlikoff 2005). In this sense, insurance companies alongside Medicare and Medicaid act as intermediaries, operating between consumers and providers in the market.

These intermediaries in the healthcare market have reduced the direct costs to consumers over the last several decades. Since World War II, health insurance enrollment has risen substantially in the United States from 12 million individuals in 1940, to 76.6 million in 1950, 158.8 million in 1970, 187 million in 1980, reaching 194.5 million in 2009 (Folland et. al. 2013). As shown in the previous section, National Healthcare Expenditures have risen dramatically since 1960, but during this time period the percentage paid directly by consumers, "out-of-pocket", has been significantly reduced. In 1960 Personal Health Care Spending as a percentage paid out-of-pocket was 55.1%. This direct expenditure has fallen over subsequent years to 14.3% in 2009 (Folland et. al. 2013). As the percentage paid directly by consumers has fallen, the percentage paid by intermediaries has risen. This change in direct costs to consumers may be one of the factors underpinning increased healthcare consumption in aggregate by American consumers.

As shown by the RAND Health Insurance Experiment, consumer demand for healthcare is highly elastic, meaning that it can be greatly influenced by the proportion of overall cost that is paid out-of-pocket (Lohr et. al. 1986). Their results showed that individuals with comprehensive health insurance, that covered most costs incurred, purchased around 40% more health care than individuals who had to pay the costs themselves (Lohr et. al. 1986). In order to better understand the effects of intermediaries on healthcare markets, the mechanics of health insurance will be examined in the next section.

The Concept of Insurance

Insurance operates through the law of large numbers in order to reduce aggregate risks. Specifically, insurance providers create large pools of individuals with varying levels of risk in order to reduce the overall variability of the pool (Folland et. al. 2013). If historical data is an accurate predictor of future outcomes, then insurance pools can mathematically quantify the risk levels of different individuals to minimize overall risk.

Consumers choose to purchase health insurance to reduce their financial exposure to unexpected events that carry a high expected financial cost, such as a heart attack or cancer diagnosis. So, consumers must exhibit a degree of risk aversion in order to purchase insurance, and they must also exhibit a diminishing marginal utility of wealth or income (Folland et. al. 2013). For these consumers, the cost of regular insurance premiums or coinsurance payments, which results in a loss of income or wealth, is worth the protection against the potential enormous financial costs of unexpected hospitalization or illness. In fact, most consumers exhibit enough risk aversion, and diminishing marginal utility of income, that they are willing to pay above the actuarial fair rate to protect themselves against such large financial losses (Manning and Marquis 1996).

Theoretically, consumer demand for health insurance will change methodically in relation to the cost of insurance and the prices of health inputs in the market. Changes in insurance premiums, expected losses from lacking insurance, and wealth, will all lead to rational reactions from consumers regarding their purchase of health insurance. When insurance premiums rise, consumers reduce their insurance coverage. When the expected losses from an unexpected health event events rise, consumers increase their insurance coverage (Folland et. al. 2013). At higher levels of wealth consumers will receive less marginal benefit from the same insurance policy, but the cost of the insurance premium also makes up a lesser amount of their total wealth. Therefore, the consumption preferences for insurance in relation to increasing wealth depend upon changes in the expected losses from not having insurance (Folland et. al. 2013).

By operating as an intermediary in the market between consumers and providers, insurance reduces the direct costs of healthcare for individuals; however, it also creates market inefficiencies and skews the allocative effect of the market for healthcare. In order to understand these inefficiencies, the problems in insurance will be examined in the next section.

Problems in Insurance

Much like the demand side of the healthcare market, insurance and other intermediaries exhibit inherent characteristics that create market inefficiencies. The presence of imperfect information, combined with the high elasticity of demand for healthcare services, leads to the manifestation of moral hazard, adverse selection, and a misallocation of resources in health insurance markets (Folland et. al. 2013, Hagist and Kotlikoff 2005).

Imperfect information in markets leads to information asymmetries between two parties in a transaction. The two parties are referred to as principles and agents. The principals are relatively uninformed compared to the other party, the agents, in relation to decision-making between the two parties. In the healthcare market, consumers are the principles, and producers are the agents. In this situation, the principal delegates a degree of decision-making power to the agent who is trusted to act in the principal's best interests. In health insurance markets, consumers are the principles, who often lack information relative to intermediaries, who are the agents. As the two parties have differing incentives to act in their own best interests, the problem of moral hazard arises. Moral hazard refers to a change in behavior by one party that is related to the actions of the other party, due to imperfect information. More specifically, the behavior of consumers may change as a result of shifting incentives due to price elasticity, as the cost of a product or service fluctuate.

Applying these concepts to the healthcare market, illustrates the foundation of the market inefficiencies. Consumers demand for healthcare is highly elastic, meaning that consumer demand for health inputs will change rapidly as their direct costs fluctuate. The direct costs to consumers for health inputs likely change as a result of either becoming insured or losing one's insurance coverage, leading to a shift in consumer demand and illustrating the problem of moral hazard (Folland et. al. 2013). Becoming insured causes consumers' marginal costs of health inputs to fall, which leads to an increase in the quantity demanded of healthcare products and services (Folland et. al. 2013). This increase in quantity demand serves the best interest of the principle, the consumer, at the expense of the best interests of the agent, the insurer. Therefore, the problem of moral hazard in healthcare markets causes the optimal level of insurance purchased by consumers to increase in relation to changes in expected losses due to illness, as the degree of moral hazard decreases (Folland et. al. 2013).

In addition to the problem of moral hazard, the presence of adverse selection and incentivized behavior in health insurance markets leads to inefficiencies in the allocation of resources. Due to adverse selection, consumers who are likely to use healthcare services at a higher rate are more likely to purchase health insurance (Folland et. al. 2013, Manning and Marquis 1996). As insurance creates pools of different individuals to reduce aggregate risk, the premiums paid by lower risk individuals are influenced by the presence of high-risk individuals, leading to a redistribution of income from healthy, low-risk consumers to unhealthy, high-risk consumers (Folland et. al. 2013). Yet, high-risk consumers are more likely to purchase health insurance, as their expected losses from becoming ill while uninsured are greater than the low-risk consumers. This dynamic underpinned by adverse selection increases insurance premiums for all individuals in the pool. Through incentivized behavior, health insurance shifts consumer demand for healthcare products and services, which can distort the allocation of resources across society (Folland et. al. 2013). Insurance subsidizes specific types of treatments and services, such as health services from professional providers and prescription drugs, but it does not subsidize alternatives that still significantly impact individual health, such as dietary nutrition and exercise (Folland et. al. 2013). Thus, consumers are incentivized to pursue certain activities regardless of the shift in resource allocation that occurs in aggregate.

The increasing demand for health insurance, combined with the inherent moral hazard and adverse selection characteristic of such insurance, may result in increasing healthcare prices beyond the theoretical competitive market rate (Feldstein 1973, Folland et. al. 2013, Manning and Marquis 1996). Insured consumers, who are not paying the full costs, purchase excess healthcare services. In this context, excess healthcare services are defined as a quantity beyond the level demanded if these consumers were uninsured or having to pay a larger proportion of the full healthcare costs out-of-pocket (Manning and Marquis 1996). As these insured consumers purchase excess healthcare services, producers can increase prices through their monopolistically competitive market position. As these prices increase, additional consumers become incentivized to purchase health insurance, and a feedback loop is developed. The feedback loop between health insurance, healthcare prices and consumers is as follows: as the price of health insurance is related to the expected loss to the consumer if they become ill, however this expected loss is related to the price of healthcare services that the consumer would need to purchase, which is itself related to the demand for health insurance (Feldstein 1973, Folland et. al. 2013).

Due to this feedback loop, it is possible that an aggregate reduction in insurance coverage could result in a net utility gain for consumers. While consumers would exhibit a utility loss due to increased risk, they would exhibit a utility gain due to reduced healthcare prices (Feldstein 1973).

Non-Market Institutions

In addition to insurance, the category of intermediaries includes the non-market institutions established by the government to serve population groups that would otherwise lack service. The following section examines the government programs of Medicare and Medicaid.

In 1965, both Medicare and Medicaid were established by the Social Security Amendments. Medicare is a federal government program that provides health insurance coverage to individuals aged 65 years or older as well as younger individuals who are permanently disabled (Medicare 2015). Medicaid is a state and federal government program that provides health insurance coverage to low-income individuals. By acting as an intermediary in the healthcare market, the programs of Medicare and Medicaid dramatically changed the role of the United States government in delivery and financing of healthcare, with over 65% of healthcare spending by elderly individuals coming from state or federal governments (Nardi et. al. 2016, Phelps 2012).

Medicare

The current Medicare program consists of four different parts: Part A, Part B, Part C, and Part D. Medicare Part A, also known as the hospital insurance, is directed to people aged 65 and older as well as anyone who receives Social Security benefits or who were permanently disabled (Phelps 2012). It covers inpatient hospitalizations, hospice care, skilled nursing facility, and home health care (Medicare 2015). The expenses of Medicare Part A are covered by the Medicare Trust Fund. While enrollment in Part A of Medicaid is mandatory, enrollment in Part B, otherwise known as Supplemental Medical Insurance, is optional. Part B enrollment is dedicated to people aged 65 and older, and it covers physician services both in hospital and nonhospital settings, services by other healthcare professions such as optometry, podiatry, dentistry, and lastly, services in outpatient clinics and emergency rooms. Together, Medicare Part A and Part B are referred to as "traditional Medicare", and almost all the people who were eligible to participate in Part A voluntarily chose to enroll in Part B as well (Folland et. al. 2013). By 1970, 97% of eligible Americans were enrolled in Medicare Part A and Part B, and that number has remained consistent ever since (Moon, M. 2001).

The other parts of Medicare, not categorized as traditional Medicare, are Medicare Part C and Part D. Also known as Medicare Advantage, Part C was established in 1996 to include dental and vision services not covered under Part A or Part B (Medicare 2015). Potential drawbacks to being enrolled in Medicare Part C instead of traditional Medicare include lack of access to certain doctors despite being in-network, being limited to specialists only referred by the primary care provider, and higher premiums than traditional Medicare (Medicare 2015). Medicare Part D was established in 2006 to offer subsidized pricing on prescription drugs. Medicare Part D is optional, and it is offered to enrollees in Medicare Part C or traditional Medicare (Medicare 2015). This portion of Medicare was enacted in response to the increasing rate of prescription drug usage by American consumers, as it provides assistance to pay for medication costs (Feke 2015). Medicare Part D covers up to $2,850 of prescription coverage before discontinuing. Coverage will resume only if the beneficiary spends another $1,700 on medications for the remainder of the year (Feke 2015). This gap in coverage is referred to as the "doughnut hole", as the out-of-pocket expenses suddenly increase until a set level of expenditures are reached, leading to financial risk for many beneficiaries. Figure 2 illustrates the payment structure of Medicare Part D and the doughnut hole in benefits. The doughnut hole was intended to serve as an encouragement for hospital providers to opt for less costly generic medications instead of prescribing brand name medications (Feke 2015). However, it has become an area of concern for individuals who need regular and expensive medications.

Figure 1. Medicare Part D
Source: Medicare, (Feke 2015).

Phase of Your Part D Plan	What You Pay	What Medicare Part D Pays
Pre-Donut Hole	Deductible Monthly premiums Copays/coinsurance	Total drug cost — copay/coinsurance
Donut Hole	Monthly premiums 47.5% cost of brand-name medications 72% of generic medications	52.5% of brand-name medications 28% of generic medications
Catastrophic Coverage	5% of drug costs or $6.35 copay for brand-name medications $2.55 copay for generic medications (whichever is greater)	95% of drug costs or Total drug cost — copay (whichever is lesser)

Medicaid

As Medicare was established to serve the elderly population who may not otherwise obtain health insurance coverage in the market, Medicaid was established to serve low-income individuals who may not be able to afford health insurance. Medicaid was also enacted through the Social Security Amendments in 1965 and is managed by both the state and federal governments, though most of the decision-making is done at the state level within federal guidelines. Under these guidelines, every state's Medicaid program must include eligibility for "most categorically needy populations, including inpatient hospital services, outpatient hospital services, prenatal care, vaccines for children, physician services, nursing facility services for persons age 21 or older, and family planning services and supplies" (Folland et. al. 2013). Moreover, the costs associated with Medicaid spending is shared between the state and federal governments. That share of government spending is known as the Federal Medical Assistance Percentage, which is determined by a specific formula based on states' average per capita income (Folland et. al. 2013).

Alongside private insurance, the non-market institutions of Medicare and Medicaid act as intermediaries in the healthcare markets. These institutions operate between consumers and providers, reducing costs to consumers, but contributing to market distortions. To understand the supply side of the healthcare market, the next section examines healthcare providers.

Providers

In investigating the supply side of the healthcare market in the United States, the third category of factors involved in the United States Healthcare system are providers. This includes the institutions that produce health inputs and provide care to consumers, as well as the dynamics of the supply of healthcare in the market. These institutions include hospitals, physicians, nursing care facilities, home health care services, and outpatient care centers (National Center for Health Statistics 2018).

In the United States, employment in the healthcare industry has grown dramatically in the last several decades, and healthcare providers now make up a large portion of the economy. From 1970 to 2009, the number of physicians in the United States rose from 334,000 to 972,000, the number of registered nurses rose from 750,000 to 2,500,000, and total employment in the healthcare industry reached 15.5 million individuals, which accounted for 11.1% of all employed adults (Folland et. al. 2013). As of 2017, employment in health and social work made up 13.4% of the total employed population in the United States, far above the OECD average of 10.1% (OECD 2019). However, the number of practicing doctors per 1,000 individuals in the population is far below the average for other OECD countries (OECD 2019).

Examining the nature of employment in the healthcare industry provides information on the supply of healthcare in the market. The overall supply of healthcare is influenced by the number of workers as well as the prices paid by consumers for healthcare services (Folland et. al. 2013). In a broad sense, the healthcare industry has two types of job roles, classified here as generalist and specialist, that exhibit very different supply characteristics. Generalist roles include jobs that support the healthcare provider business without performing healthcare services directly, such as business administration roles. These roles exhibit dramatic changes in supply in short periods of time due to low barriers to entry. Specialist roles include physicians and other types of specialists who undergo extensive education and training. These roles exhibit less variability in supply due to high barriers to entry. Such education and training represent an investment in one's human capital that is only pursued if the rate of return is higher than the rate of return for pursuing other professions.

Managed Care Organizations

In the last several decades, the American healthcare market has changed substantially regarding the overall organization of providers and re-imbursement models of intermediaries. The goal with this shift has been to reduce public expenditures and limit the increase in healthcare prices. As such, the healthcare market has exhibited a change from "fee-for-service" to managed care and value-based care. These new organizational models aim to incentivize health care providers into increasing quality and decreasing costs (Zuvekas and Cohen 2016). The costs and benefits of these different models will be explained below.

The fee-for-service model has been the historical standard for American healthcare providers. In this model a provider would receive a set payment either from the insurance company or the consumer based upon services rendered (Ginsburg 2012). However, the fee-for-service model created several market inefficiencies. Consumers were unaware of what others paid for similar services in the market due to imperfect information. This allowed providers to exhibit a degree of monopoly power in the market, as they could price discriminate between consumers. Additionally, providers under this model also had incentives to order unnecessary tests. As their remuneration was tied to the quantity of services provided, rather than the efficacy of those services (Folland et. al. 2013). However, this incentive to increase the volume of services rendered may have produced a benefit for consumers, in that providers may have produced shorter visit times across the market (Deber, Hollander, and Jacobs 2008). In moving from the fee-for-service model, managed care organizations have proliferated as the new paradigm.

Managed care organizations vertically integrate multiple functions of the healthcare market, such as both health insurance and the provision of healthcare services, with the goal of reducing production costs (Folland et. al. 2013). Managed care organizations include two types of institutions; health maintenance organizations (HMO) and preferred provider organizations (PPO). Overall production costs are reduced through reductions in administrative expenses and healthcare provision costs. This is achieved through an increased reliance on information technology and the reduction of acute hospital care for many treatments and procedures (Folland et. al. 2013). The growth of managed care has been substantial over the last several decades. In the 1980's less than 20% of the United States population was enrolled in a managed care plan; however, by 2005 around 38% of hospitals reported receiving revenue from managed care plans (Folland et. al. 2013). In addition to managed care organizations, value-based care has become another organizational model in the modern healthcare economy.

In value-based care, healthcare provider reimbursement is based on the quality of care given to patients, and this system has led to the creation of accountable care organizations. Another name for this reimbursement system is "pay for performance", as it rewards better outcomes rather than the volume of services rendered. This reimbursement model has shown an increase in patient satisfaction along with improved medical outcomes. Accountable care organizations are groups of providers, such as hospitals and physicians, that offer care to a group of beneficiaries. The ACO mission is to "manage the full continuum of care and be accountable for the overall costs and quality of care for a defined population" (Rittenhouse, Shortell, & Fisher 2009). ACOs are networks of different types of health care providers that work together to care for a patient (King et. al. 2014). An accountable care organization is rewarded if they meet the performance metrics and put patients first while also lowering healthcare costs (King et. al. 2014).

Managed care organizations and value-based accountable care organizations have proliferated in recent years with the goal of reducing healthcare costs. By vertically integrating multiple aspects of providers and intermediaries in the healthcare market, these organizations can achieve economies of scale and improved efficiency. The next section examines the managed care integration of insurance in detail.

Managed Care and Insurance

The new paradigm of managed care organizations in the American healthcare system represents a combination of intermediaries and providers in the market, as these organizations have integrated insurance into their business models. Most Americans receive health insurance through employment, employer-sponsored managed care plans make up most of the market for private health insurance. In 2009 167 million individuals had private insurance, and 150 million of those received it through employment (Folland et. al. 2013). There are a variety of employer-sponsored insurance plans, from health maintenance organizations (HMOs), preferred provider organizations (PPOs) to point-of-service (POS). HMO plans provide comprehensive care with reduced out-of-pocket expenses for individuals, but individuals are limited to receiving care from a specific network of providers and must receive authorization from a specific physician before seeking care. PPO plans incentivize the receipt of care from specific networks of providers through reduced out-of-pocket costs compared to providers outside of the network (Folland et. al. 2013). POS plans combine aspects of both HMO and PPO plans by incentivizing the receipt of care from network providers while also utilizing the authorization of a physician to reduce excessive healthcare consumption (Folland et. al. 2013).

These managed care plans create subsets of providers, known as networks, that are used to induce price competition among healthcare providers. This increase in competition between providers shifts market power to managed care organizations. Providers are unable to influence prices as they could under the fee-for-service model. Thus, managed care has lowered hospital costs in aggregate, suggesting that increased competition among hospitals can lower overall costs when there is a significant degree of managed care presence (Folland et. al. 2013).

The Economics of Managed Care

Managed care organizations are institutions that vertically integrate multiple aspects of the healthcare business in order to exert market power over providers of healthcare. They combine aspects of both providers and intermediaries to gain market power, which has led to reduced overall costs. In particular, the reductions of administrative costs by managed care organizations may be a critical component to reducing overall healthcare expenditures, as the United States exhibits significantly elevated administrative costs in healthcare relative to other advanced economies (Papanicolas et. al. 2018). However, the trade-off for consumers in exchange for these cost savings is a reduction in choice of healthcare providers. This paradigm shift in the healthcare market has led some researchers to claim that managed care exhibits characteristics of monopsony. Theoretically in monopsony, a market has only one buyer and this firm is able to exert power over suppliers. This firm is then able to influence wages and induce additional workers to enter the labor market, meaning that the labor supply curve and marginal labor cost are no longer equal.

Despite the changes in market dynamics brought about by managed care organizations, the presence of imperfect information still leads to the problem of adverse selection. It is hypothesized that higher-risk consumers with poorer health would be predisposed to choosing their own physician or healthcare provider (Cutler and Reber 1998). Therefore, higher-risk unhealthy consumers may pursue fee-for-service plans, while lower-risk healthy consumers may pursue HMO plans (Cutler and Reber 1998). This change in consumer behavior due to shifting incentives could reduce the efficacy of pooling a diverse group of individuals with varying risk profiles.

POSSIBILITIES FOR REFORM

The prior sections have outlined the current dynamics of the healthcare market in the United States; from consumer behavior and demand conditions, intermediaries and insurance, to providers and managed care organizations. The inefficiencies present in the American healthcare markets are glaring, as indicated by the high level of healthcare spending in the United States relative to other advanced countries, with no measurable gain in health outcomes. Inefficiencies exist in both the demand and supply sides of the healthcare markets, due to information problems and imperfect competition. Reforms to the healthcare system should target these inefficiencies on both sides of the market (Ellis and McGuire 1993).

On the demand-side of the market in the category of consumers, the problems of imperfect and asymmetric information combined with product differentiation lead to monopolistic competition. Reducing these information problems using information technology should be a primary goal of healthcare reform. Such improvements in public education, and the public dissemination of healthcare information, could alleviate some of the information problems found in consumer demand for healthcare. Under less asymmetric and imperfect information, consumers could make more informed decisions about healthcare purchases and prices paid. The problem of product differentiation is more difficult to solve, as the nature of human health is convoluted, and individual health status varies widely between consumers. However, steps towards increased standardization of diagnosis and treatment protocol could alleviate some of this product uncertainty, reduce the market power of providers, and lead to lower aggregate costs.

On the supply-side of the market in the category of providers, reducing production costs may facilitate a decline in overall prices paid by consumers. The United States exhibits the highest level of administrative costs in healthcare out of a group of 10 high-income economies; and it is likely these administrative costs, rather than utilization that should be targeted (Papanicolas et. al. 2018). In reducing these elevated administrative costs, the continued growth of managed care organizations shows promise.

In health insurance markets, the problems of moral hazard and adverse selection may drive a feedback loop of increasing consumer demand and rising health input costs. As consumers become insured, their demand for health inputs increases, leading monopolistically competitive providers to increase prices, thus driving more consumers towards seeking health insurance coverage. It is possible that increasing the marginal cost of health inputs for consumers could lead to an aggregate societal benefit. This would be possible through a reduction in the quantity of health inputs demanded, leading to a stagnation or reduction in prices set by providers. While many consumers would exhibit a utility loss due to increased risk of falling ill and paying out-of-pocket for treatment, the overall effect would be a reduction in healthcare prices for all consumers.

CONCLUSION

The American healthcare system is vast and complex. An examination of the healthcare system reveals the interconnectedness of various factors and the existence of market anomalies and inefficiencies. Economics provides a lens through which to view the complex relationships between these factors. An overview of the United States' healthcare system provides a view into the inter-related dynamics between three categories of factors: consumers, intermediaries and providers. Consumers demand health inputs in order to produce health status that allows them to live productive lives. Improving health status has a significant macroeconomic impact on society, which can be seen through increasing life expectancy in the United States over the last several decades. However, demand for healthcare does not behave like a normal good due to imperfect information leading to moral hazard as well as adverse selection. Intermediaries, such as insurance and government programs, reduce the direct cost of healthcare for consumers. As consumers' direct healthcare costs fall, they demand increasing amounts of healthcare, which influences both the price and supply of healthcare services and health insurance. Medicare and Medicaid aim to solve the market failures exhibited by healthcare markets by providing insurance to high-risk groups who would otherwise not be served by the insurance market. Providers, such as hospitals and physicians amongst others, have historically exhibited a degree of monopolistic power in the healthcare market. The modern trend towards managed care organizations, firms that vertically integrate multiple aspects of the healthcare market, aim to reduce costs imposed by such providers. However, managed care organizations shift the historical paradigm in healthcare markets and through a consolidation of market power lead to a degree of monopsony.

REFERENCES

Arrow, K. J. (1963). Uncertainty and the Welfare Economics of Medical Care. *The American Economic Review*, *53*(5), 941–973.

Bureau of Labor Statistics. (2019). *Employment, Hours, and Earnings from the Current Employment Statistics survey*. Author.

Cardon, J., & Hendel, I. (2001). Asymmetric Information in Health Insurance: Evidence from the National Medical Expenditure Survey. *The Rand Journal of Economics*, *32*(3), 408–427. doi:10.2307/2696362 PMID:11800005

Centers for Medicare & Medicaid Services. (2018). *National Health Accounts Historical: NHE Tables*. Author.

Cutler, D. M., & Reber, S. J. (1998). The Trade-Off Between Competition and Adverse Selection. *The Quarterly Journal of Economics*, *113*(2), 433–466. doi:10.1162/003355398555649

Cutler, D. M., Rosen, A. B., & Vijan, S. (2006). The Value of Medical Spending in the United States, 1960–2000. *The New England Journal of Medicine*, *355*(9), 920–927. doi:10.1056/NEJMsa054744 PMID:16943404

Deber, R., Hollander, M. J., & Jacobs, P. (2008). Models of funding and reimbursement in health care: A conceptual framework. *Canadian Public Administration*, *51*(3), 381–405. doi:10.1111/j.1754-7121.2008.00030.x

Ellis, R. P., & McGuire, T. G. (1993). Supply-side and demand-side cost sharing in health care. *The Journal of Economic Perspectives*, *7*(4), 135–151. doi:10.1257/jep.7.4.135 PMID:10130330

Feke, T. (2015). *Medicare*. New York: Alpha, a member of Penguin Group USA Inc.

Feldstein, M. (1973). The Welfare Loss of Excess Health Insurance. *Journal of Political Economy*, *81*(2), 251–280. doi:10.1086/260027

Folland, S., Goodman, A. C., & Stano, M. (2013). *The economics of health and health care* (7th ed.). Boston: Pearson.

Gaynor, M., & Vogt, W. B. (2000). Antitrust and competition in health care markets. In A. Culyer & J. Newhouse (Eds.), *Handbook of Health Economics* (pp. 1405–1487). New York: Elsevier Science, North-Holland.

Ginsburg, P. B. (2012). Fee-For-Service Will Remain A Feature Of Major Payment Reforms, Requiring More Changes In Medicare Physician Payment. *Health Affairs*, *31*(9), 1977–1983. doi:10.1377/hlthaff.2012.0350 PMID:22949446

Grossman, M. (1972). On the Concept of Health Capital and the Demand for Health. *Journal of Political Economy, 80*(2), 223–255. doi:10.1086/259880

Hagist, C., & Kotliko, L. J. (2006). *Who's Going Broke? Comparing Healthcare Costs in ten OECD Countries*. NBER Working Paper 11833.

King, R., Rose, R., Merritt, M., & Okray, J. (2014). *The ABCs of ACOs : a practical handbook on accountable care organizations*. Chicago, IL: ABA, Health Law Section.

Lohr, K., Brook, R., Kamberg, C., Goldberg, G., Leibowitz, A., Keesey, J., ... Newhouse, J. (1986). Use of Medical Care in the Rand Health Insurance Experiment: Diagnosis- and Service-Specific Analyses in a Randomized Controlled Trial. *Medical Care, 24*(9). PMID:3093785

Manning, W. G., & Susan Marquis, M. (1996). Health Insurance: The Tradeoff Between Risk Pooling and Moral Hazard. *Journal of Health Economics, 15*(5), 609–639. doi:10.1016/S0167-6296(96)00497-3 PMID:10164045

Miller & Grant. (2004, May 31). *The Role of Public Health Improvements in Health Advances: The 20th Century United States*. Academic Press.

Moon, M. (2001). Medicare. *The New England Journal of Medicine, 344*(12), 928–931. doi:10.1056/NEJM200103223441211 PMID:11259729

Murphy, K. M., & Topel, R. H. (2006). The Value of Health and Longevity. *Journal of Political Economy, 114*(October), 871–904. doi:10.1086/508033

Nardi, M. D., French, E., Jones, J. B., & Mccauley, J. (2016). Medical Spending of the US Elderly. *Fiscal Studies, 37*(3-4), 717–747. doi:10.1111/j.1475-5890.2016.12106 PMID:31404348

National Center for Health Statistics. (2018). Health, United States, 2017: With Special Feature on Mortality. Hyattsville, MD: Author.

Newhouse, J. P. (2002). Why Is There A Quality Chasm? *Health Affairs, 21*(4), 13–25. doi:10.1377/hlthaff.21.4.13 PMID:12117124

OECD. (2017). *Health at a Glance 2017: OECD Indicators*. Paris: OECD Publishing.

OECD. (2019). *Health at a Glance 2019: OECD Indicators*. Paris: OECD Publishing; doi:10.1787/4dd50c09-

Olsen, J. A., Smith, R. D., & Harris, A. (1999, April). *Economic Theory and the Monetary Valuation of Health Care: An Overview of the Issues as Applied to the Economic Evaluation of Health Care Programs*. Centre for Health Program Evaluation: Working Paper No. 82.

OpenStax CNX. (2016). *8.4 Efficiency in Perfectly Competitive Markets*. Retrieved from http://cnx.org/contents/69619d2b-68f0-44b0-b074-a9b2bf90b2c6@11.330

Papanicolas, I., Woskie, L. R., & Jha, A. K. (2018). Health care spending in the United States and other high-income countries. *Journal of the American Medical Association, 319*(10), 1024–1039. doi:10.1001/jama.2018.1150 PMID:29536101

Pauly, M. V., & Satterthwaite, M. A. (1981). The Pricing of Primary Care Physicians' Services: A Test of the Role of Consumer Information. *The Bell Journal of Economics, 12*(2), 488–506. doi:10.2307/3003568

Phelps, C. E. (2012). *Health Economics* (5th ed.). Pearson.

Rajaram, R., & Bilimoria, K. Y. (2015). Medicare. *Journal of the American Medical Association, 314*(4), 420. doi:10.1001/jama.2015.8049 PMID:26219069

Rittenhouse, D., Shortell, S., & Fisher, E. (2009). Primary Care and Accountable Care—Two Essential Elements of Delivery-System Reform. *The New England Journal of Medicine, 361*(24), 2301–2303. doi:10.1056/NEJMp0909327 PMID:19864649

Savedoff, D. W. (2004). 40th Anniversary: Kenneth Arrow and the Birth of Health Economics. *Bulletin of the World Health Organization, 82*(2), 139–140. PMID:15042237

Tengs, T. O., Adams, M. E., Pliskin, J. S., Safran, D. G., Siegel, J. E., Weinstein, M. C., & Graham, J. D. (1995). Five-Hundred Life-Saving Interventions and Their Cost-Effectiveness. *Risk Analysis, 15*(3), 369–390. doi:10.1111/j.1539-6924.1995.tb00330.x PMID:7604170

Viscusi, W. K., & Aldy, J. E. (2003). The Value of a Statistical Life: A Critical Review of Market Estimates throughout the World. *Journal of Risk and Uncertainty, 5*(1), 5–76. doi:10.1023/A:1025598106257

Walshe, K., & Smith, J. (2011). *Healthcare management* (2nd ed.). Maidenhead, UK: Open University Press.

Werling, J., Keehan, S., Nyhus, D., Heffler, S., Horst, R., & Meade, D. (2014). The supply side of health care. *Survey of Current Business*.

Zuvekas, S. H., & Cohen, J. W. (2016). Fee-For-Service, While Much Maligned, Remains The Dominant Payment Method For Physician Visits. *Health Affairs, 35*(3), 411–414. doi:10.1377/hlthaff.2015.1291 PMID:26953294

KEY TERMS AND DEFINITIONS

Adverse Selection: A situation where asymmetric information leads to a change in one's behavior. In insurance markets, adverse selection is exhibited when unhealthy individuals pursue more extensive health insurance than healthy individuals.

Asymmetric Information: An economic concept where parties have different amounts of information on a shared topic.

Monopolistic Competition: An economic market structure characterized by many producers selling highly differentiated products that are not substitutable. In monopolistic competition firms are price-takers.

Monopsony: An economic market structure characterized by a single buyer exerting substantial control over the market as a major purchaser of goods and services.

Moral Hazard: A change in one's behavior due to shifting incentives that reallocate risk to other parties.

Chapter 6
Maturing an Information Technology Privacy Program:
Assessment, Improvement, and Change Leadership

Mike Gregory
Community Healthcare System, USA

Cynthia Roberts
School of Business and Economics, Indiana University Northwest, USA

ABSTRACT

The Health Insurance Portability and Accountability Act of 1996 (HIPAA) was initially enacted as an administrative simplification to standardize electronic transmission of common administrative and financial transactions. The program also calls for implementation specifications regarding privacy and security standards to protect the confidentiality and integrity of individually identifiable health information or protected health information. The Affordable Care Act further expanded many of the protective provisions set forth by HIPAA. Since its implementation, healthcare organizations around the nation have invested billions of dollars and have cycled through numerous program attempts aimed at meeting these standards. This chapter reviews the process taken by one organization to review the privacy policy in place utilizing a maturity model, identify deficiencies, and lead change in order to heighten the maturity of the system. The authors conclude with reflection related to effectiveness of the process as well as implications for practice.

DOI: 10.4018/978-1-7998-2949-2.ch006

INTRODUCTION

The Health Insurance Portability and Accountability Act of 1996 (Public Law 104-191), hereafter ("HIPAA"), was initially enacted as an administrative simplification to standardize the electronic transmission of common administrative and financial transactions. The program, administered by the Department of Health and Human Services ("DHHS") and enforced by the Office for Civil Rights ("OCR"), also calls for implementation specifications regarding privacy and security standards to protect the confidentiality and integrity of individually identifiable health information or protected health information, hereafter ("PHI") (Office for Civil Rights, 2015). Although health information technology is not specifically covered in any one section of the Affordable Care Act of 2010 (Public Law 111-148), hereafter ("ACA"), it is a necessary condition to enact many of its initiatives such as streamlining services, improving access and quality of healthcare, and facilitating the analysis of large amounts of data for benchmarking best practices (Fontenot, 2013). As the use of electronic data expands, the need for assurance of privacy becomes paramount. The ACA itself references HIPAA and mentions privacy throughout the entire document.

Since its implementation, healthcare organizations around the nation have invested billions of dollars and have cycled through numerous program attempts aimed at meeting these standards. As intended, the law forced the industry at large to work together towards the same goal, that is, to increase the portability of PHI securely across the wide-open cyberspace platform. This was a tall order for an industry that had focused on making data widely available on the open market without any attempt to secure its system, programs, or data interconnected by the Internet. To date, information technology has made great progress in securing private networks by making smarter appliances to process data securely, encoding plain text with stronger cipher algorithms to prevent unauthorized exposure, and adopting best industry practices in the management of data and data systems.

Nevertheless, the assurance that information is viewed, obtained, or otherwise managed legitimately and responsibly, regardless of how secure the data is stored and transmitted, remains to be a considerable challenge. For this reason, HIPAA included the requirement to implement privacy programs for the purpose of monitoring for the proper use and disclosure of PHI. To help organizations strengthen their privacy policies, procedures, and practices, organizations such as the American Institute of Certified Public Accountants have created maturity models that have been adopted into the healthcare environment to satisfy the privacy requirements from HIPAA (AICPA, 2011). With this background in mind, this chapter presents a case example of the evaluation of a privacy program within a healthcare system in the Midwestern United States, identifies its deficiencies, and discusses the role of leadership in reinvigorating the program, heighten its maturity and meet the present demands of the organization.

The effort involved an exhaustive comparison against a known maturity model (AICPA, 2011). While the current privacy program complied with the implementation specifications outlined in HIPAA, its policies, practices, and procedures for monitoring the use of Electronic Protected Health Information ("ePHI") had remained at a standstill since the law went into effect. It is worth noting that the gaps identified in the privacy program related solely to the monitoring and enforcement of its privacy policies and procedures related to the *use* of ePHI. We conclude with reflection related to the effectiveness of the process as well as implications for practice.

BACKGROUND: PRIVACY PROTECTION AND THE HUMAN FACTOR

As a HIPAA mandate, covered entities are required to perform an annual risk assessment of all administrative, physical, and technical safeguards to identify gaps in privacy and select appropriate remediation plans for each of the environments. Most companies spend millions of dollars a year in acquiring and/or implementing technology strategies not only to comply with HIPAA regulations but to meet or exceed best industry practices. The stakes are heightened whenever a regulatory body imposes fines for the willful neglect to implement or otherwise exercise all plausible means to protect against the unauthorized use of protected health information.

Such was the case when DHHS' Office of Civil Rights recently imposed a $16 million fine on Anthem over its 2015 data breach that affected nearly 79 million people (Teichert, 2018). As part of the settlement, Anthem agreed to conduct a risk analysis and fix any deficiencies with the direct oversight of DHHS personnel. As news of the settlement began reverberating throughout the healthcare industry, OCR Director Roger Severino acknowledged that "healthcare companies are attractive targets for hacks, and they're expected to have adequate cybersecurity defenses" (Teichert, 2018).

Yet with all the cybersecurity controls and sophistication at one's disposal, none play a more vital role in cybersecurity defenses than the *human factor*. Whether by neglect or intent, human interaction with technology continues to be the weakest link in the chain of data protection or its proper use. A study on military cybersecurity defense practices reported that "one key lesson of the military's experience is that while technical upgrades are important, minimizing human error is even more crucial.

Mistakes by network administrators and users—failures to patch vulnerabilities in legacy systems, misconfigured settings, violations of standard procedures—open the door to the overwhelming majority of successful attacks" (Winnefeld, Kirchhoff, & Upton, 2015, p88).

While cyber-attacks or incidents that threaten the command and control structure of data networks in healthcare are of growing concern, human ethical violations of standard procedures, to include intentional behaviors in pursuit of unauthorized information for personal gain, remain the most unpredictable. The most common errors made include unauthorized access to medical records (snooping), emailing PHI to personal accounts, leaving electronic devices unattended, releasing patient information to an unauthorized individual, downloading PHI to unauthorized devices, and providing unauthorized access to medical records via sharing logins (HIPPAJournal, 2019). Therefore, the need for oversight in a healthcare environment where medical professionals require a trustworthy and reliable means for maintaining patient health information, participating in discussions, or otherwise collaborating on ways to protect and promote the health of the patient is vital. Therefore, a privacy program must be able to advocate and monitor for the safety and proper use of PHI as well as educate its workforce and take corrective action when necessary.

Monitoring user activity is a complicated science involving the correlation of hundreds or thousands of computer log entries per user per day from the various computer systems that are used to access or transmit PHI. In this case, the institution had already invested in an advanced computer program designed to absorb millions of computer entry logs per day to portray an accurate account of a user's activity and interaction with PHI. The computer program is aided by Artificial Intelligence ("AI") to predict activity and question whether access is appropriate under certain circumstances. However, even with the use of AI, these programs still require human intelligence and interaction to validate their algorithms and responses.

IMPROVING THE PRIVACY PRACTICE

The Annual Privacy Risk Assessment

During the preparation for the annual HIPAA risk analysis of this healthcare institution, the Information Security Officer requested an additional assessment of the privacy program to confirm observations of staff members accessing patient records without proper consent and assess all areas marked for remediation as determined by its Release of Information policies and Notice of Privacy Practices. Specific areas identified as deficient or otherwise determined as the root cause for deficiencies in the privacy program designed to monitor the use of PHI included:

- Lack of a systematic process (standards, tools, and techniques) to manage a mature user-monitoring program aimed at protecting patient information as well as educating its workforce against improper use and disclosure.

- Personnel assigned to analyze user activity lacked the fundamental understanding of the environment, the various clinical workflows, and activities generated by healthcare workers during patient care.

- Personnel lacked discipline-specific knowledge to determine whether a violation had occurred or knowledge needed to determine the root cause and complete the analysis.

- The program lacked oversight to guide its day to day activities, regularly report on its activities to governing or steering committees, and perform all analysis of user activity consistently.

- Reporting efforts focused on informing patients of a potential breach of information and reporting the same finding to authorities as required by law, but failing to recognize and report patterns to security analysts for correction.

Issues uncovered illuminated the need for a more systematic approach to privacy management that included training and development of personnel. The deficiencies uncovered were not for lack of effort. The effort exerted, however, had little to no impact in monitoring or improving the overall proper use of protected health information. The overarching root cause of this situation clearly indicated the absence of a proper framework or maturity model.

Leading Change

Although several areas of the department were in need of improvement, prior to engaging in any large change effort, one must first consider the scope, willingness and perseverance of the change agent to engage in the initiative, availability of resources, support of upper management, and the group's readiness for change (Narine & Persaud, 2003). In this case, the change process involved identifying the rationale for change, developing a strategic plan, monitoring the progress using a maturity model, creating a steering committee and forming a charter.

Identifying the Rationale for Change

Before embarking upon any change effort, one must first create a compelling reason to change as well as establish a sense of urgency (Kotter, 2007; Kerber and Buono, 2005). To gain commitment from senior management, a presentation was given that explained the initiative in terms that everyone could understand. A scenario related to the recent Anthem data breach was presented that described the root cause of the breach, the impact it had on the organization, as well as the wider effects on the rest of the healthcare industry, including the HHS' decision to impose financial penalties (Donovan, 2018). The revelation that the breach had been attributed to human error made a strong case for the need for greater security controls and monitoring data related to human activities. The Anthem breach was the catalyst needed to incite immediate response, funding, and support to improve the security posture, and ultimately, to drive the privacy program to the desired maturity level. The meeting concluded with a directive to form a committee and bring back a strategic plan for final approval.

Developing a Strategic Plan

After considerable research into privacy law, similar programs in comparable healthcare systems, implementation strategies, and maturity models, a one-sheet agenda outlining the plan was developed that included the rationale, benefits, resources needed, timeline, and personal commitment required for a successful outcome. Legal counsel was also obtained to solidify the case. Utilizing Ashford and Detert's suggestions (2015), the message was tailored for the audience (by first understanding their goals, values, and knowledge levels) and was positioned in a manner that aligned with the company's strategic objectives. In addition, planning for possible sources of resistance in advance enabled us to anticipate and readily address objections, engage others in the conversation and provide transparency to the process (Kotter & Schlesinger, 2008).

To ensure that all colleagues understood the scope and complexity of the problem, key terms written in the law were explicitly defined for them. Under the terms of the HIPAA Privacy Rule, "Protected Health Information ("PHI") referred to "individually identifiable health information" held or transmitted by a covered entity or its business associate, in any form or medium, whether electronic, on paper, or oral. Protected health information is information, including demographic information, which related to:

- the individual's past, present, or future physical or mental health or condition,
- the provision of health care to the individual, or
- the past, present, or future payment for the provision of health care to the individual, and that identifies the individual or for which there is a reasonable basis to believe can be used to identify the individual. Protected health information includes many common identifiers (e.g., name, address, birth date, Social Security Number) when they can be associated with the health information listed above" (Office for Civil Rights, 2015).

Privacy, on the other hand, was defined as "the rights and obligations of individuals and organizations with respect to the collection, use, retention, disclosure, and disposal of personal information" (2011). Therefore, the focus of the plan was to measure and monitor the lifecycle and usage of PHI, in all of its forms, and to handle inconsistencies appropriately and effectively.

Monitoring Progress Using A Maturity Model

To measure the effectiveness of the new plan, the leadership team studied several maturity models before settling on the one most appropriate for our environment. By definition, maturity models are recognized means by which organizations can measure their capability based on established benchmarks. They also provide a pathway by which an entity can transform to higher levels of performance (Rajteric, 2010). We developed criteria beforehand to evaluate and select the model most appropriate for this setting. Criteria included:

- Easily understandable and relatable to upper management
- Affordable to implement and maintain
- Offered reasonable flexibility for adoption
- Clearly defined metrics which were reasonably achievable

In addition to reviewing the model criteria, leadership prepared the following outline to demonstrate the value of working towards a mature privacy program.

- Maintaining the privacy of information is the reason for implementing security standards
- Demonstrating compliance allows the business to receive reimbursements from government programs
- Low privacy complaints allow the business to maintain accreditation and financing
- Privacy advocacy helps the business to maintain its reputation and be trusted by the community
- An active privacy program increases interdepartmental communication
- Skillful privacy monitoring promotes employee awareness and deterrence

The committee reviewed several maturity models from a variety of sources to include American Institute of Certified Public Accountants (2011), Accident Compensation Corporation of New Zealand (2016), Perkins and Company (2012), West Virginia University (2017), Veriato (2019), and International Association of

Privacy Professionals (2019). The final model adopted was the result of a compilation of elements that would be most applicable to our healthcare environment. The model contained five stages or levels of maturity defined as follows:

- **Ad hoc:** resources are allocated on an 'as needed' basis to address privacy issues.
- **Reactive:** procedures exist; results are reproduced but affect only a small group.
- **Proactive:** personnel with responsibility or accountability are empowered with appropriate authority and resources.
- **Predictive:** management ensures adequate qualified privacy resources and results are proven, credentialed, and trustworthy.
- **Optimized:** management annually reviews its privacy program and seeks ways to improve the program's performance, including assessing the adequacy, availability, and performance of resources.

The model served as the basis for a rubric which we used to measure the state of seventy-three generally accepted privacy principles against the five maturity levels. A small committee was formed to align each of the privacy principals with the objectives of our program. This activity allowed us to select the principles to which we could commit, and subsequently, assign to several implementation phases. The group ultimately committed to improving eleven areas and three phases of remediation over three years. The first phase identified maturing the Accountability and Management, Incident Breach Response, and Policy Administration areas of the model. Specific objectives and related activities were included in the plan to provide clarity, employing both qualitative and quantitative analysis.

Creating A Steering Committee and A New Position

For change to be successful, a guiding coalition of representatives from multiple stakeholders must be on board to support, commuunicate, and help keep progress on track (Kotter, 2007; Tesch, Kloppenborg & Frolick, 2007). Selecting a steering committee, however, involves careful planning and considerable persuasion in order to select the right people to advance the initiative. The primary goal was to include a mix of people with significant authority and influence within the organization. A group of thirty-two upper and middle managers responsible for direct patient care were selected to join the committee. Also, based on suggestions from colleagues within the department, others who were believed to be advocates for privacy and change were asked to join. After many phone calls and casual conversations, the committee had representation from all clinical areas as well as upper management, including physician advocates and human resource professionals. Although sharing ideas with a group this large could prove to be difficult at times, the involvement early on was necessary to ensure a higher probability of adoption and successful implementation (Kotter & Schlesinger, 2008; Lapointe, Lamothe, & Fortin, 2006).

During the development of this change initiative, a vacancy in a key position arose. It provided a unique opportunity to review the current job description and revise it to articulate the most important outcomes needed for an employee to perform effectively within the new system. In order to create the position description, we reviewed commonly used employment websites for comparable positions and then tailored the position to meet our needs. A panel of three colleagues also provided feedback, perspectives, and considerations. The final description:

In collaboration with the Information Security Officer and the Vice President of Compliance, Quality and Risk Management, the Privacy Analyst is responsible for the day to day privacy investigation and privacy regulatory compliance program for the Healthcare System. In addition, the Privacy Analyst develops new methods to identify areas of privacy risk and best practices for risk remediation. The Privacy Analyst is responsible for managing the investigations team, and the ongoing development of an efficient and effective investigatory and regulatory response process within the evolving state and federal regulatory framework for complex compliance and privacy issues.

Candidate qualifications for the position included a BA/BS degree in business, pre-law, technology, information security, or related field; 4 years of experience working in a health care organization, or a combination of experience in healthcare with significant experience managing privacy or privacy related programs; working knowledge of the laws that affect privacy with specific application to healthcare or government institutions; and experience in project management, data mining, analysis and reporting. In addition, we required excellent interpersonal skills, as well as the ability to work effectively with diverse skill sets and personalities, and to manage difficult, sensitive, and confidential situations with integrity and professionalism.

Forming a Charter

The next stage for developing the implementation plan consisted of writing the plan's charter to lend credibility and purpose for the committee, define objectives and tie the outcomes to healthcare mandates and best practices (Tesch, Kloppenborg & Frolick, 2007). First, the criteria for selecting the topics for discussion were developed. Secondly, a framework for problem resolution was defined. Several sections were dedicated to clarifying terminology used in the HIPAA Privacy Rule, providing examples of required implementation specifications, outlining a roadmap to reach the desired maturity level, and codifying membership expectations. The final edition of the charter included the following topics:

- The objective was to provide an anchor to HIPAA Security and Privacy Rules mandate and best practices. Furthermore, industry best practices will be tied to those of the National Institution of Standards and Technology (NIST). The standards will then serve as talking points for staff education.
- Topics for educational programming will be directly connected to Privacy, specifically, the handling of privacy in healthcare
- Roadmaps for compliance to HIPAA and NIST standards must be clearly defined, prioritized, and funded before approval. They will serve as levers for garnering commitment to change business practices and company culture.
- Support for programs and technology that secure the organization, prevent employees from violating policies, and fund educational efforts.
- Sanctions related to policy violation must be fully developed, then supported by the human resources department before approval.

IMPLEMENTATION: THE HUMAN FACTOR

Part of the challenge of implementing advanced technology lies within the expertise of the personnel appointed to use it. They may not be fully aware of the purpose or intended use of the system or the extent of its full potential. In addition, in order to formulate desirable outcomes, programs aided by Artificial Intelligence require that the user or its input interface provide accurate information into the decision making process. This technology is also known as "predictive analytics," a process for analyzing data using a set of sophisticated statistical tools to predict the likely behavior of individuals or what the environment will do in the future. It has been utilized in healthcare to mitigate risk, improve operations, identify best practices, and gain a broad understanding of future trends (Wang, Kung, & Byrd, 2018).

The privacy monitoring software selected in this case relies on information that can describe the user's current role, work schedule, geographical location, and the expected patient workflow. Based on these values, the computer program establishes a baseline behavioral profile for each user by which it judges all future interaction with the system. When users stray from their known behavioral profile, the software creates a case that must be investigated more deeply to confirm whether a violation had actually taken place or not. It is during the case investigation where the informed analyst gives feedback to the system to confirm whether the case is a violation or simply a change in user behavior. The interaction between the analyst and the computer program forms the basis for predictive analytics as the machine learns what is acceptable or not acceptable in a given workflow. Therefore, having the right person in this position with an appropriate skill set, having substantial knowledge in clinical workflow and expertise in analytical reporting, was crucial for crafting a reliable predictive strategy going forward (Tesch, Kloppenborg & Frolick, 2007). The implementation phases included a significant amount of communication to establish a sense of urgency, garner support, and minimize uncertainty. Part of the plan included presentation of evidence confirming the value and utility of the new technology. One must also establish systems to reinforce new behavior.

Communication

An essential element of any change program is effective communication (Kotter, 2007, Kash, et al., 2014, Fickenscher & Bakerman, 2011). It helps to build trust and engender commitment, which is essential when working through any major change. It can also reduce resistance by assuaging uncertainty. The core of this initiative also centered on proper communication throughout the various levels of the organization. It was necessary to alter communication styles based on the audience to ensure that the message was received and understood (Ashford & Detert, 2015; Fickenscher & Bakerman, 2011).

When it came to selecting the technology, the primary change leader relied on his technical expertise to steer the conversation and decision-making process. When forming the steering committee, however, considerable time was spent by the change agent to talk with colleagues on a one-to-one basis to convey importance and urgency, as well as to garner support. Members of the committee were shown statistics and milestones related to progress on the maturity model, focusing on increasing maturity and decreasing risk. They were also shown published Federal and State penalties from comparable healthcare organizations who had violated privacy law. In most cases, penalties were imposed on organizations for not operationalizing the controls they have available – which directly relates to the maturity of their privacy program. The *HIPAA Journal*, an online journal that provides comprehensive information, advice, and best practices, was a useful source from which to glean recent cases and settlements. Fines for violations found during 2018 ranged from $100,000 to $16,000,000. The data presented made a case for the need to change and proved to be very informative and persuasive.

Communicating with other members of the organization required a more collaborative and tailored approach. In most institutions, members serving in higher levels of management are typically more concerned with high-level information and less interested in the minutia or complexity associated with the operation of the technology. In this case, it was best to emphasize program goals and objectives, show progress along the way to meeting those goals, and most importantly, clearly illustrate the benefits of the program to sustain support and buy-in. Achieving widespread user acceptance in a large organization, however, requires a more strategic and persistent approach to communication. The change leader must adopt the role of a salesperson on occasion to ensure support. Sharing examples of personalized consequences such as termination, sanction from professional boards, and criminal charges including fines and imprisonment (*HIPAA Journal*, 2018) also helped to underscore to everyone the importance of the program.

Presenting Confirmatory Evidence

Shortly after hiring an analyst with the requisite skill set, we began examining cases and categorizing the violations. We created a template that guided how to present the findings to the steering committee and upper management. The Privacy Maturity Framework and Phase 1 of the plan were presented at each of the hospital's executive committees. A historical timeline of the results uncovered by the previous ad hoc reporting system over the past twelve months was presented alongside the cases recently produced using the new system. The differences were readily apparent and truly highlighted the value and significance of the new process. With the aid of this new tool, it was now possible to show with a high degree of certainty how users were interacting with the electronic medical record in their respective workflows. Moreover, it was possible to reproduce the same analytical results in cases marked for violation. The presentation also included comparable metrics from other organizations – essential in justifying efforts for this program. The benefits presented included:

- Suspected privacy violations would be presented to the analysts for confirmation, thus eliminating the need to search manually through logs for anomalies
- The program would get 'smarter' with time as user cases were validated
- All violation cases were fully documented and archived for reference
- Violation results served as material for privacy education, to drive changes in assigned security access, and the evaluation of third-party contractual agreements
- A way to measure improvement

Reinforcing New Behavior

To fully integrate any change within an organization, in addition to providing significant communication and training, one must also consider revising current performance management policy to support and reinforce the change (Roberto &

Levesque, 2005). Rolling out this plan throughout the organization required several additional considerations. The Corporate Compliance and Human Resources department developed, approved, and adopted a privacy audit matrix that outlines possible infractions classified by severity, examples of infractions and their potential impact on the patient and organization, and suggested sanctions. Additionally, we created notification templates by risk-based category to be used when corresponding to the workforce member and their supervisor. Standard messages alerting the individual of an infraction were developed for each level of severity. This process served as a way to maintain consistency as well as provide further clarity around new expectations.

RESULTS AND REFLECTIONS

The first phase of the Privacy Model Framework, focused primarily on upper management activities related to Accountability and Management, Policies and Procedures, and Incident Breach Response. As of this writing, the system is measuring the overall effectiveness of this first phase, and preliminary results are quite encouraging. The progress we have made in each of the three areas to date:

Accountability and Management

- PHI Identification and Classification. Baseline 60%; data collection in progress.
- Review and approval. Baseline 50% currently approaching 80%.
- Risk Assessment processes. Goal is to reach 100% by June 2020.
- Infrastructure and system management protocols in place. Now 100%.

Policies and Procedures

- Contracts with affiliates and vendors in compliance. Baseline 80%, now 100%.
- Policy Documentation. Baseline 40%, now at 60%. Target is 100% by end of year.
- Privacy Awareness and Training. Baseline 30%, piloting user group. Target 50% by Dec 2019.
- Cybersecurity and Privacy Budget. Baseline 50% funded. Target 100% in next fiscal cycle, June 2020.
- Data Security/Access Control policies. Baseline 25%, currently 50%. Target is 100% by June 2020.

Incident Breach Response

Incident Response Plan Started. 50% complete. On target to reach 100% by end of Dec 2019.

We have also observed increases in senior management participation during the steering committee meetings, better collaboration with Human Resources, and an overall increase in privacy awareness and activity. The feedback received related to the implementation was better than expected, especially from several colleagues on the steering committee. As a result of this process, we have experienced a closer working relationship in common areas of interest.

The need to hire a privacy analyst during this process was challenging at first but proved to be an opportunity in the long-run. It allowed us to review the current job responsibilities and revise them to reflect the skills needed in the new environment. It was paramount to bring the right person on board (Tesch, Kloppenborg & Frolick, 2007). Considerable time was spent writing a new job description and updating qualifications for the privacy analyst position. To date, the revision to this position and the selection of a qualified analyst has helped foster the success of the implementation.

IMPLICATIONS FOR PRACTICE

Overall the movement of our PHI monitoring operation to a higher level of performance utilizing a maturity model was a considerable undertaking. To facilitate a large-scale change such as this, we offer several suggestions for practice.

Prior to beginning any large scale change effort, one must obtain the support of upper management to garner resources, advocate for change, mitigate resistance, and facilitate implementation (Kotter, 2007; Kotter & Schlesinger, 2008). Change may be impossible if one does not have senior-level sponsorship (Kerber & Buono, 2005). In this project, the immediate credibility and financial support received from senior management were crucial to success.

Developing a plan and charter can provide the necessary framework for progress. The scope must be defined as well as the roles of the participants (Kash, Spaulding, Johnson & Gamm, 2014; Roberto & Levesque, 2005). Establishing benchmarks for measurement allows one to keep focused on the progress to improvement. In this case, considerable time was spent researching and collaboratively developing a maturity model and corresponding rubric that met the needs of the organization. We included a section in the Maturity Framework to analyze reportable activities. A scorecard was developed to monitor and trend results over time.

Implementing new technologies or administrative programs and educating others continues to be a challenge in multi-disciplinary environments. Effective communication throughout the process is paramount to its success (Kotter, 2007; Kash, et al., 2014; Fickenscher & Bakerman, 2011). Being heard requires engaging the audience, promoting common interests, and building a reputation as a trusted source of information, all of which takes time. For this project, getting people on board with the plan was the biggest challenge, and tailoring the message to each stakeholder group proved to be an effective mechanism to do so (Ashford & Detert, 2015). Sharing rationale for change as well as consequences for non-compliance can also serve as a powerful motivator. Education efforts will continue throughout the program's lifecycle. To ensure the expected change in behavior will become permanent, new performance management parameters must be established as well (Roberts & Levesque, 2005). The vision is to continue growing the program as well as expand the staff to educate and mitigate situations before they become punitive. In the case the infractions do occur however, we established a very detailed matrix that identifies infractions, messages, and consequences, which has helped to provide clarity and consistency of enforcement.

Although there has been no noticeable resistance to the newly implemented privacy program, this is not the case in many other institutions undergoing significant change. Change can create anxiety, fear, and discomfort. Resistance may surface in the form of disruptive behavior or disengagement that can impede the efficiency of operations, create additional work, and decrease motivation, which will, in turn, diminish any anticipated benefit. Ford and Ford (2009) suggest that managing this process effectively through openness and dialogue can help provide clarity, open a space to explore additional opportunities for improvement, and foster buy-in of the change initiative. It can also build participation and engagement, ultimately improving the change process.

CONCLUSION

Healthcare continues to remain in a state of rapid change and turmoil. As of the writing of this chapter, there are many questions about the future of the Affordable Care Act. Regardless of the legislation, electronic data and the need for transferability across institutions will continue to increase. Maintaining the privacy of protected health information will continue to be paramount. This chapter sets forth a process for improving how an organization monitors the use of private data to ensure that it remains secure. Selecting a maturity model and utilizing it concurrently with principles of effective change leadership can help move an organization to a higher level of security.

REFERENCES

Accident Compensation Corporation of New Zealand. (2016). *ACC Privacy Maturity Plan 2016/17*. Retrieved from https://www.acc.co.nz/

AICPA/CICA Privacy Maturity Model. (2011). Retrieved from https://iapp.org/media/pdf/resource_center/aicpa_cica_privacy_maturity_model_final-2011.pdf

Ashford, S. J., & Detert, J. (2015). Get the boss to buy-in. *Harvard Business Review*, *93*(1/2), 72–79.

Donovan, F. (2018, August 22). *Judge Gives Final OK to $115M Anthem Data Breach Settlement*. Retrieved from https://healthitsecurity.com/news/judge-gives-final-ok-to-115m-anthem-data-breach-settlement

Fickenscher, K., & Bakerman, M. (2011). Change management in health care IT. *Physician Executive*, *37*(2), 64–67. PMID:21465898

Fontenot, S. F. (2013). The affordable care act and electronic health care records. *Physician Executive*, *39*(6), 72–76. PMID:24354149

Ford, J., & Ford, L. (2009). Decoding resistance to change. *Harvard Business Review*, 99–103.

Henderson, J., & Cavalancia, N. (2019) Insider Threat Program Maturity Model. *Techvangelism & Insider Threat Defense*. Retrieved from https://www.veriato.com/docs/default-source/collateral-assets/insider-threat-maturity-report.pdf

HIPAA Journal. (2018). *What Happens if UPi Break HIPAA Rules*. Retrieved from https://www.hipaajournal.com/what-happens-if-you-break-hipaa-rules/

HIPAA Journal. (2019). *The Most Common HIPAA Violations You Should Be Aware Of*. Retrieved from https://www.hipaajournal.com/common-hipaa-violations/

Hulet, M. (2012). *Privacy Risk Assessments. Nov. 2012 Perkins and Company*. Retrieved from: http://perkinsaccounting.com/wp-content/uploads/ISACA-Privacy-Risk-Assessmentv7.pdf

International Association of Privacy Professionals. (2019). *Overview of Privacy Maturity Models*, Retrieved from https://iapp.org/resources/tools/

Kash, B. A., Spaulding, A., Johnson, C. E., & Gamm, L. (2014, January/February). Success Factors for Strategic Change Initiatives: A Qualitative Study. *Journal of Healthcare Management*, *59*(1), 65–82. doi:10.1097/00115514-201401000-00011 PMID:24611428

Kerber, K., & Buono, A. (2005, Fall). Rethinking organizational change: Reframing the Challenge of Change Management. *Organization Development Journal, 23*, 3.Kotter, J. P. (2007). Leading Change: Why Transformation Efforts Fail. *Harvard Business Review, 85*(1), 96–103.

Kotter, J. P., & Schlesinger, L. A. (2008). Choosing Strategies for Change. *Harvard Business Review, 86*(7/8), 130–139. PMID:10240501

Lapointe, L., Lamothe, L., & Fortin, J. (2006). The Dynamics of IT Adoption in a Major Change Process in Healthcare Delivery. In T. Spil & R. Schuring (Eds.), *E-Health Systems Diffusion and Use: The Innovation, the User and the Use IT Model* (pp. 107–127). Hershey, PA: IGI Global. doi:10.4018/978-1-59140-423-1.ch007

Narine, L., & Persaud, D. D. (2003). Gaining and maintaining commitment to large-scale change in healthcare organizations. *Health Services Management, 16*(3), 179–187. doi:10.1258/095148403322167933 PMID:12908992

Office for Civil Rights. (2015, November 6). *Methods for De-identification of PHI.* Retrieved from https://www.hhs.gov/hipaa/for-professionals/privacy/special-topics/de-identification/index.html

Rajteric, I. H. (2010). Overview of business intelligence maturity models. *Journal of Contemporary Management Issues, 15*(1), 47–67.

Roberto, M. A., & Levesque, L. C. (2005). The art of making change initiatives stick. *MIT Sloan Management Review, 46*(4), 53.

Teichert, E. (2018, October 16). *Anthem to pay $16M in record data breach settlement.* Retrieved from https://www.modernhealthcare.com/article/20181016/NEWS/181019927

Tesch, D., Kloppenborg, T. J., & Frolick, M. N. (2007). IT Project Risk Factors: The Project Management Professionals Perspective. *Journal of Computer Information Systems, 47*(4), 61–69.

Timsina, P., Liu, J., & El-Gayar, O. (2016). Advanced analytics for the automation of medical systematic reviews. *Information Systems Frontiers, 18*(2), 237–252. doi:10.100710796-015-9589-7

Wang, Y., Kung, L. A., & Byrd, T. A. (2018). Big data analytics: Understanding its capabilities and potential benefits for healthcare organizations. *Technological Forecasting and Social Change, 126*, 3–13. doi:10.1016/j.techfore.2015.12.019

West Virginia University. (2017). *Privacy Program Maturity Template*. Retrieved from: https://library.educause.edu/resources/2017/8/privacy-program-maturity-template

Winnefeld, J. A., Jr., Kirchhoff, C., & Upton, D. M. (2015). Cybersecurity's Human Factor: Lessons from the Pentagon. *Harvard Business Review*, *93*(9), 86–17.

ADDITIONAL READING

Carvalho, J. V., Rocha, Á., & Abreu, A. (2016). Maturity models of healthcare information systems and technologies: A literature review. *Journal of Medical Systems*, *40*(6), 131. doi:10.100710916-016-0486-5 PMID:27083575

Ghazvini, A., & Shukur, Z. (2016). Awareness training transfer and information security content development for healthcare industry. *International Journal of Advanced Computer Science and Application*, *7*(5), 361–370. doi:10.14569/IJACSA.2016.070549

Kotter, J. (2012). *Leading Change*. Harvard Business Review Press.

Liginlal, D. (2015). HIPAA and Human Error: The Role of Enhanced Situation Awareness in Protecting Health Information. In A. Gkoulalas-Divanis & G. Loukides (Eds.), *Medical Data Privacy Handbook*. Cham: Springer. doi:10.1007/978-3-319-23633-9_25

Murphy, S. (2015). *Healthcare Information Security and Privacy*. McGraw-Hill Publishing.

KEY TERMS AND DEFINITIONS

Change Leadership: A comprehensive and systematic process designed to strategically introduce and implement large scale organizational change in a manner that ensures the changes will take hold.

HIPAA: Health Insurance Portability and Accountability Act of 1996, a federal law in the United States that provides rules and regulations for health care providers and health insurance in order to ensure the privacy of personal health information.

Maturity Model: A business tool that facilitates change or improvement by providing a framework based on certain performance parameters designed to assess the current capabilities of an organization as well as provide a path for improvement.

Predictive Analytics: A process for analyzing data in a manner that seeks to predict a likely future scenario or outcome. It can be used to improve decision making, mitigate risk, improve operations, and identify best practices.

Privacy Monitoring Software: Technology designed to detect privacy breach events due to unauthorized access of patient records.

Chapter 7

Healthcare Reform:
A Dire Need to Retool the System

Abburi Anil Kumar
Prairie View A&M University, USA

ABSTRACT

The healthcare system in the U.S. is very fragmented in its structure. It is generally agreed that it needs to be reformed. This chapter addresses this issue from an organizational point of view with specific reference to cancer, a disease termed "The Emperor of All Maladies." The basic tenet of this chapter is that any healthcare system should be designed so as to maximize the benefit to all the stakeholders involved, while incorporating the newer advances in technologies, but above all, must be patient-centered. Solving a complex adaptive problem requires different approaches compared to solving a simple technical challenge. Especially, when it comes to dealing with cancer—a very intelligent, continually adapting, rule breaking, self-sustaining disease—simple technical solutions are insufficient without an understanding of how to change the system. After discussing the current healthcare system in the U.S., a proposal is made as to how to reform the system.

DOI: 10.4018/978-1-7998-2949-2.ch007

INTRODUCTION

In the past quarter century, the American medical system has stopped focusing on health or even science. Instead it attends more or less single-mindedly to its own profits.

Everyone knows the healthcare system is in disarray. We've grown numb to huge bills. We regard high prices as an inescapable American burden. We accept the drugmakers' argument that they have to charge twice as much for prescriptions as in any other country because lawmakers in nations like Germany and France don't pay them enough to recoup their research costs. But would anyone accept that argument if we replaced the word prescriptions with cars or films? (Rosenthal, 2018)

So begins the book, *An American Sickness by Elisabeth Rosenthal*, with the subtitle, How Healthcare Became Big Business and How You Can Take it Back. The healthcare system in the U.S. is somewhat of a misnomer, since it is very fragmented in its structure. It seems to have become even more complicated than the system it is created for and expected to support – the human body. It is generally agreed that the healthcare system in the U.S. is to be reformed. This paper addresses this issue from an organizational point of view with a specific reference to cancer, a disease termed by the physician Siddhartha Mukherjee, "The Emperor of All Maladies." The reason for choosing cancer as an example is because it is perhaps the most complex set of diseases known to us. To put it in simple terms, cancer is: (i) intelligent, in the sense that it can sustain itself by establishing its own lifeline at the expense of its host; (ii) rebellious, in the sense that it does not obey the natural laws of cell apoptosis; (iii) diverse, in the sense that there are more than 200 types of cancer known thus far; (iv) its evolution – how it metastasizes and colonizes distant parts of the body; (v) its ability to tunnel through the blood-brain barrier. For any healthcare system to provide proper care for such a complex disease, there should be a confluence of factors addressed by both public and private agencies. Public refers to federal and local governments, private refers to medical industry as well as medical professionals. An entirely public system, in terms of the government providing universal healthcare, or an entirely private system, where, by necessity, different services are provided by different organizations is not tenable since it does not have the interests of all the stakeholders – governing bodies, industry, medical professionals, and most importantly, the patient. The basic tenet of this paper is that any healthcare reform in a capitalist society should be designed so as to maximize the benefit to all the stakeholders involved, while incorporating the newer advances in technologies, but above all, must be patient-centered. As always, solving a complex adaptive problem requires different approaches compared to solving a simple technical challenge.

Especially, when it comes to dealing with cancer – a very intelligent, continually adapting, rule breaking, self-sustaining disease – simple technical solutions are insufficient without an understanding of how it works.

This chapter is divided into five sections. The first section, Status of Healthcare in the U.S., provides the most recent data on the benefits and costs of healthcare, along with some international comparisons. The second section, The Case of Cancer-Emperor of all Maladies, discusses the subject of cancer, what it is, what is known about it, a few of the novel efforts in dealing with it along with the costs. The third section, Aiming for the Best Healthcare System, raises the question of what an ideal healthcare system should like. A proposal is then made as to how to reform the system. The fourth section, Future Research Directions, lists a set of innovation and innovative carried out across the globe. The final section, Conclusions, summarizes the chapter. The viewpoint presented herein should be taken as from the vantage point of someone who is a trained scientist and a practicing engineer, who is outside the medical field but as a former cancer patient himself, who is a concerned citizen and who has studied organizational structures in profit and non-profit settings.

STATUS OF HEALTHCARE IN THE U.S.

Relevant Data and International Comparisons

The title of this paper reflects the general frustrations among most Americans in regards to the existing health care system in the U.S. The U.S. Healthcare System is decentralized and fragmented, with insurers, both public and private, operating mostly independently of each other. There is a large number of health insurance companies, in addition to the Federal Medicare program and other public programs. The primary function of health insurance, like other types of insurance, is to protect individuals against unexpected financial risk. However, due to a lack of universal health insurance coverage to its citizens, individuals in different age groups and varying economic status receive varying levels of coverage.

A Pew study published in Fall 2018 found that 6 in 10 Americans say that it is the federal government's responsibility to guarantee health care coverage for all Americans (Kiley, 2018). Having a well-developed public health system is one of nine attributes used to develop the Quality of Life sub-ranking in the 2019 Best Countries report. The survey is based on a study that surveyed more than 20,000 global citizens from four regions to assess perceptions of 80 countries on 75 different metrics. Of the top 10 countries viewed to have the best public health systems, Finland was rated 1st, UK 10th, while the U.S. ranked 19th.

In another study, the U.S. ranked last on performance overall and ranked nearly last on the Access, Administrative Efficiency, Equity, and Health Care Outcomes domains (Schneider, Sarnak, Squires, Shah and Doty, 2017). The top-ranked countries overall were the U.K., Australia, and the Netherlands. Based on a broad range of indicators, the U.S. health system is an outlier, spending far more but falling short of the performance achieved by other high-income countries. The results suggest the U.S. health care system should look at other countries' approaches if it wants to achieve an affordable high-performing health care system that serves all Americans.

In a 2010 study by World Health Organization (WHO) Ranking of the World's 100 Best Health Systems 2010, US ranks 37th ("World Health Organization," 2017). As reported in the U.S. Health Care System: An International Perspective:

The U.S. health care system is unique among advanced industrialized countries. The U.S. does not have a uniform health system, has no universal health care coverage, and only recently enacted legislation mandating healthcare coverage for almost everyone. Rather than operating a national health service, a single-payer national health insurance system, or a multi-payer universal health insurance fund, the U.S. health care system can best be described as a hybrid system. In 2014, 48 percent of U.S. health care spending came from private funds, with 28 percent coming from households and 20 percent coming from private businesses. The federal government accounted for 28 percent of spending while state and local governments accounted for 17 percent. Most health care, even if publicly financed, is delivered privately.

In 2014, 283.2 million people in the U.S., 89.6 percent of the U.S. population had some type of health insurance, with 66 percent of workers covered by a private health insurance plan. Among the insured, 115.4 million people, 36.5 percent of the population, received coverage through the U.S. government in 2014 through Medicare (50.5 million), Medicaid (61.65 million), and/or Veterans Administration or other military care (14.14 million) (people may be covered by more than one government plan). In 2014, nearly 32.9 million people in the U.S. had no health insurance.

Cost of Healthcare in the U.S.

According to a study from a team led by a Johns Hopkins Bloomberg School of Public Health, based on an analysis of health care use and spending in the U.S. and the other industrialized countries that are members of the Organization for Economic Cooperation and Development (OECD), the United States, on a per capita basis, spends much more on health care than other developed countries; the chief reason is not greater health care utilization, but higher prices. (U.S. Health Care Spending, 2019). In the U.S., the per capita health care spending was $9,892 in 2016, more than double the $4,559 the U.S. spent per capita on health care in 2000. A comparison with the second-place Switzerland's healthcare shows that this figure is about 25 percent higher, $7,919. It was also 108 percent higher than Canada's $4,753, and 145 percent higher than the OECD median of $4,033. The late Princeton health care economist Uwe Reinhardt, came to the same conclusion in their well-known 2003 study, "It's the prices, stupid: why the United States is so different from other countries."

The results of this study yield the following data that might provide a glimpse into the needed reform in the healthcare system in the U.S.:

- The higher overall health care spending in the U.S. was due mainly to higher prices—including higher drug prices, higher salaries for doctors and nurses, higher hospital administration costs and higher prices for many medical services.
- Not only does the U.S outspend other OECD countries, on the whole it has less access to many health care resources. The researchers found that in 2015, the most recent year for which data were available in the U.S., there were only 7.9 practicing nurses and 2.6 practicing physicians per 1,000 population, compared to the OECD medians of 9.9 nurses and 3.2 physicians. (U.S. Health Care Spending, 2019)
- Similarly, the U.S. in 2015 had only 7.5 new medical school graduates per 100,000 population, compared to the OECD median of 12.1, and just 2.5 acute care hospital beds per 1,000 population compared to the OECD median of 3.4.
- A widening of the gap between what public insurers and private insurers pay for the same health care services.
- Although the U.S. ranked second in the numbers of MRI machines per capita and third in the numbers of CT scanners per capita—implying a relatively high use of these expensive resources—Japan ranked first in both categories, yet was among the lowest overall health care spenders in the OECD in 2016.
- Overall U.S. health spending increased at an average rate of 2.8 percent annually between 2000 and 2016, which is greater than the OECD median annual increase of 2.6 percent. Per capita, inflation-adjusted spending on pharmaceuticals also increased much more quickly in the U.S.—at a rate of 3.8 percent per year, compared to just 1.1 percent for the OECD median.

Similar data has been reported in Forbes (McCarthy, 2019) and Centers for Medicare and Medicaid Services (CMS, 2019)

There are three major reasons why costs are so high. First, most of the cost comes from treating people over the first 10 days and last 10 days of their life. A lot of progress has been made in terms of medical procedures that save premature babies and extend the life expectancy of the elderly. But these innovative procedures are very expensive. Some other countries limit that high level of care. They refuse the procedure if it has a low chance of success. In the United States, such care is given even if the prognosis is poor. (Amadeo, 2019).

The second reason for high health care costs is the rise of malpractice lawsuits. Doctors often over-test, ordering $1,000 MRIs and $1,500 colonoscopies. They do this even if they do not think those procedures are needed. Practicing highly preventive type of medicine protects healthcare professionals from getting sued, yet evidently contributes to the higher cost in healthcare services.

The third reason is that there is less price competition in health care than in other industries, such as consumer electronics. Most people don't pay for their own health care. Patients only pay a set fee or co-pay, while the insurance company pays the rest. As a result, patients don't price-shop for doctors, lab tests, or procedures as they would for computers or television sets.

THE CASE OF CANCER: THE EMPEROR OF ALL MALADIES

To make ideas more precise, this section addresses cancer – termed the Emperor of All Maladies – by the physician Siddhartha Mukherjee, in his book with the same title. (Mukherjee, 2012). Cancer is an excellent example of a subject that demonstrates several aspects that need to be addressed before providing for an efficient approach towards its control and cure. These aspects include: multiplicity of treatments that are expensive but in many cases unnecessary; an inadequate understanding of the disease; a lack of clear focus on its treatment; and in the author's opinion, a lack of consensus among different research groups on the origins and the metastasis of the primary tumors. In the next section we address these aspects from a personal example.

Every sixth death in the world is due to cancer, making it the second leading cause of death (second only to cardiovascular diseases). In 2017, 9.6 million people are estimated to have died from the various forms of cancer. The Institute for Health Metrics and Evaluation (IHME) put relatively small error margins around this global figure: the lower and upper estimates extend from 9.2 to 9.7 million. (How many people in the world die from cancer? (n.d.)).

Cancers are defined by the National Cancer Institute (NCI) as a collection of diseases in which abnormal cells can divide and spread to nearby tissue. As this definition suggests, cancers can arise in many parts of the body and in some cases spread to other parts of the body through the blood and lymph systems via a process termed metastasis. When broken down by cancer type globally, breast cancer is the most prevalent form, followed by prostrate and colon & rectum cancer. (Roser & Ritchie, 2015).

More data can be found at Cancer Data and Statistics (2019).

Current Costs of Cancer Cure

The financial costs of cancer are high for both the person with cancer and for society as a whole. The Agency for Healthcare research and Quality (AHRQ) estimates that the direct medical costs (total of all health care costs) for cancer in the US in 2015 were $80.2 billion. (American Cancer Society [ACS], 2018):

- 52% of this cost is for hospital outpatient or doctor office visits
- 38% of this cost is for inpatient hospital stays

The potency, complexity and innovative nature of cancer treatments are noteworthy. But so was the price. Each cost more than$100,000 per person when taken for a year — a rarity at the time for oncology drugs. The prices seemed staggering to doctors, patients and health-care providers alike. But quickly, they became normal. By 2014, the average cost of a new orally administered cancer medicine exceeded $135,000 a year — up to six times the cost of similar drugs approved in the early 2000s, after adjusting for inflation, 2017 brought the most eye-popping price tag in oncology yet: a one-time cost of $475,000 per patient for a personalized cell-based therapy for childhood leukaemia. (Dolgin, 2018).

The estimates of national expenditures for cancer care (in millions of dollars) are shown in table below. For a full list of cancer types see ("Financial Burden of Cancer Care," 2019)

A case in point, a study presented at the American Society of Clinical Oncology's annual meeting in Chicago in 2018, reported that Americans paid twice as much as Canadians did for health care, but they didn't get twice the benefit. The study addressed patients with advanced colorectal cancer who lived, in some cases, mere miles from each other. The patients had similar diagnoses, levels of education, financial situations and other demographics that commonly affect health outcomes and mortality. Some of their ages were different, but the biggest difference between them is on which side of the border they live. (Christensen, 2018).

Table 1. Financial Burden of Cancer Care

	2010	2014	2018
Female Breast	$16,499.8	$18,116.6	$19.700.0
Colorectal	$14,140.5	$15,280.2	$16,630.9
Prostate	$11,848.1	$13,426.1	$15,299.2

For instance, using data from hospitals, Dr. Todd Yezefski of Fred Hutchinson Cancer Research Center in Washington found that a total of about $12,345 was spent a month on the cancer patients in his study who lived in western Washington, whereas the monthly spending for British Columbia patients was $6,195.

Care varied slightly for the two groups. American doctors ordered chemotherapy more often than the Canadian doctors did, but that may have been because the US patients were a little younger as a group than the Canadian patients, Yezefski said. But most everything else was the same, and while American patients' treatment was twice as expensive, these patients didn't live any longer than the Canadians.

One reason for this is that, in Canada, the government sets the prices for what they pay for chemotherapy and for the drugs involved, while in the US, price is really set by the market and what pharmaceutical companies are charging. If Medicare, the largest payer for medication, could negotiate drug prices, the cost could go down overall, even for what private insurance pays. However, under current policy, the US Health and Human Services secretary is explicitly forbidden from negotiating directly with drug makers on behalf of people enrolled in Medicare Part D, the program's prescription plan. (Panner, 2019).

What We Know of Cancer So Far

A report (Geeta & Barad, 2018), rather succinctly, summarizes the situation about cancer – *"A game whose rules we don't even understand, so we play checkers while cancer is playing chess."*

- Cancer cells are less specialized than normal cells – whereas normal cells mature into very distinct cell types with specific functions, cancer cells do not. They continue to divide without stopping.
- Cancer cells are able to ignore signals that normally tell cells to stop dividing or that begin a process known as programmed cell death, or apoptosis.
- Cancer cells may be able to influence the normal cells, molecules, and blood vessels that surround and feed a tumor—an area known as the microenvironment.
- Cancer cells are able to evade the immune system.
- Tumors can also use the immune system to stay alive and grow. For example, with the help of certain immune system cells that normally prevent a runaway immune response, cancer cells can actually keep the immune system from killing cancer cells.

Success Stories Regarding Cancer

There have been a few success stories regarding cancer (Simon, 2019):

- Lung cancer death rates declined 48% from 1990 to 2016 among men and 23% from 2002 to 2016 among women. From 2011 to 2015, the rates of new lung cancer cases dropped by 3% per year in men and 1.5% per year in women. The differences reflect historical patterns in tobacco use, where women began smoking in large numbers many years later than men and were slower to quit. However, smoking patterns do not appear to explain the higher lung cancer rates being reported in women compared with men born around the 1960s.
- Breast cancer death rates declined 40% from 1989 to 2016 among women. The progress is attributed to improvements in early detection.
- Prostate cancer death rates declined 51% from 1993 to 2016 among men. Routine screening with the PSA blood test is no longer recommended because of concerns about high rates of over-diagnosis (finding cancers that would never need to be treated). Therefore, fewer cases of prostate cancer are now being detected.
- Colorectal cancer death rates declined 53% from 1970 to 2016 among men and women because of increased screening and improvements in treatment. However, in adults younger than age 55, new cases of colorectal cancer have increased almost 2% per year since the mid-1990s.

As the data shows, early detection of cancer can reduce the risk of increased sickness and even of death. However, some cancers such as the ovarian cancer are not easily detectable till later in stage. However, as the quotes from a few physicians below show, the approach to cancer cure needs reform.

*I'll be the first to admit that despite all the billions put into cancer research, **the end results of preventing cancer and treating advanced cancer have been disappointing**. Unlike reducing deaths from heart attacks and stroke, progress in reducing deaths from cancer has been disappointingly slow. Sure, we've had our breakthrough drugs like Gleevec, the targeted drug for chronic myelogenous leukemia, and Herceptin for a certain type of breast cancer. **But for a lot of other cancers, the treatments aren't giving us bang for the buck.** Spending $100,000 to $200,000 a year to **extend life for an additional three to six months** may be very important to those individuals with cancer, but are **a very poor return on investment for society.** It's* *not sustainable, and that's why a lot of national health care programs won't pay for drugs like Avastin, Sutent, Yervoy, and Provenge. – David Chan, MD, Oncologist (Contributor, 2013)*

More than 40 years after the war on cancer was declared, we have spent billions fighting the good fight. The National Cancer Institute has spent some $90 billion on research and treatment during that time. Some 260 nonprofit organizations in the United States have dedicated themselves to cancer — more than the number established for heart disease, AIDS, Alzheimer's disease, and stroke combined. Together, these 260 organizations have budgets that top $2.2 billion. (Cuomo, 2012).

When it comes to treating cancer, we seem to be in a holding pattern. We are still relying on surgery, chemotherapy and other anticancer drugs, and radiation, just as we did 40 years ago. We are stuck in a paradigm of treatment. And our treatments are not working. – Ronald Herberman, MD, the former director of the University of Pittsburgh Cancer Institute. (Cuomo, 2013).

Simply put, we have not adequately channeled our scientific know-how, funding, and energy into a full exploration of the one path certain to save lives: prevention. That it should become the ultimate goal of cancer research has been recognized since the war on cancer began. When I look at NCI's budget request for fiscal year 2012, I'm deeply disappointed, though past experience tells me I shouldn't be surprised. It is business as usual at the nation's foremost cancer research establishment. More than $2 billion is requested for basic research into the mechanism and causes of cancer. Another $1.3 billion is requested for treatment. And cancer prevention and control? It gets $232 million altogether. – From A World Without Cancer by Dr. Margaret Cuomo (Cuomo, 2013).

"Patients and politicians anxiously await and increasingly demand a 'cure' for cancer. But trying to control the disease may prove a better plan than striving to cure it." – From "A change of strategy in the war on cancer."(Gatenby, 2009).

A Conference of New Ideas in Cancer: Challenging Dogmas

Sponsored by the Tata Memorial Centre to celebrate its 75th anniversary, a major conference was held during February 26 - 28, 2016, in Mumbai, India. The three-day meeting, supported by *Lancet Oncology*, the American Association of Cancer Research (AACR) and the US National Cancer Institute, hosted a diverse body of 1000 delegates from 23 countries (Gandhi & Jalali, 2017, Geeta & Barad, 2018).

The brief the organizers had given to the speakers was simple:

- *We are unhappy with the little that has been achieved against the scourge of cancer;*

- *We find it difficult to sit complacently with this 'rah–rah' scientific culture, amplified in public media by headlines of war-cry-like rhetoric enshrined by the ever so sexy 'moonshot'.*
- *A leitmotif that ran through this meeting was that there is a crisis in mainstream biology. The linear, deterministic computer models that grew out of our cultural fascination with the genetic code, beginning with the discovery of the DNA structure in early 1950s, no longer serve us well as explainers and predictors of modern biology and cancer. Yet no better alternative has yet emerged to make sense of things.*
- *Cancer is a defect of tissue architecture, and that the predominant theories that see it as a cell-based disease could therefore be leading us up the wrong path. There is a need for the "tissue organization field theory."*
- *There is a need for a new model which focuses on the patho-physiological role played by circulating fragments of DNA and chromatin, which act as DNA damaging agents when they are freely uptaken by healthy cells.*
- *These circulating fragments are released into the blood from dying cells during the programmed cell death process, apoptosis. The causal link proposed between these bits of biological detritus and DNA damage could throw new light on what causes cancer and open up potential new avenues for prevention and treatment.*

Novel Approaches to Cancer

In 2008, the National Cancer Institute (NCI) convened a series of strategic Think Tanks to investigate approaches to more effectively engage the physical sciences in cancer research. (Physical Sciences in Oncology [PS-ON], 2018).

Think Tank participants identified a number of scientific areas where physical sciences perspectives could inform cancer research and concluded that integrated transdisciplinary teams were best suited to overcoming the traditional barriers and silos that have separated these two scientific communities.

In the fall of 2009, the NCI launched the PS-OC Program, a Network of 12 Centers investigating complex and challenging questions in cancer research from a physical sciences perspective.

- Explore and uncover the physics and physical sciences principles underlying cancer-relevant perturbations.
- Develop an understanding of the initiation and evolution of cancer at all length-scales (sub-molecular, molecular, cellular, tissues, organisms, and populations) based on the physical principles and laws that define the behavior of matter.

- Thematic areas of emphasis supported by the PS-ON include:
- understanding the physics and physical dynamics of cancer;
- exploring and understanding evolution and evolutionary theory in cancer with experimental approaches from the physical sciences;
- understanding the coding, decoding, transfer, and translation of information in cancer; and
- deconvoluting the complexity of cancer using computational physics approaches.

A Few of The Novel Ways of Perceiving Cancer

- Seeing cancer not as a disease but as a systematic *response* to a damaging environment (davis, 2018).
- Cancer is not a *product* of damage but a systematic *response* to a damaging environment – a primitive cellular defense mechanism. Cancer is a cell's way of coping with a bad place.
- Cancer may be *triggered* by mutations, but its root cause is the self-activation of a very old and deeply embedded toolkit of emergency survival procedures.
- A helpful analogy is a computer that suffers an insult, such as corrupted software, and starts up in safe mode.
- This is a default program enabling the computer to run on its core functionality even when defective.
- In the same way, we think, cancer is a default state in which a cell under threat runs on *its* ancient core functionality, thereby preserving its vital functions, of which proliferation is the most ancient, most vital and best preserved.
- Seeing cancer as an applied ecological system: the parallels between cancerous cells and invasive species suggest that the principles for successful cancer therapy might lie not in the magic bullets of microbiology but in the evolutionary dynamics of applied ecology.
- Dispersal, proliferation, migration and evolution — analogous to the processes that allow cancer cells to spread from a primary tumor into adjacent tissues or to new locations in the body via the lymphatic system or blood vessels.
- Ability of tumor cells to adapt to a wide range of environmental conditions, including to toxic chemicals, is very similar to the evolutionary capacities shown by invasive species.
- Lessons learned in dealing with exotic species, combined with recent mathematical models of the evolutionary dynamics of tumors, indicate that eradicating most disseminated cancers may be impossible.

- Just as invasive species consistently adapt to pesticides, regardless of concentration or cleverness of design, so too do cancerous cells adapt to therapies.

Two Specific Instances of Cancer Care

Two cases are reported here based on personal experience. A friend of the author, a professor and a senior deacon in his church, was diagnosed with kidney cancer that spread very aggressively to the entire body, resulting in death in two months after initial diagnosis, despite a lengthy stay in the hospital and intense medical care. His family physician lamented that if only a body scan was performed at the right time, the disease would have been caught in its early stages, thereby providing the necessary treatment in time, thus achieving success on several accounts: saving the person's life and increasing the quality of his life, considerable reduction in associated costs such as hospital stay, medical staff assistance, medicines and reduced trauma for the patient as well as his family. However, such full body scans are not permitted by the insurance companies. This cancer was very aggressive.

The author was diagnosed with colorectal cancer Stage III, just on the verge of becoming Stage IV. His case was treated with timely care, employing a new form of therapy, termed neoadjuvant therapy, which consisted of chemotherapy coupled with radiation treatment followed by tumor removal through surgery, in turn followed by another extensive chemotherapy. The recommended post-surgery treatment was a repeat of chemotherapy tablets as well as chemotherapy by chemical infusion every other week – intravenous fluorouracil or its oral equivalent, capecitabine. However, consultation with the surgeon and supported by research from European oncology studies, showed that post-surgery chemotherapy was not necessary in cases where neo-adjuvant therapy was done before the tumor removal. A compromise was reached with the author receiving reduced tablet intake and the elimination of infusion. Evidence-based therapy and personalized medicine is a novel idea that should be pursued.

In both cases mentioned above, the recommended approaches to curing cancer were almost identical. Both were based on hospital stay with radiation and chemotherapy – oral as well as infusion. The primary difference in the second case was treating the tumor to reduce in size first so as to minimize the extent of resection. The recommended post surgery treatment however, was in strict alignment with the standard approach to treatment. "We are stuck in a paradigm of treatment." (Herberman, quoted in Promoting a More Balanced Approach to Cancer Prevention and Treatment. (n.d.)), rather than assessing the treatment needed based on the individual need as well as on available research. The second case drastically reduced the post-surgery treatment costs via the elimination of expensive chemo-infusion and reduced chemotherapy tablets.

AIMING FOR THE BEST HEALTHCARE SYSTEM

The Question: What Does an Ideal Healthcare System Look Like?

A natural question that arises is: What does an ideal healthcare system look like? (Jha, 2017). There are multiple models of healthcare systems, none of which is perfect in any given environment. One model assumes that a market-based system, a free enterprise system, is the solution because it relies on competition, customized care for individuals, keeping prices down, and allowing the highest quality providers to flourish. Such a system has been proven to be effective in the area of consumer electronics for instance, and is the basis of the system in the U.S., however without the benefit of increased return on investment to the consumer. Another model is a government-run, single-payer system where everyone has equal access, gets comparable quality, and patients are not concerned about costs because the government has the total control in setting prices as well as providing transparency. While each model is an extreme example, a third set of models might be based on a combination of aspects of the two. A change in mindset from "one size fits all" to "no size fits all" is needed. But the overarching principle should be that, any healthcare reform in a capitalist society should be designed so as to maximize the benefit to all the stakeholders involved, while incorporating the newer advances in technologies, but above all, must be patient-centered.

Most developed countries control costs, in part, by having the government play a stronger role in negotiating prices for healthcare. Their healthcare systems don't require the high administrative costs that drive up pricing in the U.S. These governments have the ability to negotiate lower drug, medical equipment and hospital costs. They can influence the mix of treatments used and patients' ability to go to specialists or seek more expensive treatments. However, the tax rate in these countries is very high. For instance, in Switzerland the rate is 42%, Sweden 60%, U.K. 47%, Finland 58%. The highest tax rate in the U.S. is about 37%, even that for individuals making over half a million dollars a year.

In contrast, in the U.S., there has been a lack of political support for the government taking a larger role in controlling healthcare costs. The Affordable Care Act focused on ensuring access to healthcare but maintained the status quo to encourage competition among insurers and healthcare providers. This means there will be multiple payers for the services and less control over negotiated pricing from providers of healthcare services.

Attempt to Design and Build a Fairer Healthcare System

When a system is so broken, it makes sense to get back to the basics and ask the most fundamental question, "What is the system in place for? How can it be modified to serve the purpose it was created for?" Additionally, ask: "What would a fair system of healthcare look like?" Fair in the sense that all stakeholders – patients, service providers, insurance agencies and the government – are served to maximize their own interests.

Changing Environment in Healthcare

The questions posed above are designed to be a fair and impartial point of view that is to be adopted in our reasoning about fundamental principles of healthcare reform. Imagine ourselves in the position of free and equal entities who jointly agree upon and commit themselves to principles of such a fair healthcare for all. Each stakeholder is presented with a list of needed aspects of reform and is assigned the task of choosing the best option that best advances their own interests in establishing conditions so they can pursue their final ends – superior healthcare for the patient, profits for the drug manufacturers and the service providers, enhanced trust in the governing bodies.

In the U.S., just as the case is with education, most healthcare is not provided by the government. A somewhat socialistic approach has been developed wherein an organization (group insurance) is created that charges all participants a fee every month, and the collective sum, through various investments, grows into a pool from which an individual with an illness gets partial support towards its cure. The underlying assumption is that the percentage of people falling ill is relatively small, or the illness is not very serious, so the insurance organization maintains its profits without doling out a large amount of funds, thus minimizing any risks.

The above description is somewhat simplistic, but is a good representation of the current healthcare system in the U.S. The disadvantages include: costs of administration in the insurance organization, competition with other such agencies, lack of control on drug prices, inadequate, at best, oversight, among others. More importantly, as the theory of systems shows, each organization begins to develop an identity of its own with its own need for its long-term sustainability, resulting in reduced services to the patient, sometimes even rejecting any claim in cases of serious illness. The institution's survivability takes precedent over supporting the patient, thus effectively removing the patient from the center of attention, for whom the organization was created in the first place. The "system" ends up having so many stakeholders that it ends up being no longer patient-centric.

Hence the need to seek answers for the questions posed above.

Perhaps what we need to do is, instead of trying to fix the existing system, travel to the future, say 2025, think about what we would like to see and create it. Wasn't it President Lincoln who said, "The best way to predict a future is to create it?" Specific questions to ask: "How can you change the patient-doctor interface? How can we make the medical documents understandable to patients? How can we control the spiraling costs? How can we measure outcomes? Can we integrate all the services needed for a specific patient in one setting? Over all, how can we make the patient the center of attention and an equal shareholder?

Essential Elements of any Healthcare System

Any healthcare framework is expected to provide the following four environments: (i) Access (timeliness, proximity); (ii) Affordability (cost transparency, reasonable price for service, financial assistance); (iii) Patient Education (preventive care, web-based access to test results and suggestions for follow-up); and (iv) Continuous Quality Improvement (incorporation of technologies into physician knowledge updates, use of Artificial Intelligence in scanning publications and provide alternate treatment suggestions). In the following we discuss each of these factors.

Access: In the landmark Institute of Medicine report *Access to Health Care in America*, access to health care was defined as "the timely use of personal health services to achieve the best possible health outcomes." This definition encompasses both the ability of individuals to obtain needed medical services and the potential for those medical services to improve health. Such care depends upon the severity of the disease but on a continuing bases for several years, it is imperative throughout the "cancer control continuum, including primary care, with providers who discuss cancer risk factors and encourage healthy lifestyles, implement cancer screening, ensure early recognition of and timely response to symptoms, encourage adherence to medical treatments, and coordinate survivorship care. Access to palliative care is increasingly recognized as an important component of high-quality care at the time of diagnosis as well as at the end of life." (Milman, 1993).

Affordability: In the United States, as discussed in a previous section, the main reason for reforming health care is high costs. Also the main reason limited lower class citizens access to health care. Such costs can be minimized by having health care providers and practices affiliated with multiple hospitals, networks, and insurance plans. Importantly, care should be explicitly coordinated across these multiple insurers, plans, hospitals, and practices. Medical records and patient data should reside in multiple places, readily accessible to patients and service providers alike. Such an integration of data should result in coordination of services, reduction or even elimination of ineffective care, proper use of effective care, and appropriate use of health care services. The recent set-up of MyChart in the Baylor College of Medicine and its accessibility across multiple major service providers is a great example in that regard.

Patient Education: The patient should play an important role in making a choice of the type of care he/she needs. In second case discussed above, the standard post-surgery treatment consisted of six more months of chemotherapy – tablets and infusion. But a consultation with the surgeon on wanting to know more about that approach revealed that such an approach is not always necessary. Based on that consultation and existing research from Europe, a decision was made to cut down the extent of treatment drastically. Service providers should advise their patients of such available research and treatments so the patient, properly educated, can decide on the type of follow-up care he/she needs. Such education, on a personalized basis, can be made available through web-based access.

Continuous Quality Improvement (CQI): Several service providers, large such as the Baylor College of Medicine, and small such as individual or small groups of physicians, have created web-based access for communicating with their patients. Such access provides the patients with anytime-anywhere information of their health status and keeps them apprised of upcoming appointments, needed prescription refills, reasonable communication with their physicians and nurses for responses to any after-care, non-urgent inquiries. The system should be improved to include real time diagnoses of simple illnesses such as common colds as well as communicating self-conducted tests that should eliminate unnecessary visits to the provider's locations, thus increasing access to physician consulting, reducing administrative costs and reducing time spent in the waiting rooms. The recent introduction of at home colon cancer screening test is a step in the right direction.

An important element of CQI is staying in tune with current research and technology improvements. A single cancer patient can generate nearly one terabyte of biomedical data, consisting of routine diagnostic data as well as all the patient's clinical data. It is the equivalent to storing more than 300,000 photos or 130,000 books. Alongside patient history and diagnostic imaging data, genetic data has become a key tool in the battle against cancer. As the cost of DNA sequencing has plummeted over the last two decades, the gathering of detailed genetic information on both the patient and the tumor has become far more commonplace, rapidly increasing the volume of data available to scientists. Today, researchers not only look at the genetic code of the cancer cells that were the original source of the disease, they can also compare them with the DNA of metastases, or secondary tumors, that develop.

By the end of 2017, it was estimated that research based around genome sequencing of patients generated one exabyte of data annually – that's a million terabytes (the equivalent of 130 billion books – a thousand times more than have ever been published). (Bayer, 2018).

FUTURE RESEARCH DIRECTIONS

A Few Innovations Across the Globe

A fairly comprehensive list of top ten healthcare innovations is listed in an article by Copeland (Copeland, 2018): Next-generation sequencing, 3D-printed devices, Immunotherapy, Artificial intelligence, Point-of-care diagnostics, Virtual reality, Leveraging social media to improve patient experience, Biosensors and trackers, Convenient care and Telehealth.

Other innovations occurring across the globe are as follows:

1. Telehealth: 10 Paths to Innovation in Health Care Delivery A collection of original content from NEJM Catalyst (Paths to Innovation in Health Care Delivery, 2019).
2. What can payers do to reduce costs? (MedCity News, n.d.).
3. Artificial Intelligence could improve health care for all – unless it doesn't (Hsu, 2019).
4. Principles for Health Care Payment Reform to Improve Cancer Care Quality ("Principles for Health Care," n.d.).

Additionally, in the author's opinion, the following are the directions in research that have the highest potential for improving healthcare.

- Develop a comprehensive website – Medicopedia – that maintains updated information on various diseases, available treatments, available service locations, cost of treatment. A website with the name MedicOpedia from India has a presence on the web. However, the website is still in its infancy and has very little information, but it does provide a viable platform for patient education and other vital information listed earlier. The website may be maintained under a collaboration among universities, health centers, industry and medical experts. The web currently hosts several such sites, for instance WebMD, however they are not comprehensive, possess (sometimes) widely diverse information, generally not easy to navigate and never contain relevant information relating to the available experts, locations, and most importantly, cost of treatment.

- Currently, a lot of cancer research is conducted among established groups with little to inadequate communication among such groups. An effort such as previously mentioned PS-ON center based research is needed, but with a 360^0 view of cancer.

- Drug development, testing and evaluation can be done more effectively and cost-effectively when big pharma works in collaboration with start-ups and academic research centers. Such a collaboration has the potential to drastically bring down the costs of drugs, speed up the testing and evaluation process, and receive more timely approvals from relevant agencies. A Mentor-Protégé type collaboration is an example of such effort.

- Multi-disciplinary research centers such as ADM Biopolis in Singapore with focus on complex diseases should be established in the U.S.

CONCLUSION

This paper is an attempt to suggest a new framework for healthcare reform in the U.S. Since the existing healthcare system is too fragmented, it is suggested that, a "Retooling the System" approach be adopted by asking the question, "What does a reasonable healthcare system look like, that maximizes benefits to all the stakeholders concerned, but which is patient centered?" A specific case of cancer is discussed, both from experts' point of view as well as from a personal experience. While the concept of a universal healthcare is attractive and welcome, its actual structure has to depend upon the socioeconomic infrastructure in the country. The author feels that no reform will be possible unless some change in the mindsets occurs – on the part of the service receiver (patient) to realize that some tax increases might be unavoidable and on the part of the service providers that profits must be balanced against quality and speed of healthcare provided. As the Nobel Laureate John Nash proved, the best system is one in which each participant/stakeholder does what is best for him as well as for everyone else. The current system, skewed towards the pharma industry, is neither patient-centered nor sustainable.

REFERENCES

ADM Biopolis core expertise is finding, designing and developing microorganisms for industrial and health-related purposes. To develop ground-breaking products, our R&D is based on a series of harmonized, interconnected research platforms. (n.d.). Retrieved from http://biopolis.es/

Amadeo, K. (2019, August 22). *4 Reasons Why We Need Healthcare Reform.* Retrieved from https://www.thebalance.com/why-reform-health-care-3305749

Bayer. (2018). *Finding a cure for cancer – is big data the solution?* Retrieved from https://www.canwelivebetter.bayer.com/innovation/finding-cure-cancer-big-data-solution#the-data-mountain

Cancer Data and Statistics. (2019, July 9). Retrieved from https://www.cdc.gov/cancer/dcpc/data

Christensen, J. (2018, June 4). *Same cancer, worse results and twice the cost in the US. CNN.* Retrieved from https://www.cnn.com/2018/06/01/health/us-canada-health-care-spending-study/index.html

Contributor, Q. (2013, February 7). *Where Do the Millions of Cancer Research Dollars Go Every Year?* Retrieved from https://slate.com/human-interest/2013/02/where-do-the-millions-of-cancer-research-dollars-go-every-year.html

Copeland, B. Bill, & US Life Sciences & Health Care. (2018, January 18). *Top 10 health care innovations: Deloitte US.* Retrieved from https://www2.deloitte.com/us/en/pages/life-sciences-and-health-care/articles/top-10-health-care-innovations.html

Cuomo, M. I. (2012, October 2). *Are We Wasting Billions Seeking a Cure for Cancer?* Retrieved from https://www.thedailybeast.com/are-we-wasting-billions-seeking-a-cure-for-cancer

Cuomo, M. I. (2013). *World without cancer: the making of a new cure and the real promise of prevention.* New York: Rodale.

Davis, P. (2018, December 5). *A new theory of cancer.* Retrieved from https://www.themonthly.com.au/issue/2018/november/1540990800/paul-davies/new-theory-cancer

Dolgin, E. (2018). Cancer's cost conundrum. *Nature, 555*(7695). doi: 10.1038-d41486-018-02483-3

Financial Burden of Cancer Care. (2019, February). National Cancer Institute. Retrieved from https://progressreport.cancer.gov/after/economic_burden

Gandhi, V., & Jalali, R. (2017, January 15). *A Conference of New Ideas in Cancer-Challenging Dogmas.* Retrieved from https://www.ncbi.nlm.nih.gov/pubmed/28062401

Gatenby, R. (2009). A chance of strategy in the way on cancer. *Nature, 459.*

Geeta, S. M., & Barad, T. (2016, November 18). *Challenging cancer dogma in Mumbai.* Retrieved from https://cancerworld.net/cutting-edge/challenging-cancer-dogma-in-mumbai/

Historical. (2019, December 17). *Centers for Medicare & Medicaid Services.* Retrieved from https://www.cms.gov/Research-Statistics-Data-and-Systems/Statistics-Trends-and-Reports/NationalHealthExpendData/NationalHealthAccountsHistorical

How many people in the world die from cancer? (n.d.). Retrieved from https://ourworldindata.org/how-many-people-in-the-world-die-from-cancer

Hsu, J. (2019, July 31). *Artificial intelligence could improve healthcare for all-unless it doesn't.* Retrieved from https://www.fastcompany.com/90384481/artificial-intelligence-could-improve-health-care-for-all-unless-it-doesnt

Jha, A. (2017, September 20). *What Does an Ideal Healthcare System Look Like?* Retrieved from https://thehealthcareblog.com/blog/2017/09/20/what-does-an-ideal-healthcare-system-look-like/

Kiley, J. (2018, October 3). *60% in US say health care coverage is government's responsibility.* Retrieved from https://www.pewresearch.org/fact-tank/2018/10/03/most-continue-to-say-ensuring-health-care-coverage-is-governments-responsibility/

McCarthy, N. (2019, August 8). How U.S. Healthcare Spending Per Capita Compares With Other Countries [Infographic]. *Forbes.* Retrieved from https://www.forbes.com/sites/niallmccarthy/2019/08/08/how-us-healthcare-spending-per-capita-compares-with-other-countries-infographic/#37dfa6fd575d

Medicopedia. (n.d.). Retrieved from https://medicopedia.co/

Millman, M. (1993). *18 Institute of Medicine Committee on Monitoring Access to Personal Healthcare Services. In Access to Healthcare in America.* Washington, DC: National Academies Press.

Mukherjee, S. (2012). *The emperor of all maladies a biography of cancer.* Detroit, MI: Gale, Cengage Learning. doi:10.5005/jp-journals-10028-1025

Panner, M. (2019, March 25). *Cancer Treatment Costs Imperil Patients. Forbes.* Retrieved from https://www.forbes.com/sites/forbestechcouncil/2019/03/25/cancer-treatment-costs-imperil-patients/#1e91a53f2b6f

PAR-19-101: Physical Sciences-Oncology Network (PS-ON): Physical Sciences-Oncology Projects (PS-OP) (U01 Clinical Trial Optional). (n.d.). Retrieved from https://grants.nih.gov/grants/guide/pa-files/PAR-19-101.html

10 . Paths to Innovation in Health Care Delivery. (2019, October). *NEJM Catalyst.* Retrieved from https://cdn2.hubspot.net/hubfs/558940/Event_October_2019/Landing/10-Paths-to-Innovation-in-Health-Care-Delivery.pdf

Physical Sciences in Oncology. (2018). Retrieved from https://physics.cancer.gov/

Principles for Health Care Payment Reform to Improve Cancer Care Quality. (n.d.). Retrieved from https://www.canceradvocacy.org/cancer-policy/principles-for-health-care-payment-reform-to-improve-cancer-care-quality/

Promoting a More Balanced Approach to Cancer Prevention and Treatment. (n.d.). Retrieved from https://www.ascopost.com/issues/december-15-2012/promoting-a-more-balanced-approach-to-cancer-prevention-and-treatment/

Rose, M., & Ritchie, H. (2015, July 3). *Cancer.* Retrieved from https://ourworldindata.org/cancer

Rosenthal, E. (2018). *An American sickness: how healthcare became big business and how you can take it back.* New York: Penguin Books.

Schneider, E., Sarnak, D., Shah, A., & Doty, M. (2017). *Mirror, Mirror 2017: International Comparison Reflects Flaws and Opportunities for Better U.S. Health Care.* Retrieved from https://interactives.commonwealthfund.org/2017/july/mirror-mirror/

Simon, S. (2019, January 8). *Facts & Figures 2019: US Cancer Death Rate has Dropped 27% in 25 Years.* American Cancer Society. Retrieved from https://www.cancer.org/latest-news/facts-and-figures-2019.html

The U.S. Health Care System: An International Perspective. (n.d.). Retrieved from https://dpeaflcio.org/programs-publications/issue-fact-sheets/the-u-s-health-care-system-an-international-perspective/

U.S. Health Care Spending Highest Among Developed Countries. (2019, January 7). Retrieved from https://www.jhsph.edu/news/news-releases/2019/us-health-care-spending-highest-among-developed-countries.html

What can payers do to reduce costs? (n.d.). Retrieved from https://medcitynews.com/2019/08/what-can-payers-do-to-reduce-costs-start-by-simplifying-how-they-verify-provider-data/?rf=1

World Health Organization's Ranking of the World's Health Systems. (n.d.). Retrieved from http://thepatientfactor.com/canadian-health-care-information/world-health-organizations-ranking-of-the-worlds-health-systems/

Chapter 8
Telemedicine Adoption Opportunities and Challenges in the Developing World

Khondker Mohammad Zobair
Griffith University, Australia

Louis Sanzogni
Griffith University, Australia

Kuldeep Sandhu
Griffith University, Australia

Md Jahirul Islam
Bangladesh Planning Commission, Ministry of Planning, Bangladesh

ABSTRACT

Mapping opportunities and challenges of telemedicine adoption in an emerging economy has always been presumptive due to the scarcity of empirical evidence. Only recently the potential influencing factors of both issues in the rural context of emerging economies (using Bangladesh as a cases study) were investigated. Analysis of existing literature identified seven broad categories of challenges (e.g., deficient organisational commitment, inadequate technological infrastructure, insufficient resource allocations, deficient service quality, clinicians demotivation, patients' dissatisfaction, and patients' distrust) and six broad categories of opportunities (e.g., service usefulness, service assurance, secured patient privacy, adequacy of services, peer influence on use of services, and environmental conditions) concerning telemedicine adoption. Their significance is outlined. These findings contribute to the literature by distinguishing significant factors, which can positively favour or deter telemedicine implementation in developing countries and similar settings.

DOI: 10.4018/978-1-7998-2949-2.ch008

INTRODUCTION

Providing equally efficient and systematised healthcare services in rural areas of developing or developed countries poses many challenges. For example sustainability, one of the substantial challenges in rural healthcare systems has widened its complexity in public administration, leading to high interest in adopting information and communications technology-mediated healthcare services (Celdrán, Pérez, Clemente, & Pérez, 2018; Zobair, 2019). Rural and remote communities are mostly reliant on primary care physicians because specialist physicians rarely practice in rural areas (Leaming, 2007), highlighting the necessity for innovation in the service delivery of health care. Despite growing demand for telemedicine, the implementation rate is below expectation (Kim, Gellis, Bradway, & Kenaley, 2018). An abundance of published studies investigating the challenges and opportunities associated with telemedicine adoption are reviewed, and guidelines to gain insight on how to optimise successfully sustainable telemedicine in underdeveloped contexts are put forward.

It is anticipated that without a commitment to recognise opportunities and challenges, the substantial promise of telemedicine as an innovative health care system, may not be evidently understood and therefore remain underutilised. The prevalent objective is to gain a clear understanding of the opportunities and challenges of telemedicine adoption in the rural context of emerging economies. This can provide valuable insights for government, policymakers, and stakeholders with the added benefit of informing/developing appropriate policy strategies for the improvement of rural healthcare in underdeveloped areas (Zobair, Sanzogni, & Sandhu, 2019). This research has undertaken a comprehensive, in-depth review of the literature (journal articles, conferences, and reports) including some recent direct experiences to the application of telemedicine, e-health, telehealth, and m-Health projects in both developed and developing countries contexts. These narrative proceeds as follows:

- Definition and scope of telemedicine services.
- Socioeconomic impact of telemedicine services.
- Emerging challenges for telemedicine services.
- Promoting adoption opportunities for telemedicine services.
- Conclusion.

DEFINITION AND SCOPE OF TELEMEDICINE SERVICES

A growing body of published studies is attempting to define telemedicine (R. Bashshur, Shannon, Krupinski, & Grigsby, 2011; R. L. Bashshur, 1995). The first formal published definition of telemedicine refers to 'the practice of medicine without the usual physician-patient confrontation via an interactive audio-video communication system' (R. L. Bashshur, Reardon, & Shannon, 2000, p. 614). According to the World Health Organization (WHO) "Telemedicine is the delivery of healthcare services, where distance is a critical factor, by all healthcare professionals using information and communication for the exchange of valid information for diagnosis, treatment, and prevention of disease and injuries, research and evaluation, and for continuing education of healthcare providers, all in the interests of advancing the health of individuals and their communities"(Organization, 1998).

Rapid Information and Communication Technology (ICT) developments have considerably widened the scope of telemedicine services (Sood et al., 2007). Although the successful initialisation of telemedicine necessitates a broad set of talents, including technologists, researchers, scientists, engineers, clinicians, and practitioners (Sood et al., 2007). Telemedicine has enormous potential to address many of the challenges facing today's healthcare industries (R. L. Bashshur et al., 2016) particularly in emerging economies (Zobair et al., 2019). For instance, telemedicine healthcare services offer a multiplicity of health facilities including evaluation, diagnosis, treatment, monitoring, triage, consultation, and follow-up without the necessity to travel (Swanson Kazley, McLeod, & Wager, 2012). A recent study by Demaerschalk et al. (2017) recommended that telemedicine should be extended well in advance to include numerous additional new health deliveries, including wellness, remote monitoring, disease prevention, and sub-acute health management. The broader concepts of telemedicine (see Figure 1) are often used interchangeably and could be a source of the problem (Van Dyk, 2014).

Under the banner of e-Health, 'telemedicine' refers to the use of computers, cameras, speakers, high-speed internet and other ICT to administer and facilitate healthcare delivery over distance as an alternative to face-to-face interactions between caregivers and care seekers (Yallah, 2014). Telemedicine is a rapidly growing technology that enables timely healthcare delivery at a distance, increased efficiency and data quality, reduction of bottlenecks, and provision of continuing education and adherence in the form of health programs and plans (Doswell, Braxter, Dabbs, Nilsen, & Klem, 2013; Joos et al., 2016). Telemedicine is an emerging technology-based healthcare system and serves as a means for generating value-added services for health providers and seekers (Evans, 2015; Van Dyk, 2013). Telemedicine's contemporary iterations include teleradiology (Evans, 2015; Van Dyk, 2013) telehealth (Evans, 2015), teleimaging (Evans, 2015), teledermatology ((Evans, 2015; Van Dyk, 2013), teleoperations (Evans, 2015), telerobotics (Evans, 2015) (Evans, 2015), telepsychiatry (Evans, 2015; Van Dyk, 2013), teleorthodontics (Evans, 2015), teleorthopaedics (Evans, 2015) and telepharmacy (Van Dyk, 2013). Two studies revealed that telemedicine improves patient health, particularly for those with chronic diseases such as cardiovascular, hyperglycaemia, and hyperlipidaemia

Figure 1. Telemedicine, e-Health, telehealth, telecare and m-Health.
Adapted from Van Dyk (2014). Terms and conditions of the Creative Commons Attribution license
(http://creativecommons.org/licenses/by/3.0).

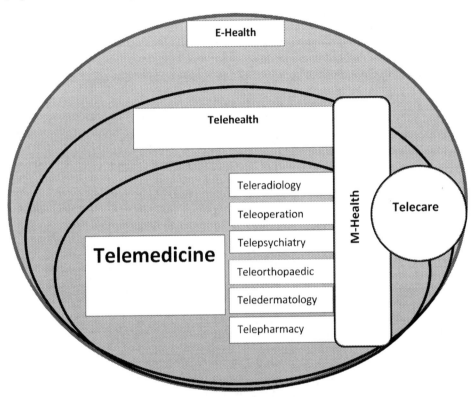

(Li, Li, Deng, & Zhu, 2018), diabetes mellitus, hypertension, and cancer including many other diseases by reducing medical costs (Rho, young Choi, & Lee, 2014).

The modern telemedicine era began in 1968 when the United States (US) based Massachusetts General Hospital offered remote clinical support to travellers and airport staff at Logan International Airport (Ronald S. Weinstein, Krupinski, & Doarn, 2018). For unclear reasons, it disappeared by 1980 but resumed in 1990 due to the speedy growth of the internet, telecommunication technologies (i.e., smartphones), and cost reduction of technologies, all of which reinforced telemedicine innovations (Ronald S. Weinstein et al., 2018). Similar findings voiced by Aranda-Jan, Mohutsiwa-Dibe, and Loukanova (2014) revealed that reduction of ICT-related costs and improved network coverage offered large-scale opportunities for e-Health, telemedicine and mobile healthcare systems (m-Health) deployment in many developing countries.

From a patients perspective, there are a range of platforms (i.e., telemedicine, e-Health, and m-Health) that facilitate health seekers' access to health providers, and when and where they wish to access them (Menvielle, Audrain-Pontevia, & Menvielle, 2017). Due to the significant shortage of highly qualified health professionals, there has been an increasing demand for telemedicine in many developed and developing countries, with the most prevalent needs in rural areas (Ahmed, Evans, Standing, & Mahmud, 2013). Another study by Leaming (2007) reported that less than 4% of American medical graduates plan to practice in rural areas, heightening concerns for future access to healthcare services in rural America. Additionally, both supply-side and demand-side determinants (Krämer & Schreyögg, 2019) play a significant role in the access problem. These reported issues give impetus to the present research.

SOCIOECONOMIC IMPACT OF TELEMEDICINE SERVICES

Worldwide, stakeholders are looking at ways to make healthcare services more sustainable to enhance citizens' health and wellbeing and minimise health discrimination (Coopers, 2013). To address these challenges, many developed and developing countries' healthcare systems are focusing on making healthcare more patient-centric to empower patients in managing their healthcare demands (Zobair, 2019). For example, Schweitzer and Synowiec (2010) acknowledged that ICT is evidently powerful instrument to reinforce healthcare delivery, particularly in the context of both developed and developing countries' rural counterparts. Telemedicine healthcare services influence patients' behaviour to enhance their lifestyle, enable remote treatment of chronic health conditions with minimal cost, minimise the demand for healthcare, and would allow caregivers to make optimum clinical decisions (Coopers, 2013).

E-Health (i.e., telemedicine) service has the potential to not only to reduce health-related costs but provide transformative alternatives to increase healthcare productivity (Schweitzer & Synowiec, 2010). Within the telehealth context, Bagayoko et al. (2014) found that telehealth services contributed to improving the medical diagnoses of cardiology and obstetrics by 92.6% in low and middle income countries. A study by Jennett et al. (2004) confirmed that chronic heart failure, chronic obstructive pulmonary disease, diabetes, asthma, anxiety, and wound care could follow such health treatment methods by significantly reduce costs and in-person interactions. Another study by Coopers (2013) found that through e-Health, telemedicine and m-Health care systems, chronic and elderly patients could manage their diseases better and minimise their severity, thereby lowering associated healthcare expenses.

Dávalos, French, Burdick, and Simmons (2009) outlined the socioeconomic benefits of telemedicine for remotely located cardiovascular and diabetes patients, or those who have inadequate accessibility to specialty care, through the transmission of echocardiograms for faster expert diagnosis via telephone or videoconferencing. They (Dávalos et al., 2009) confirmed that in dermatology and ophthalmology, video conferencing and image transmission allow for long-distance medical consultation with a specialised physician for prompt diagnosis and medication while avoiding needless travel costs and effort for care seekers and their families. Another study by Jennett et al. (2003) confirmed that through paediatric tele-echocardiography, some socioeconomic benefits are attained namely, fewer neonatal hospital transfers decreased length of stay in neonatal intensive care, and increased efficiency and quality of care. Although, Dávalos et al. (2009) argued that telemedicine service providers sometimes bear the heavy economic pressure during the implementation process, since fixed costs, such as specialised equipment purchases, can be very expensive.

Russo et al. (2017) revealed that telemedicine is viable for multiple aspects of medical specialities such as cardiology, neurology, surgery, dermatology, ophthalmology, radiology and paediatrics treatments. In terms of socioeconomic effectiveness, telemedicine is found to be highly cost-effective for intensive care patients. For example, in a high-income country context, Scott Kruse et al. (2018) found that in the US, telemedicine saved patients an average of 145 miles of travel and 142 minutes per visit, while a tele-neurology patient saved approximately two hours of travel time and US$70 per visit, and orthopaedic telemedicine saved US$5,538,120 for 921 remote patients over 5.5 years. Contextually, in low-income countries/areas Sorwar, Rahamn, Uddin, and Hoque (2016) recognised that telemedicine has the potential to reduce patient waiting times and health systems operation costs, enhance inter-departmental and inter-hospital communications and collaborations and enhance sharing of health information among health practitioners. Another recent study by Lee and Lee (2018) acknowledged that telemedicine is a cost effective healthcare service for diabetes management. However, Bain (2006) argued that it is challenging to confirm socio-economic benefits, in particular the cost effectiveness of telemedicine, due to substantial lack of research concerning clinical outcomes related to telemedicine applications. More importantly, the cost-effectiveness of telemedicine research is critical to examine the complex and rapidly growing telemedicine deployment (Koenig, 2019).

EMERGING CHALLENGES FOR TELEMEDICINE ADOPTION

Lewis, Synowiec, Lagomarsino, and Schweitzer (2012) examined major e-Health adoption issues in low- and middle-income countries and determined that these countries are continuing to face significant challenges in providing high-quality, affordable and universally accessible healthcare facilities. Within a developing country's context, Andaleeb, Siddiqui, and Khandakar (2007) for example, asserted that the quality of healthcare services is the primary concern in Bangladesh and has led to the loss of faith in public and private health facilities. A recent study by Roy, van der Weijden, and de Vries (2017) echoed that the most apparent reason for health seekers' dissatisfaction lay in the disparate funding of the country's public and private healthcare organisations. Roy et al. (2017) noted that 72% of Bangladesh's population are rural dwellers, of which 35.2% are below the poverty line; thus, the burden of health-related costs is a critical concern in Bangladesh.

Despite significant advantages and benefits, challenges to telemedicine adoption in developed and developing countries slow its diffusion (Scott et al., 2018). For example, Scott Kruse et al. (2018) classified country-specific challenges, organisation-specific challenges, patient-specific challenges and medical-staff and programme-specific challenges. Within the North American context, Bain (2006) revealed that these challenges significatly affect telemedicine adoption in clinical settings. Some empirical evidence suggested that legislation, organisational infrastructure, societal factors (Boonstra & Broekhuis, 2010; Van Dyk, 2014) and strategic planning (Modi, Portney, Hollenbeck, & Ellimoottil, 2018; Scott & Mars, 2013) have also been reported as challenges of telemedicine adoption.

The challenges for successful implementation of telemedicine services in rural settings identified in this study emerged in seven popular categories of challenges adapted from various prior studies on e-Health, telemedicine and m-Health namely, deficient organisational commitment, inadequate technological infrastructure, insufficient resource allocations, clinician demotivation, deficient service quality, patients' dissatisfaction, and patients' distrust. Figure 2 demonstrates the common and popular categories of challenges associated with telemedicine adoption in emerging economies' rural settings.

Deficient Organisational Commitment

Evidence suggests that organisational commitment is a significant factor for the successful implementation of technology-mediated services (Cresswell and Sheikh (2013). A study by Alaboudi et al. (2016) revealed that many organisations face common challenges in implementing telemedicine with a considerable degree of variation. For example, Hsia, Chiang, Wu, Teng, and Rubin (2019) revealed that

Figure 2. Telemedicine Adoption Challenges

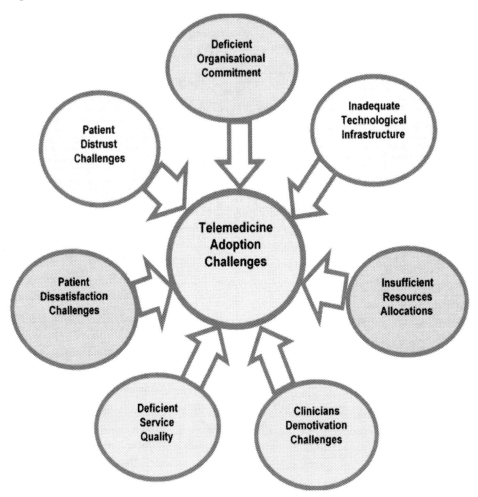

external institutional pressure significantly affects enterprise information systems, including top management's team behaviours. In the context of telemedicine services, organisational commitment (i.e., effectiveness) refers to the development of supportive organisational structures, the implementation of patient care procedures and protocols by professionals, and enrolment of cooperative groups that facilitate patients and physicians, integrating with telemedicine platforms effectively (Boonstra & Broekhuis, 2010; Evans, 2015; Kifle, Mbarika, Tsuma, Wilkerson, & Tan, 2008; Whittaker, Aufdenkamp, & Tinley, 2009). Some studies found that strategic, regulatory infrastructure, legislation, change management and governance issues support organisational challenges to telemedicine adoption (Boonstra & Broekhuis, 2010; Modi et al., 2018; Scott & Mars, 2013; Van Dyk, 2014) in many developed and developing countries. Successful e-Health (i.e., telemedicine) adoption in organisations has been shown to be challenging and demanding at various levels (Hage, Roo, van Offenbeek, & Boonstra, 2013) particularly in rural settings. Most often cited organisational challenges: insufficient investment, lack of systems accessibility, skilled clinicians unavailability, reduced clinical efficacy, poor quality of services, negative attitudes of clinicians, and inadequate support from top management (Dünnebeil, Sunyaev, Blohm, Leimeister, & Krcmar, 2012) negatively influence organizational effectiveness (i.e., commitment) in telemedicine services.

Inadequate Technological Infrastructure

Multimedia technology improvements and expansion of internet access have facilitated increased accessibility to online services, including convenient alternatives to traditional hospital-based services (Nord Garrison, 2019) such as telemedicine. Telemedicine is a technology-mediated healthcare delivery service contributing to better, and safe health management by integrating ICT, clinics, and the internet to deliver teleconsultation between physicians and patients (Vincent M Kiberu, Mars, & Scott, 2017). Inadequate ICT infrastructure, unavailability and unaffordability of ICT resources (e.g., hardware and software), and insufficient power supply are considered to be impediments to implementing telemedicine services (Vincent Micheal Kiberu, Scott, & Mars, 2019). Van Dyk (2014) found that integrated and sustainable technologies (e.g., usability, interoperability and privacy and security issues) are necessary to secure telemedicine services adoption. In the context of Bangladesh for instance, M. R. Hoque, Mazmum, and Bao (2014) found that internet access and power supply are inadequate to successfully implement e-Health (i.e., telemedicine) services. Similar findings echoed by Hossain, Quaresma, and Rahman (2019) revealed that erratic power supply causing computer crashes is a common phenomenon in Bangladesh. These are some critical challenges related to inadequate technological infrastructure (Lewis et al., 2012) for the adoption of telemedicine health care services in developing countries. Another study by Hoque, Bao, and Sorwar (2017) further revealed that many users are reluctant to adopt ICT-supported healthcare services in Bangladesh because of their negative perception related to efficacy and effectiveness.

Insufficient Resources Allocations

Many low and middle income countries lack sufficient financial resources to adopt telemedicine services (Khan, Shahid, Hedstrom, & Andersson, 2012). A growing body of evidence suggests that insufficient funds (Miller, 2010), insufficient resources allocation (Boonstra & Broekhuis, 2010), insufficient ICT and medical equipment (Kruse et al., 2018), high equipment costs (Kiberu et al. 2017) and insufficient allocation of expert human resources (Fanta, Pretorius, & Erasmus, 2015) are considered challenges to telemedicine adoption. In the context of developing countries, M. R. Hoque et al. (2014) found that insufficient funding resources become a dominant impediment to adopting e-Health (i.e., telemedicine) in Bangladesh. Evidence suggests that challenges to telemedicine adoption of similar characteristics are also well-founded in high-income countries. Ronald S Weinstein et al. (2014) for instance, demonstrated that the cost, allocation of funding for equipment, and recruitment of physicians are some dominant challenges to telehealth adoption in the United States. Similar findings acknowledged by Berry (2019) found that the U.S. is experiencing the highest healthcare costs in the world on a per capita basis, nearing 20% of the gross domestic product.

Clinicians Demotivation Challenges

Clinicians motivation refers to the degree to which a clinician is willing to accomplish allotted responsibilities to achieve organisational goals (Franco, Bennett, & Kanfer, 2002), and found to be a vital question facing many developing countries (Jayasuriya, Jayasinghe, & Wang, 2014). Deficiency of clear benefits, incentive and support for clinicians, shortcomings in facilities and a strong sense of mission, and deficient organisational commitment are established critical issues tied to clinicians' motivation (Boonstra & Broekhuis, 2010; Jayasuriya et al., 2014; Miller, 2010). Financial incentives could be a crucial factor influencing clinicians' motivation since health services are undeniably labour intensive (Franco et al., 2002). A recent study by Lagarde, Huicho, and Papanicolas (2019) for example, revealed that in high-income settings financial incentives had improved the quality of services; and in low-income settings the clinicians were found to be demotivated. Vishwanath and Scamurra (2007) for example, noted that if clinicians do not observe personal benefits from their services, they will not be motivated to change their usual working habits. Within the context of health provision, Berry (2019) acknowledged that caregivers hold most of the power, more precisely in the cases of severe sickness when anxious patients become highly dependent on them. Consistent with this situation, financial incentives to health staff could lead to quality improvement, intensifying telemedicine service adoption. A recent study by Faulkner, Dale, and Lau (2019) further revealed that a financial incentives policy reduced health costs in Canada.

Deficient Service Quality

To achieving health goals, service quality must be a high standard, yet there is rising evidence that the quality of health services delivered to communities in many low and middle income countries is deficient (Lagarde et al., 2019). Service quality is considered consumers' comparative evaluation between service expectations and service performance, reflecting how much they like or dislike the services after experiencing them (Woodside, Frey, & Daly, 1989). Within the healthcare context, quality is a critical issue of the right to health (Mgawadere, Smith, Asfaw, Lambert, & van den Broek, 2019). Deficient service quality in health delivery is considered to be one of the most significant challenges in developing countries and attributed to the low motivation of health professionals (Chandler, Chonya, Mtei, Reyburn, & Whitty, 2009). M. S. Akter, Upal, and Hani (2008) noted that patients' satisfaction concerning quality assurance has continuously been neglected in many developing countries, while their satisfaction corroborates organisational performance in hospital settings (Koné Péfoyo & Wodchis, 2013). Another study by Boonstra and Broekhuis (2010) further indicated that physician-patient relationship interference is a prominent challenge to implement electronic medical records in hospital settings.

Patient Dissatisfaction Challenges

Easy accessibility to telemedicine services contributes to increasing patients perceptions of service satisfaction (Gustke, Balch, West, & Rogers, 2000). Patients' satisfaction is critical to healthcare quality assessment and establishes organisational loyalty; it has received significant recognition related to the healthcare industry's survival (Tuzkaya, Sennaroglu, Kalender, & Mutlu, 2019). Evidence suggests that patients satisfaction is considered to be one of the most reliable indicators of service quality measurement (Gustke et al., 2000) in healthcare provision. For example, Hage et al. (2013) revealed that telemedicine services that do not meet requirements and have lack of accessibility lead to patient dissatisfaction. Martin, Probst, Shah, Chen, and Garr (2012) claimed that patients expect high service satisfaction from health service providers. Conversely, poor-availability and accessibility to healthcare services contribute to patient dissatisfaction. Boonstra and Broekhuis (2010) for instance, noted that medical malpractice, unclear legislation about telemedicine practices, and varying virtual medical devices at rural healthcare centres are dominant impediments plaguing telemedicine health provision.

Patients Distrust Challenges

Service quality, satisfaction, and behavioural intention are strictly interrelated factors that serve as a foundation of theoretical frameworks (Woodside et al., 1989) for explaining customer behaviour. Customers' perceived satisfaction/dissatisfaction in service delivery (Woodside et al., 1989) contribute to building trust/distrust regarding the service. In the context of telemedicine Cutts (2017) for example, revealed that trust and commitment were found to be the antecedent factors that influence users' intention to use telemedicine healthcare services. Within the health context, a study by S. Akter, D'Ambra, and Ray (2011) further indicated that trustworthiness plays a critical role in forming patients' confidence and their continuing intentions to reuse the systems/services. Some empirical studies recognised that inadequate monitoring, lack of usefulness (Vishwanath & Scamurra, 2007) and patient privacy, security, and confidentiality (Chang, 2015) led to patients' distrust of telemedicine services. Alongside, some other challenges to telemedicine services adoption are a lack of management support, security standards, and clear patient benefits (Vishwanath & Scamurra, 2007), all established as the foundation components of patients' distrust of the services.

PROMOTING SUCCESSFUL ADOPTION OPPORTUNITIES FOR TELEMEDICINE SERVICES

Rapid development in digital technologies and advancements in Internet speed and capacity appear to promote the viability of health delivery at a distance, contributing to patient satisfaction with telemedicine (Waller & Stotler, 2018). Rural patients' demand, particularly for specialty health services, has been increasing, and telemedicine has been promoted as a way to address these issues (Bain, 2006). The growing demand for health care services and the anticipated health workforce shortage in rural areas contribute to the conditions necessary for the perfect choice of telemedicine services (Leaming, 2007).

Determining individuals' acceptance or rejection of technology, such as computers, appears to be one of the most challenging factors in information systems research (Davis et al., 1989). Telemedicine by all accounts, appears to be well accepted by rural patients in many developed countries (Bros et al., 2018). Conversely, it's acceptance by rural patients in many developing countries; however, this could be based on different factors that influence their behavioural intention (Lin & Chang, 2018).

Six broad categories of opportunities related to telemedicine adoption were evaluated namely, service usefulness, service assurance, secured patients privacy, adequacy of telemedicine services, peer influence on the use of telemedicine services, and environmental conditions. These were adapted from prior studies on telemedicine namely, e-Health, and m-Health adoption associated with the technology acceptance model. The TAM is a popular model for explaining users' technology acceptance (Venkatesh, 2000; Venkatesh & Davis, 2000) and has been successfully used in the healthcare context (Dutot, Bergeron, Rozhkova, & Moreau, 2019). Figure 3 illustrates the common and popular categories of opportunities associated with telemedicine adoption.

Figure 3. Telemedicine Adoption Opportunities

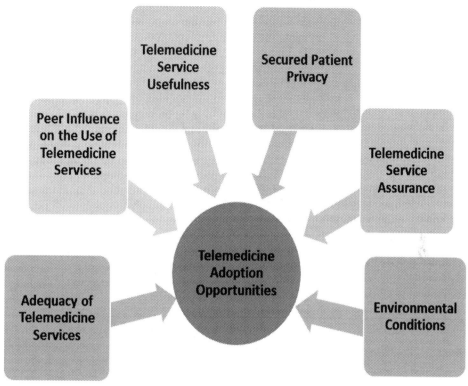

Telemedicine Service Usefulness

The usefulness of ICT based system/service has been found significant in all healthcare related TAM studies (Dünnebeil et al., 2012). Perceived usefulness refers to the degree to which an individual believes that using a system will improve his/her job performance (Venkatesh, 2000; Venkatesh & Davis, 2000). In the context of telemedicine services, Rho et al. (2014) noted that perceived service usefulness influences the patient's behavioural intention to use telemedicine services. Or et al. (2011) further indicated that patients would be more likely to accept health services if they believe the system is useful to meet their health needs. Holden and Karsh (2010), for example, noted that perceived usefulness has a substantial effect on users' behavioural intention to use services. Therefore, it is predicted that when a patient's perception of the usefulness of telemedicine is high, the patient is more likely to use telemedicine. More importantly, in Bangladesh' context, observations indicate that patients believe that telemedicine via videoconferencing, rather than local general health services, will provide better, secure specialised care to improve their health while they remain in rural areas. This is a vivid indication that patients are more likely to increase their acceptance of, and intention to use telemedicine if their perceived usefulness of telemedicine is significant.

Telemedicine Service Assurance

Precise measurement of quality of services, as perceived by patients, is indispensable for sustaining healthcare organisations (Woodside et al., 1989). Service quality assurance is considered to be an essential strategy for the critical success of an organisation (Zeithaml, Berry, & Parasuraman, 1996). The service quality agenda has shifted to its highest priority (Zeithaml et al., 1996) in the modern era. In the healthcare context, patients' perceived service satisfaction is important to determine whether patients continue to use these services or move to other health providers (Hill & Doddato, 2002). For example, Zeithaml et al. (1996) found that customers' service quality assessments favourably influence their behavioural intentions.

Similarly, Woodside et al. (1989) revealed that customers' satisfaction strongly influences their behavioural intention to return to the services. Within the context of telemedicine, patients' perceived service quality refers to the extent of their understanding of the nature and reality of telemedicine services. For example, patients are directly involved in the health process, and their future behavioural intention entirely depends on their present perception of how current services perform. This indicates that patients perceived high service quality assurance has a strong effect on their behavioural characteristics to accept telemedicine services. These findings are consistent. For example, Oriade and Schofield (2019) confirmed a significant relationship between service quality assurance and behavioural intentions in the UK.

Secured Patient Privacy

Patients' health privacy and data security issues have been found noticeable in recent research (Esmaeilzadeh, 2019). Innovative ICT mediated health technologies offer a promising health solution to many of the challenges facing the USA' health care systems (Hale & Kvedar, 2014). Although, many Americans remain interested in using telehealth (i.e., telemedicine) services despite their health-related privacy and confidentiality (Hale & Kvedar, 2014). Esmaeilzadeh (2019) for instance, revealed that prior empirical studies emphasise significant evidence concerning patients' privacy violations in healthcare services such as unauthorised access to patients' information, or stolen medical data. Health information sensitivity may strengthen privacy and security concerns and risk perceptions and weaken consumers intention to ratify health information exchange (Esmaeilzadeh, 2019). For example, Appari and Johnson (2010) and Hoque et al. (2017) revealed that patients might not be confident in disclosing information related to their diseases (e.g., HIV), psychiatric behaviour, genetics and sexual preference with a third party, due to fear of social discrimination. Another study (Dünnebeil et al., 2012) found that data security is a major concern over ICT mediated healthcare services in Germany.

Adequacy of Telemedicine Services

Venkatesh and Davis (2000) revealed that perceived ease of use (i.e., adequacy of telemedicine services) is a strong determinant of behavioural intention to use a system. In the context of telemedicine services, patients' behavioural intention to use telemedicine is augmented when they perceive it is easier to use relative to their disease concerns, wants, and needs. Dünnebeil et al. (2012) noted that 12 healthcare studies employing TAM, identified that perceived ease of use has a substantial positive effect on perceived usefulness. Further, a study investigating patients' acceptance of web-based interactive self-management technology found that perceived ease of use has a positive impact on users' acceptance by mediating perceived usefulness (Or et al., 2011). However, Klingberg, Sawe, Hammar, Wallis, and Hasselberg (2019) found that perceived ease of use or adequacy of use has a weak effect on behavioural intention. In the context of telehealth (i.e., telemedicine) a recent study by Tsai, Cheng, Tsai, Hung, and Chen (2019) found that perceived easy to use (i.e., adequacy of telemedicine services) significantly influence patients' acceptance intention.

Peer Influence on the Use of Telemedicine Services

Social norms/peer influence and interpersonal communications play a significant role contributing to accepting a decision by an individual (Mun, Jackson, Park, & Probst, 2006). In ICT context, social/peer influence can be defined as 'the degree to which an individual perceives that important others believe he or she should use the new system' (Venkatesh, Morris, Davis, & Davis, 2003, p. 451). Dutot et al. (2019) revealed that social influence (i.e., peer influence) has positive effects on behavioural intention to use e-Health services. Mun et al. (2006) confirmed that people are inclined to follow an action/behaviour, if highly perceived referents believe they should. This indicates that individuals might be influenced by superiors or peers to accept a particular innovation (i.e., system/service) if they perceive the usefulness of the change (i.e., system/services) (Mun et al., 2006). More precisely, in telemedicine's context, patients' decisions to accept telemedicine healthcare services could be strongly influenced by their family members, friends, physicians, social media and political awareness. These are consistent with prior studies. For example, BenMessaoud, Kharrazi, and MacDorman (2011) revealed that social influence (i.e., peer influence) proved significant in the understanding of users' acceptance decision to use the technology.

Environmental Conditions

Facilitating conditions (i.e., environmental conditions) refers to the extent and type of support provided to an individual that influence his/her use of the technology (Lu, Yu, & Liu, 2005). Facilitating conditions have positive effects on behavioural intention to use a system/service (Dutot et al., 2019). Facilitating conditions (i.e., environmental conditions) incorporates both resources and technologies that positively influence successful implementation of ICT-based systems (Aggelidis & Chatzoglou, 2009). Within the e-Health context, Hossain et al. (2019) for example, indicated that facilitating conditions have a significant impact on behavioural intention to use e-Health (i.e., telemedicine) services. A study by Lu et al. (2005) revealed that facilitating conditions have been demonstrated significant, affecting information systems adoption. For example, Ajjan and Hartshorne (2008), found that in e-learning adoption, faculty members' awareness related to the benefits (i.e., environmental conditions) of Web 2.0 technologies could improve students' learning, interaction with faculty and peers, writing abilities, and satisfaction with the courses. This indicates that the better the facilitated conditions in an e-learning environment (i.e., better access to course materials, interactions with instructors and peers, teaching and learning), the more likely there was to be a decision from faculty members to adopt Web 2.0 technologies for students (Ajjan & Hartshorne, 2008).

CONCLUSION

This study explored a range of challenges to telemedicine adoption in rural areas of emerging economies, using Bangladesh's current public projects as a case study. Through prior robust investigations on telemedicine, e-Health, and m-Health, this study investigated the challenges and opportunities of telemedicine adoption. This study analysed and found that deficient organisational commitment, inadequate technological infrastructure, insufficient resource allocations, deficient service quality, clinicians demotivation, patients' dissatisfaction, and patients' distrust are the dominant challenges of telemedicine adoption. These challenges present considerable threats to sustainable telemedicine ventures but are believed to be manageable for policymakers, stakeholders and implementers.

Similarly, the opportunities for telemedicine adoption lead to the exploration of the factors that influence patients' acceptance and adoption of the technology mediated telemedicine services. The contribution of this study is the identification of six significant factors concerning telemedicine (e.g., service usefulness, service assurance, secured patient privacy, adequacy of services, peer influences and environmental conditions) that strongly influence patients' behavioural intentions, translating into telemedicine adoption opportunities. These findings are consistent with prior studies carried out in developing and developed countries. The findings will also be useful in developing appropriate policy guidelines for the betterment of healthcare industries in a similar setting.

These empirical findings may help to build telemedicine into an institutionalised health infrastructure for providing better quality patient care with greater flexibility through modernised, specialised healthcare support for medically underprivileged rural communities in emerging economies as well as other similar settings (Zobair et al., 2019). Also, they could advance an enhanced realistic picture of how to sustain telemedicine health care services in rural settings in both developed and developing countries. These findings may shed light on the profound challenges and highlight the opportunities of telemedicine in areas such as rural USA and significant increases in aged population seeking health services are forthcoming.

REFERENCES

Aggelidis, V. P., & Chatzoglou, P. D. (2009). Using a modified technology acceptance model in hospitals. *International Journal of Medical Informatics*, *78*(2), 115–126. doi:10.1016/j.ijmedinf.2008.06.006 PMID:18675583

Ahmed, E., Evans, T. G., Standing, H., & Mahmud, S. (2013). Harnessing pluralism for better health in Bangladesh. *Lancet*, *382*(9906), 1746–1755. doi:10.1016/S0140-6736(13)62147-9 PMID:24268003

Ajjan, H., & Hartshorne, R. (2008). Investigating faculty decisions to adopt Web 2.0 technologies: Theory and empirical tests. *The Internet and Higher Education*, *11*(2), 71–80. doi:10.1016/j.iheduc.2008.05.002

Akter, M. S., Upal, M., & Hani, U. (2008). Service quality perception and satisfaction: A study over sub-urban public hospitals in Bangladesh. *Journal of Services Research*, 125.

Akter, S., D'Ambra, J., & Ray, P. (2011). Trustworthiness in mHealth information services: An assessment of a hierarchical model with mediating and moderating effects using partial least squares (PLS). *Journal of the Association for Information Science and Technology, 62*(1), 100–116.

Alaboudi, A., Atkins, A., Sharp, B., Balkhair, A., Alzahrani, M., & Sunbul, T. (2016). Barriers and challenges in adopting Saudi telemedicine network: The perceptions of decision makers of healthcare facilities in Saudi Arabia. *Journal of Infection and Public Health, 9*(6), 725–733. doi:10.1016/j.jiph.2016.09.001 PMID:27649882

Andaleeb, S. S., Siddiqui, N., & Khandakar, S. (2007). Patient satisfaction with health services in Bangladesh. *Health Policy and Planning, 22*(4), 263–273. doi:10.1093/heapol/czm017 PMID:17545252

Appari, A., & Johnson, M. E. (2010). Information security and privacy in healthcare: current state of research. *International Journal of Internet and Enterprise Management, 6*(4), 279-314.

Aranda-Jan, C. B., Mohutsiwa-Dibe, N., & Loukanova, S. (2014). Systematic review on what works, what does not work and why of implementation of mobile health (mHealth) projects in Africa. *BMC Public Health, 14*(1), 188. doi:10.1186/1471-2458-14-188 PMID:24555733

Bagayoko, C. O., Traoré, D., Thevoz, L., Diabaté, S., Pecoul, D., Niang, M., ... Geissbuhler, A. (2014). Medical and economic benefits of telehealth in low-and middle-income countries: Results of a study in four district hospitals in Mali. *BMC Health Services Research, 14*(1), S9. doi:10.1186/1472-6963-14-S1-S9 PMID:25080312

Bain, D. M. (2006). *The Influences on Physician Attitudes Toward the Use of Telemedicine for the Delivery of Patient Care*. ProQuest.

Bashshur, R., Shannon, G., Krupinski, E., & Grigsby, J. (2011). The Taxonomy of Telemedicine. *Telemedicine Journal and e-Health, 17*(6), 484–494. doi:10.1089/tmj.2011.0103 PMID:21718114

Bashshur, R. L. (1995). On the definition and evaluation of telemedicine. *Telemedicine Journal, 1*(1), 19–30. doi:10.1089/tmj.1.1995.1.19 PMID:10165319

Bashshur, R. L., Howell, J. D., Krupinski, E. A., Harms, K. M., Bashshur, N., & Doarn, C. R. (2016). The empirical foundations of telemedicine interventions in primary care. *Telemedicine Journal and e-Health, 22*(5), 342–375. doi:10.1089/tmj.2016.0045 PMID:27128779

Bashshur, R. L., Reardon, T. G., & Shannon, G. W. (2000). Telemedicine: A new health care delivery system. *Annual Review of Public Health, 21*(1), 613–637. doi:10.1146/annurev.publhealth.21.1.613 PMID:10884967

BenMessaoud, C., Kharrazi, H., & MacDorman, K. F. (2011). Facilitators and barriers to adopting robotic-assisted surgery: Contextualizing the unified theory of acceptance and use of technology. *PLoS One, 6*(1), e16395. doi:10.1371/journal.pone.0016395 PMID:21283719

Berry, L. L. (2019). Service innovation is urgent in healthcare. *AMS Review*, 1-15.

Boonstra, A., & Broekhuis, M. (2010). Barriers to the acceptance of electronic medical records by physicians from systematic review to taxonomy and interventions. *BMC Health Services Research, 10*(1), 231. doi:10.1186/1472-6963-10-231 PMID:20691097

Celdrán, A. H., Pérez, M. G., Clemente, F. J. G., & Pérez, G. M. (2018). Sustainable securing of Medical Cyber-Physical Systems for the healthcare of the future. *Sustainable Computing: Informatics and Systems*.

Chandler, C. I. R., Chonya, S., Mtei, F., Reyburn, H., & Whitty, C. J. M. (2009). Motivation, money and respect: A mixed-method study of Tanzanian non-physician clinicians. *Social Science & Medicine, 68*(11), 2078–2088. doi:10.1016/j.socscimed.2009.03.007 PMID:19328607

Chang, H. (2015). Evaluation framework for telemedicine using the logical framework approach and a fishbone diagram. *Healthcare Informatics Research, 21*(4), 230–238. doi:10.4258/hir.2015.21.4.230 PMID:26618028

Coopers, P. W. (2013*). Socio-economic impact of mHealth*. An assessment report for the European Union.

Cresswell, K., & Sheikh, A. (2013). Organizational issues in the implementation and adoption of health information technology innovations: An interpretative review. *International Journal of Medical Informatics, 82*(5), e73–e86. doi:10.1016/j.ijmedinf.2012.10.007 PMID:23146626

Cutts, H. (2017). *An Investigation of Circumstances Affecting Consumer Behavioral Intentions to Use Telemedicine Technology: An Interpretative Phenomenological Study*. Northcentral University.

Dávalos, M. E., French, M. T., Burdick, A. E., & Simmons, S. C. (2009). Economic evaluation of telemedicine: Review of the literature and research guidelines for benefit–cost analysis. *Telemedicine Journal and e-Health, 15*(10), 933–948.

Demaerschalk, B. M., Berg, J., Chong, B. W., Gross, H., Nystrom, K., Adeoye, O., ... Whitchurch, S. (2017). American telemedicine association: Telestroke guidelines. *Telemedicine Journal and e-Health*, 23(5), 376–389. doi:10.1089/tmj.2017.0006 PMID:28384077

Doswell, W. M., Braxter, B., Dabbs, A. D., Nilsen, W., & Klem, M. L. (2013). mHealth: Technology for nursing practice, education, and research. *Journal of Nursing Education and Practice*, 3(10), 99. doi:10.5430/jnep.v3n10p99

Dünnebeil, S., Sunyaev, A., Blohm, I., Leimeister, J. M., & Krcmar, H. (2012). Determinants of physicians' technology acceptance for e-health in ambulatory care. *International Journal of Medical Informatics*, 81(11), 746–760. doi:10.1016/j. ijmedinf.2012.02.002 PMID:22397989

Dutot, V., Bergeron, F., Rozhkova, K., & Moreau, N. (2019). Factors Affecting the Adoption of Connected Objects in e-Health: A Mixed Methods Approach. *Systèmes d'Information et Management*, 23(4), 3.

Esmaeilzadeh, P. (2019). The effects of public concern for information privacy on the adoption of Health Information Exchanges (HIEs) by healthcare entities. *Health Communication*, 34(10), 1202–1211. doi:10.1080/10410236.2018.147133 6 PMID:29737872

Evans, P. R. (2015). *An exploration of the perceptions of a US Midwest acute care hospital organization regarding the adoption and acceptance of telemedicine.* Capella University.

Fanta, G. B., Pretorius, L., & Erasmus, L. (2015). An evaluation of eHealth systems implementation frameworks for sustainability in resource constrained environments: A literature review. *IAMOT 2015 Conference Proceedings*.

Faulkner, G., Dale, L. P., & Lau, E. (2019). Examining the use of loyalty point incentives to encourage health and fitness centre participation. *Preventive Medicine Reports*, 14, 100831. doi:10.1016/j.pmedr.2019.100831 PMID:30886815

Franco, L. M., Bennett, S., & Kanfer, R. (2002). Health sector reform and public sector health worker motivation: A conceptual framework. *Social Science & Medicine*, 54(8), 1255–1266. doi:10.1016/S0277-9536(01)00094-6 PMID:11989961

Gustke, S. S., Balch, D. C., West, V. L., & Rogers, L. O. (2000). Patient satisfaction with telemedicine. *Telemedicine Journal*, 6(1), 5–13. doi:10.1089/107830200311806

Hage, E., Roo, J. P., van Offenbeek, M. A., & Boonstra, A. (2013). Implementation factors and their effect on e-Health service adoption in rural communities: A systematic literature review. *BMC Health Services Research*, *13*(1), 19. doi:10.1186/1472-6963-13-19 PMID:23311452

Hale, T. M., & Kvedar, J. C. (2014). Privacy and security concerns in telehealth. *The Virtual Mentor*, *16*(12), 981. PMID:25493367

Hill, M. H., & Doddato, T. (2002). Relationships among patient satisfaction, intent to return, and intent to recommend services provided by an academic nursing center. *Journal of Cultural Diversity*, *9*(4), 108–112. PMID:12674887

Holden, R. J., & Karsh, B.-T. (2010). The technology acceptance model: Its past and its future in health care. *Journal of Biomedical Informatics*, *43*(1), 159–172. doi:10.1016/j.jbi.2009.07.002 PMID:19615467

Hoque, B., Bao, Y., & Sorwar, G. (2017). Investigating factors influencing the adoption of e-Health in developing countries: A patient's perspective. *Informatics for Health & Social Care*, *42*(1), 1–17. doi:10.3109/17538157.2015.1075541 PMID:26865037

Hoque, M. R., Mazmum, M., & Bao, Y. (2014). e-Health in Bangladesh: Current status, challenges, and future direction. *Int Tech Manag Rev*, *4*(2), 87–96. doi:10.2991/itmr.2014.4.2.3

Hossain, A., Quaresma, R., & Rahman, H. (2019). Investigating factors influencing the physicians' adoption of electronic health record (EHR) in healthcare system of Bangladesh: An empirical study. *International Journal of Information Management*, *44*, 76–87. doi:10.1016/j.ijinfomgt.2018.09.016

Hsia, T.-L., Chiang, A.-J., Wu, J.-H., Teng, N. N., & Rubin, A. D. (2019). What Drives E-Health Usage? Integrated Institutional Forces and Top Management Perspectives. *Computers in Human Behavior*, *97*, 260–270. doi:10.1016/j.chb.2019.01.010

Jayasuriya, R., Jayasinghe, U. W., & Wang, Q. (2014). Health worker performance in rural health organizations in low- and middle-income countries: Do organizational factors predict non-task performance? *Social Science & Medicine*, *113*, 1–4. doi:10.1016/j.socscimed.2014.04.042 PMID:24820407

Jennett, H., Hall, L. A., Hailey, D., Ohinmaa, A., Anderson, C., Thomas, R., ... Scott, R. E. (2003). The socio-economic impact of telehealth: A systematic review. *Journal of Telemedicine and Telecare*, *9*(6), 311–320. doi:10.1258/135763303771005207 PMID:14680514

Jennett, S., Scott, R. E., Affleck Hall, L., Hailey, D., Ohinmaa, A., Anderson, C., ... Lorenzetti, D. (2004). Policy implications associated with the socioeconomic and health system impact of telehealth: A case study from Canada. *Telemedicine Journal and e-Health, 10*(1), 77–83. doi:10.1089/153056204773644616 PMID:15104919

Joos, O., Silva, R., Amouzou, A., Moulton, L. H., Perin, J., Bryce, J., & Mullany, L. C. (2016). Evaluation of a mHealth data quality intervention to improve documentation of pregnancy outcomes by health surveillance assistants in Malawi: A cluster randomized trial. *PLoS One, 11*(1), e0145238. doi:10.1371/journal.pone.0145238 PMID:26731401

Khan, S. Z., Shahid, Z., Hedstrom, K., & Andersson, A. (2012). Hopes and fears in implementation of electronic health records in Bangladesh. *The Electronic Journal on Information Systems in Developing Countries, 54*(1), 1–18. doi:10.1002/j.1681-4835.2012.tb00387.x

Kiberu, V. M., Mars, M., & Scott, R. E. (2017). Barriers and opportunities to implementation of sustainable e-Health programmes in Uganda: A literature review. *African Journal of Primary Health Care & Family Medicine, 9*(1). doi:10.4102/phcfm.v9i1.1277 PMID:28582996

Kiberu, V. M., Scott, R. E., & Mars, M. (2019). Assessing core, e-learning, clinical and technology readiness to integrate telemedicine at public health facilities in Uganda: A health facility–based survey. *BMC Health Services Research, 19*(1), 266. doi:10.118612913-019-4057-6 PMID:31035976

Kifle, M., Mbarika, V. W., Tsuma, C., Wilkerson, D., & Tan, J. (2008). A telemedicine transfer model for Sub-Saharan Africa. *Hawaii International Conference on System Sciences, Proceedings of the 41st Annual*. 10.1109/HICSS.2008.41

Kim, E., Gellis, Z. D., Bradway, C., & Kenaley, B. (2018). Key determinants to using telehealth technology to serve medically ill and depressed homebound older adults. *Journal of Gerontological Social Work*, 1–24. doi:10.1080/01634372.2018.1499575 PMID:30040598

Klingberg, A., Sawe, H. R., Hammar, U., Wallis, L. A., & Hasselberg, M. (2019). mHealth for burn injury consultations in a low-resource setting: An acceptability study among health care providers. *Telemedicine Journal and e-Health*, tmj.2019.0048. doi:10.1089/tmj.2019.0048 PMID:31161967

Koenig, M. A. (2019). *Telemedicine in the ICU*. Springer. doi:10.1007/978-3-030-11569-2

Koné Péfoyo, A. J., & Wodchis, W. P. (2013). Organizational performance impacting patient satisfaction in Ontario hospitals: A multilevel analysis. *BMC Research Notes*, *6*(1), 509–509. doi:10.1186/1756-0500-6-509 PMID:24304888

Krämer, J., & Schreyögg, J. (2019). Demand-side determinants of rising hospital admissions in Germany: The role of ageing. *The European Journal of Health Economics*, 1–14. PMID:30739296

Kruse, C. S., Atkins, J. M., Baker, T. D., Gonzales, E. N., Paul, J. L., & Brooks, M. (2018). Factors influencing the adoption of telemedicine for treatment of military veterans with post-traumatic stress disorder. *Journal of Rehabilitation Medicine*, *50*(5), 385–392. doi:10.2340/16501977-2302 PMID:29700551

Lagarde, M., Huicho, L., & Papanicolas, I. (2019). Motivating provision of high quality care: It is not all about the money. *BMJ (Clinical Research Ed.)*, *366*, l5210. doi:10.1136/bmj.l5210 PMID:31548200

Leaming, L. E. (2007). *Barriers to physician adoption of telemedicine and best practices for overcoming these barriers*. Medical University of South Carolina.

Lee, J. Y., & Lee, S. W. H. (2018). Telemedicine Cost–Effectiveness for Diabetes Management: A Systematic Review. *Diabetes Technology & Therapeutics*.

Lewis, S., Synowiec, C., Lagomarsino, G., & Schweitzer, J. (2012). E-health in low-and middle-income countries: Findings from the Center for Health Market Innovations. *Bulletin of the World Health Organization*, *90*(5), 332–340. doi:10.2471/BLT.11.099820 PMID:22589566

Li, Y., Li, Y., Deng, Z., & Zhu, Z. (2018). *A Collaborative Telemedicine Platform Focusing on Paranasal Sinus Segmentation*. Paper presented at the International Conference on Intelligent Interactive Multimedia Systems and Services.

Lu, J., Yu, C.-S., & Liu, C. (2005). Facilitating conditions, wireless trust and adoption intention. *Journal of Computer Information Systems*, *46*(1), 17–24.

Martin, A. B., Probst, J. C., Shah, K., Chen, Z., & Garr, D. (2012). Differences in readiness between rural hospitals and primary care providers for telemedicine adoption and implementation: Findings from a statewide telemedicine survey. *The Journal of Rural Health*, *28*(1), 8–15. doi:10.1111/j.1748-0361.2011.00369.x PMID:22236310

Menvielle, L., Audrain-Pontevia, A.-F., & Menvielle, W. (2017). *The digitization of healthcare: New challenges and opportunities*. Springer. doi:10.1057/978-1-349-95173-4

Mgawadere, F., Smith, H., Asfaw, A., Lambert, J., & van den Broek, N. (2019). "There is no time for knowing each other": Quality of care during childbirth in a low resource setting. *Midwifery*, *75*, 33–40. doi:10.1016/j.midw.2019.04.006 PMID:30986692

Miller, E. (2010). *Telemedicine and the provider-patient relationship: What we know so far.* Report prepared for the Nuffield Council's Working Party on Medical Profiling and Online Medicine.

Modi, P. K., Portney, D., Hollenbeck, B. K., & Ellimoottil, C. (2018). Engaging telehealth to drive value-based urology. *Current Opinion in Urology, 28*(4), 342–347. PMID:29697472

Mun, Y. Y., Jackson, J. D., Park, J. S., & Probst, J. C. (2006). Understanding information technology acceptance by individual professionals: Toward an integrative view. *Information & Management*, *43*(3), 350–363. doi:10.1016/j.im.2005.08.006

Or, C. K., Karsh, B.-T., Severtson, D. J., Burke, L. J., Brown, R. L., & Brennan, P. F. (2011). Factors affecting home care patients' acceptance of a web-based interactive self-management technology. *Journal of the American Medical Informatics Association, 18*(1), 51–59. doi:10.1136/jamia.2010.007336 PMID:21131605

Organization, W. H. (1998). A Health Telematics Policy in Support of WHO'S Health-For-All Strategy for Global Development: Report of the WHO Group Consultation on Health Telematics 11-16 December, Geneva, 1997. World Health Organization.

Oriade, A., & Schofield, P. (2019). An examination of the role of service quality and perceived value in visitor attraction experience. *Journal of Destination Marketing & Management, 11*, 1–9. doi:10.1016/j.jdmm.2018.10.002

Rho, M. J., Choi, I., & Lee, J. (2014). Predictive factors of telemedicine service acceptance and behavioral intention of physicians. *International Journal of Medical Informatics*, *83*(8), 559–571. doi:10.1016/j.ijmcdinf.2014.05.005 PMID:24961820

Roy, A., van der Weijden, T., & de Vries, N. (2017). Predictors and consequences of rural clients' satisfaction level in the district public-private mixed health system of Bangladesh. *Global Health Research and Policy, 2*(1), 31.

Russo, L., Campagna, I., Ferretti, B., Pandolfi, E., Carloni, E., D'Ambrosio, A., ... Tozzi, A. E. (2017). What drives attitude towards telemedicine among families of pediatric patients? A survey. *BMC Pediatrics, 17*(1), 21. doi:10.118612887-016-0756-x PMID:28095894

Schweitzer, J., & Synowiec, C. (2010). The economics of eHealth. *Health, 29*(2), 235–238.

Scott, R. E., & Mars, M. (2013). Principles and framework for eHealth strategy development. *Journal of Medical Internet Research, 15*(7), e155. doi:10.2196/jmir.2250 PMID:23900066

Scott Kruse, C., Karem, P., Shifflett, K., Vegi, L., Ravi, K., & Brooks, M. (2018). Evaluating barriers to adopting Telemedicine worldwide: A systematic review. *Journal of Telemedicine and Telecare, 24*(1), 4–12. doi:10.1177/1357633X16674087 PMID:29320966

Sood, S., Mbarika, V., Jugoo, S., Dookhy, R., Doarn, C. R., Prakash, N., & Merrell, R. C. (2007). What is telemedicine? A collection of 104 peer-reviewed perspectives and theoretical underpinnings. *Telemedicine Journal and e-Health, 13*(5), 573–590. doi:10.1089/tmj.2006.0073 PMID:17999619

Sorwar, G., Rahamn, M. M., Uddin, R., & Hoque, M. (2016). Cost and time effectiveness analysis of a telemedicine service in Bangladesh. *Studies in Health Technology and Informatics, 231*, 127–134. PMID:27782024

Swanson Kazley, A., McLeod, A. C., & Wager, K. A. (2012). Telemedicine in an international context: definition, use, and future. In *Health Information Technology in the International Context* (pp. 143–169). Emerald Group Publishing Limited. doi:10.1108/S1474-8231(2012)0000012011

Tsai, J.-M., Cheng, M.-J., Tsai, H.-H., Hung, S.-W., & Chen, Y.-L. (2019). Acceptance and resistance of telehealth: The perspective of dual-factor concepts in technology adoption. *International Journal of Information Management, 49*, 34–44. doi:10.1016/j.ijinfomgt.2019.03.003

Tuzkaya, G., Sennaroglu, B., Kalender, Z. T., & Mutlu, M. (2019). Hospital service quality evaluation with IVIF-PROMETHEE and a case study. *Socio-Economic Planning Sciences, 68*, 100705. doi:10.1016/j.seps.2019.04.002

Van Dyk, L. (2013). *The development of a telemedicine service maturity model.* Stellenbosch: Stellenbosch University.

Van Dyk, L. (2014). A review of telehealth service implementation frameworks. *International Journal of Environmental Research and Public Health, 11*(2), 1279–1298. doi:10.3390/ijerph110201279 PMID:24464237

Venkatesh, V. (2000). Determinants of perceived ease of use: Integrating control, intrinsic motivation, and emotion into the technology acceptance model. *Information Systems Research, 11*(4), 342–365. doi:10.1287/isre.11.4.342.11872

Venkatesh, V., & Davis, F. D. (2000). A theoretical extension of the technology acceptance model: Four longitudinal field studies. *Management Science, 46*(2), 186–204. doi:10.1287/mnsc.46.2.186.11926

Venkatesh, V., Morris, M. G., Davis, G. B., & Davis, F. D. (2003). User acceptance of information technology: Toward a unified view. *Management Information Systems Quarterly, 27*(3), 425–478. doi:10.2307/30036540

Vishwanath, A., & Scamurra, S. D. (2007). Barriers to the adoption of electronic health records: Using concept mapping to develop a comprehensive empirical model. *Health Informatics Journal, 13*(2), 119–134. doi:10.1177/1460458207076468 PMID:17510224

Waller, M., & Stotler, C. (2018). Telemedicine: A primer. *Current Allergy and Asthma Reports, 18*(10), 54. doi:10.100711882-018-0808-4 PMID:30145709

Weinstein, R. S., Krupinski, E. A., & Doarn, C. R. (2018). Clinical Examination Component of Telemedicine, Telehealth, mHealth, and Connected Health Medical Practices. *The Medical Clinics of North America, 102*(3), 533–544. doi:10.1016/j.mcna.2018.01.002 PMID:29650074

Weinstein, R. S., Lopez, A. M., Joseph, B. A., Erps, K. A., Holcomb, M., Barker, G. P., & Krupinski, E. A. (2014). Telemedicine, telehealth, and mobile health applications that work: Opportunities and barriers. *The American Journal of Medicine, 127*(3), 183–187. doi:10.1016/j.amjmed.2013.09.032 PMID:24384059

Whittaker, A. A., Aufdenkamp, M., & Tinley, S. (2009). Barriers and facilitators to electronic documentation in a rural hospital. *Journal of Nursing Scholarship, 41*(3), 293–300. doi:10.1111/j.1547-5069.2009.01278.x PMID:19723278

Woodside, A. G., Frey, L. L., & Daly, R. T. (1989). Linking sort/ice anlity, customer satisfaction, and behavioral intention. *Journal of Health Care Marketing, 9*(4), 5–17. PMID:10304174

Yallah, A. (2014). *A Correlational Study of the Technology Acceptance Model and Georgia Behavioral Healthcare Provider Telemedicine Adoption.* ERIC.

Zeithaml, V. A., Berry, L. L., & Parasuraman, A. (1996). The behavioral consequences of service quality. *Journal of Marketing, 60*(2), 31–46. doi:10.2307/1251929

Zobair, K. M. (2019). *Barriers, facilitators and expectations of telemedicine healthcare services adoption in rural public hospital settings in Bangladesh* (Unpublished Thesis). Retrieved from http://hdl.handle.net/10072/388646

Zobair, K. M., Sanzogni, L., & Sandhu, K. (2019). Expectations of telemedicine health service adoption in rural Bangladesh. *Social Science & Medicine, 238*, 112485. doi:10.1016/j.socscimed.2019.112485 PMID:31476664

Section 3

Chapter 9

Interprofessionality:
A Pathway to a More Sustainable National Healthcare System

Chidiebele Constance Obichi

https://orcid.org/0000-0002-7527-9187
Indiana University Northwest, USA

April D. Newton
Indiana University, USA

Ukamaka Marian Oruche
Indiana University, USA

ABSTRACT

Preventable medical errors (PME) is the third leading cause of death in the United States with an incidence range of 210,000 to 400,000 deaths per year and an estimated cost of $19.5 billion to $958 billion per year. Despite advances in patient safety, PME persists across the nation. An unmarked extremity, a soft sponge, medication dose, poor communication, etc. are possible precursors of PME that may lead to death. Preventable medical errors such as wrong-patient or wrong-site surgery, botched transplants, and death from myocardial infarction or septic shock following a discharge from the emergency department are frequently reported. According to the Institute of Medicine, most PME in the healthcare system are caused by poor team collaboration and care coordination, particularly when patient care was provided by independent providers. Therefore, the healthcare workforce must work within interprofessional teams for safe, cost-effective, and quality care delivery significant to sustainable healthcare reform.

DOI: 10.4018/978-1-7998-2949-2.ch009

INTRODUCTION

The healthcare system is like an orchestra. The orchestra combines instruments from different families which are unified by a set tempo that shapes the sound of the ensemble. These instruments must be in sync to produce the harmonious and satisfying sound that offers the patron an opportunity to experience the power and passion of classical music.

Preventable medical errors (PME) is the third leading cause of death in the United States (US) (Makary & Daniel, 2016; Robertson & Long, 2018) with an incidence range of 210,000 to 400,000 deaths per year (Andel, Davidow, Hollander, & Moreno, 2012; James, 2013; Makary & Daniel, 2016). The cost of PME is estimated at $19.5 billion to $958 billion per year (Patient Safety Movement, n.d). Despite advances in patient safety, PME persists across the nation.

An unmarked extremity, a soft sponge, medication dose, poor communication are possible precursors of PME that lead to patient injuries or death. Preventable medical errors that are frequently reported include: wrong-patient or wrong-site surgery; botched transplants, and death from myocardial infarction or septic shock following a discharge from the emergency department (Wachter & Gupta, 2019). According to a multicenter study led by researchers from Boston Children's Hospital (Starmer et al., 2014), poor communication and hand-off errors are the most reported PME in hospitals across the US. Starmer et al., (2014) reported a relationship between communication, hand-offs, and PME. Hence PME decreased by 30 percent if improvements were made in verbal and written communication between healthcare providers during patient hand-offs. Similarly, PME decreased in the operating room through the use of 'time-outs' - when a procedure can be interrupted to confirm patient identification and surgical site selection (Altpeter et al., 2007).

Preventing PME has become the responsibility of the entire healthcare team. According to the Institute of Medicine (Wakefield, 2000), most PME in the healthcare system are caused by poor team collaboration and care coordination, particularly when patient care was provided by independent providers (Wakefield, 2000). Hence, effective collaborative interprofessional teamwork may serve to avoid and mitigate medical errors (Thomas, Sherwood, & Helmreich, 2003).

The healthcare industry looked toward aviation to determine how teamwork was instilled in the crew members to similarly inform healthcare teams. Following the tragic collision of two 747s on a foggy morning in Tenerife and other similar accidents, aviation began a series of training programs, generally called "crew resource management" or "cockpit resource management" programs, designed to train diverse crews in communication and teamwork (Wachter & Gupta, 2019). Some of the training programs utilized the Situation, Background, Assessment, and Recommendations (SBAR) technique - commonly used in healthcare - for communication strategies and briefing/debriefing techniques (Wachter & Gupta, 2019). The aviation industry acknowledged that these communication and teamwork-based programs were in large part responsible for improving the culture of aviation and the remarkable safety record of commercial airlines over the years (Wachter & Gupta, 2019). The dynamics of the airplane cockpit are similar to those of the operating room. Therefore, operating room services were selected to pilot-test the aviation model of safety training in healthcare (Rivers, Swain, & Nixon, 2003).

The experience of teamwork and crew members in the aviation industry has substantiated the need for teamwork and a focus on improving safe and quality patient care within the healthcare system. Healthcare providers must train and work within interprofessional teams for safe and quality care delivery to patients. However, current healthcare professions' curricula are lacking with regards to interprofessionality. Traditional curricula do not address the necessary interprofessional aspects that equip learners with the tools they need to provide optimally safe and quality care (Alper, Rosenberg, O'Brien, Fischer, & Durning, 2009; Thom, 2016). Hence, the on-going reform of the healthcare system is warranted.

According to Berwick et al. (2008), the current healthcare system is broken. Berwick et al. reported that the most powerful team members: patients, family members, and community partners are not asked to be on the healthcare team. There is no consciousness of interaction among healthcare professionals and healthcare professions students; and there is little awareness of interdependence among the healthcare professions and the healthcare workforce. Consequently, healthcare delivery systems and education systems are fragmented. This lack of coordination produces inadequate quality of care and high cost of healthcare that results in tremendous suffering among patients, families, and the society in general. Hence, the urgent need for healthcare reform (Berwick et al., 2008; Healthcare Reform Roundtable [Part I], 2009; Emanuel & Orszag, 2010) that is founded on the principles of interprofessionality and collaborative practice across health professions and other disciplines. According to D'amour and Oandasan (2005), interprofessionality is a response to the realities of the fragmentation within the US healthcare system. It is the "process by which professionals reflect on and develop ways of practicing that provides an integrated and cohesive answer to the needs of the client, family or the population" (p.9). This process involves professionals from diverse disciplines who gather to: reconcile their differences and opposing views, establish shared goals, and address patient care issues to optimize care.

Increasingly, there is growing recognition that complex public health problems require interprofessional solutions (Lakhani, Benzies, & Hayden, 2012; Lee, McDonald, Anderson, & Tarczy-Hornoch, 2009). Leading research funding agencies in the US including the National Institutes of Health (NIH) require researchers from different professions or disciplines working together in interprofessional teams to produce effective and sustained solutions to myriad of complex and multifaceted health care problems (Nagarajan, Kalinka, & Hogan, 2013). Yet, most models of research training for health professions students at both undergraduate and graduate levels still operate in silos (Little et l., 2017) – which hinders preparation of a collaborative practice-ready biomedical or biobehavioral research workforce (World Health Organization [WHO], 2010). We need an interprofessional and collaborative research workforce for the effective generation of knowledge to advance population health, reduce healthcare costs, and patient health-related outcomes (Little et al., 2017; Nelson-Brantley & Warshawsky, 2018). This chapter aims to present the current state of interprofessional education (IPE), interprofessional collaborative practice (IPCP), and collaborative research training, challenges, solutions, and future and emerging trends for the way forward.

BACKGROUND

The Institute of Medicine ([IOM], 2001) examined the state of the current US healthcare system and identified strategies to achieve substantial improvements in the quality of healthcare. In the report (2001), IOM recognized the benefits of IPE and recommended that training for health professions students should be redesigned to include more opportunities for interprofessional training (Institute of Medicine, 2001). Further, in an address at the 2011 annual meeting of the American Psychology Association, Rozensky (2012) emphasized the importance of interprofessional education and collaborative practice (IPECP) towards the delivery of cost effective and quality healthcare.

Following the IOM report (2001), synergistic efforts have emerged among academic educators, health professions students, and healthcare providers to increase awareness and understanding of IPECP (Retchin, 2008; Zwarenstein, Goldman, & Reeves, 2009; Kirsh, Schaub, & Aron, 2009; Khan, Louie, Reicherter, & Roberts, 2016). In another IOM report (2015), three major barriers to the advancement of IPECP were identified which includes: 1) misalignment between education and health delivery systems; 2) lack of a conceptual model that provides a common taxonomy and framework to guide studies that examine the influence of IPE on systems outcomes; and 3) scarcity of research that examine associations of IPECP and patient, population, and health system outcomes. Additionally, the IOM (2015) developed the interprofessional learning continuum (IPLC) model to guide IPE evaluation from education to practice and health and systems outcomes. Although this model can be adapted in multiple settings, the model has not been empirically tested (IOM, 2015). Creating innovative strategies to address these barriers will provide the evidence that funders and policy makers require to support a redesign of the US healthcare system (Cox, Cuff, Brandt, Reeves, & Zierler, 2016).

Consistent with the WHO framework on IPE (2010), investigators including Little and colleagues (2017) agree that interprofessional collaborative research practice occurs when practitioners from more than one health profession engage in scientific inquiry to jointly create and disseminate new knowledge to health professionals in order to provide the highest quality of care to improve patient-level and population-level health outcomes (p.15). Although, interprofessional collaborative research practice is widely implemented, interprofessional collaborative research training for students at all educational levels has lagged behind (Interprofessional Education Collaborative [IPEC] Expert Panel, 2011; Little et al., 2017). Yet, NIH - the nation's leading authority on health research funding - requires and funds research studies conducted by interprofessional collaborative research teams. While some researchers without formal interprofessional collaborative research training might be able to figure out how to function, a workforce trained through IPE is more likely to work better in teams to deliver better health outcomes to the patient populations served (Green & Johnson, 2015; IPEC Expert Panel, 2011). Potential barriers to interprofessional collaborative research training may include lack of knowledge of effective models of training (Lutfiyya et al., 2019) and challenges inherent in collaborative process. Collaborative process may be hindered by differences in health professions' (e.g., medicine and nursing) unique knowledge and skills for managing patients' health care problems; differences in hierarchy and knowledge generation, and available resources among different professions (Green & Johnson, 2015; Little et al., 2017). Therefore, different health professionals must have not only mutual respect for one another's professions but also work cooperatively and transparently to foster equitable sharing of responsibilities and decision-making (Bridges et al., 2011; Hall, 2005). The next section of the chapter will focus on solutions and recommendations in dealing with issues related to interprofessionality in education, clinical practice, and research in addition to future and emerging trends for the way forward.

MAIN FOCUS OF THE CHAPTER

Interprofessionality and Education

Interprofessional education and collaborative practice (IPECP) encompasses IPE and interprofessional collaborative practice (IPCP). Interprofessional education occurs when individuals from multiple professions learn about, from, and with each other to enable effective collaborative interactions that may improve health outcomes.

Interprofessional education involves initiatives and structured interprofessional educational activities that impact learner outcomes (D'amour & Oandasan, 2005; Levett-Jones et al., 2018). Interprofessional collaborative practice involves healthcare professionals working together to improve the quality and safety of patient care using complementary knowledge and skills with respect for each other's expertise (Rogers et al., 2017). Ultimately, the goal is to enhance patient outcomes; however, the opportunity for collaborative practice depends on the team members' ability to bond, mutually trust one another, and understand each other's role in patient care. Consequently, collaborators must know each other's educational model, professional cultural values, and roles and responsibilities (D'amour & Oandasan, 2005) in providing care to patients in acute and primary care settings.

With on-going developments to redesign primary care, US health systems and institutions of higher learning are challenged in educating students in the classroom, simulations, and clinical settings in ways that may release collaborative-minded healthcare professionals into the workforce. The majority of the current healthcare workforce were trained in silos. Consequently, many healthcare providers may lack the skills required to practice in an interprofessional, team-based environment. To develop interprofessional team-based health professionals, a paradigm shift is imperative to generate collaborative team-based characteristics among health professions students as well as healthcare providers. A workforce prepared to function in a collaborative team-model emerges from IPE training experiences (Green & Johnson, 2015).

To further advance IPECP in the US, accreditation bodies for the health professions programs have developed accepted standards for curricula in medicine, nursing, …, and pharmacy programs. For example, undergraduate nursing curricula elements for IPE have been clearly stated in The Essentials of Baccalaureate Education for Professional Nursing Practice which stated that "…interprofessional education enables the baccalaureate graduate to enter the workplace with baseline competencies and confidence for interactions and communication skills, that will improve practice, thus yielding better patient outcomes . . . interprofessional education optimizes opportunities for the development of respect and trust for other members of the healthcare team" (American Association of Colleges of Nursing, p. 22, 2008). Given that the elements of IPECP curriculum in nursing have been provided and that many nursing programs have implemented this IPECP as a pedagogical approach, it is pertinent that studies are conducted that evaluate IPECP programs across the US education and health systems.

Issues Related to Interprofessional Education. Research has indicated that challenges to the systemic integration of IPECP include: 1) absence of evidence base regarding the specific interprofessional education and training for all learners (Lutfiyya et al., 2016; Cox, Cuff, Brandt, Reeves & Zierler, 2016); 2) identifying facilities where interprofessional clinical competencies and learning objectives can be achieved and the tools for assessing site readiness (Gilligan, Outram, & Levett-Jones, 2014); 3) healthcare workforce planning disconnected from an interprofessional team-based orientation; differences in accreditation requirements and competencies across the health professions (Schuetz, Mann, & Everett, 2010); 4) ill-prepared faculty members being assigned to deliver interprofessional curriculum (Hall & Zierler, 2015); and 5) identifying the best approaches for implementing IPECP during workforce training and the expected outcomes that should be achieved (Reeves, Perrier, Goldman, Freeth, & Zwarenstein, 2013).

Major barriers encountered in IPECP are the existence of silos, prevalent stereotypes and minimal interaction among the health professions (D'amour & Oandasan, 2005; Berwick et al., 2008; Schuetz, Mann, & Everett, 2010; Gilligan et al., 2014). Health professions students receive profession-specific training and have the tendency to practice in silos. For example, inadequate interaction between: 1) students of the health professions and 2) students of the health professions and students of other disciplines (Meleis, 2016).

Interprofessionality and Clinical Practice

According to Green and Johnson (2015), IPCP is the future for delivering quality healthcare in the US, specifically, in the management of chronic diseases such as asthma, type 2 diabetes, cardiovascular disease, hypertension, mood disorders and other complex health conditions. The expectation is that team members in IPCP must be well informed and effective when collaborating in practice to improve clinical outcomes.

Issues Related to Interprofessional Clinical Practice. The management of chronic diseases and complex health conditions require a variety of health services. However, health professionals encounter difficulties when collaborating in delivering care. The barriers are related to "imbalances of authority, limited understanding of others' roles and responsibilities, and professional boundary friction" (Reeves, Pelone, Harrison, Goldman, & Zwarenstein, 2017, p.7).

The task of creating an efficient standard IPCP model for the US healthcare system is an on-going process. The use of IPCP among innovative healthcare systems has increased over the last decade via a variety of models, most notably in chronic disease management (Southerland, Webster-Cyriaque, Bednarsh, & Mouton, 2016). The Chronic Care Model (CCM) is the most well-known model in chronic disease management which was designed to transform acute and reactive care to proactive, planned, and population-based care (Wagner, 1998). However, Cherry Health and *CHI Health* are two emerging IPCP CCM models with outcome data to support their roles in IPCP care.

Cherry Health. This Federally Qualified Health Center (FQHC) was established in 1988. It is the largest independent, non-profit FQHC system in the state of Michigan serving seven counties in more than 20 locations. Cherry Health clinics provide services that include: primary care, women's health, pediatrics, dental, vision, behavioral health, mental health, correctional health, five school-based health centers and employee assistance for employers (Hardin, Kilian, & Spykerman, 2017). The *Cherry Health Durham Clinic* (CHDC), created a high-need, high frequency patient integrated primary care model. Patients receive services in one location from all team members with a primary focus of providing high quality healthcare services to those who have little or no access to healthcare, regardless of income or insurance status. The CHDC incorporates care with a primary care physician, physician assistant, psychiatrist, nurses, health coaches, and supports coordinator in one office (Hardin, Kilian, & Spykerman, 2017).

In 2012, CHDC *and Mercy Health Saint Mary's* (MHSM) decided to investigate an inter-organizational collaborative practice between the healthcare systems to improve patient outcomes and quality of patient care, to reduce healthcare costs while improving clinical outcomes, and to address fragmentation in the patients' plans of care contributing to patterns of high utilization (Hardin, Kilian, & Spykerman, 2017). The inter-organizational collaborative practice had 19 patients with 396 hospital visits (emergency department [ED]; Inpatient [IP]; and outpatient) during the 12 months prior to the intervention. The outcomes of the inter-organizational collaborative practice 12 months post-intervention included a decrease in: average ED visits by 28%; IP admissions by 50%; length of stay days by 49%; computerized axial tomography scans by 67%; gross charges in the population by 51%; and direct expenses by 54%. Despite decrease in hospital visits, operating margin increased by $84,774, representing a 71% increase in operating margin (Hardin, Kilian, & Spykerman, 2017).

CHI Health. In 2017, *CHI Health - Creighton University Medical Center – University Campus* re-opened its doors as an IPCP ambulatory care clinic (ACC) located in a family medicine residency and faculty practice at a new ACC (Guck et al., 2019). The IPCP clinic serves high-risk patients by integrating family medicine, pediatrics, women's health, psychiatry, pharmacy, and physical therapy in a one-stop location (Creighton University, 2017). To integrate the IPCP team with each other, the team attended three conflict engagement sessions before and after opening; the team attends daily huddles before morning and afternoon clinic; teamlets collaborate on patient care throughout the day; and all ACC patients are introduced to the IPCP team with handoffs from the primary care physician or medical assistant (Creighton University, 2017).

The patient outcomes and costs for the IPCP ACC were compared before the clinic opened in 2016 and after it opened as an IPCP ACC in 2017. The outcomes included a decrease of: 16.7% in ED visits; 17.7% in hospital visits; and a decrease of 0.8% in patients' hemoglobin A_{1C} levels. Total patient charges decreased from $18,491 to $9,572 representing a 48.2% decrease in total patient charges (Creighton University, 2017).

Further, two hospital-based models awaiting final outcomes provide IPCP clinical education experiences for health professions students. The models are: 1) The Vanderbilt Program in Interprofessional Learning (VPIL) which is a longitudinal continuity experience for health professions students assigned to a clinic for two years and 2) The Veterans Health Administration Patient Aligned Care Team (VHA-PACT) which is a provider and health professions students model designed to promote patient-centric care in a variety of clinical services (Vanderbilt University, 2019; VHA, 2019).

The VPIL Clinic. This is a model for health professions students from five universities in the middle Tennessee region. This model includes students from nursing, medicine, pharmacy, and social work who spend one half-day per week in either clinics or classroom settings working in interprofessional teams. The clinic provides one half-day each week for students to deliver care to a panel of patients under the supervision of multi-professional attending providers. As the learners advance in their pre-licensure program, their clinic roles also advance and differentiate. Learners also provide a breadth of services to their patients including health coaching and medication counseling. The learners also have the opportunity to arrange for laboratory and imaging studies, contact consultants, and access community resources, when necessary. In addition, one half-day each month the teams meet for a variety of classroom-based activities. Teams have the opportunity to debrief using reflective exercises, assess team performances, and review patient outcomes and ongoing needs. The ultimate goal for the experience is to prepare health professions students for a collaborative-practice-ready workforce (Vanderbilt University, 2019).

The VHA-PACT. In this model, transformation begins with primary care and permeates into other areas of the health care system to include specialty care, women's health care, and geriatrics. The PACT focuses on partnerships with veterans, access to care using diverse methods, coordinated care among team members, and team-based care, with Veterans at the center of the team. The PACT considers all aspects of the veterans' health, with an emphasis on prevention and health promotion through a team-based collaboration with all providers and learners. The PACT members have defined roles with a focus on forging trusted personal relationships with the veterans (VHA, 2019).

As IPCP models evolve, the US health care systems and institutions of higher learning must; 1) partner to develop new educational environments for IPECP; 2) share new ideas and novel innovations in practice designs; and 3) partner to generate evidence-based knowledge for IPECP via research (Earnest & Brandt, 2014).

Interprofessionality and Research

Issues Related to Interprofessional Research. Although there are funded research training programs, most are traditionally limited to a single profession. One example is the National Research Service Awards (NRSA), which is funded by several institutes within NIH including National Institute of Nursing Research (NINR). The National Institute of Nursing Research, grants the Ruth Kirschstein Research Service Award to institutions or individual pre-doctoral or post-doctoral students or fellows (NIH, n.d.). Fellows include one-profession group, in this case nursing only. Fellows meet together regularly with their program directors for seminars. Fellows are expected to have a health or health-related non-nursing mentor. However, there is no expectation to train together with students from other professions. Yet, as a future biomedical or biobehavioral research workforce, they are expected to conduct interprofessional research projects. This is a missed opportunity for preparation of a collaborative practice-ready research workforce (World Health Organization [WHO], 2010). Hence, the need for an interprofessional and collaborative research workforce for the effective generation of knowledge to advance population health, reduce healthcare costs, and improve patient health-related outcomes (Little et al., 2017; Nelson-Brantley & Warshawsky, 2018).

SOLUTIONS AND RECOMMENDATIONS

Despite the challenges, creative strategies that target adequate implementation of IPECP continue to emerge. These strategies include: extracurricular activities that involve informal social interaction that will help break down the preconceptions, stereotypes, and silos of the health professions; scheduling and provision of co-curricular activities that involve actual intellectual interaction among interprofessional students in lectures and simulations, and clinical settings; initiatives that necessitate healthcare professionals interacting with one another in new ways that may improve patient outcomes (Gordon, Lasater, Brunett, & Dieckmann, 2015; Lutfiyya et al., 2016).

According to Meleis (2016), it is well documented in the literature that medicine as a discipline claims hierarchical supremacy over other healthcare professions. Consequently, we must be reminded that effective teams: 1) respect and complement each other with no privilege or feelings of supremacy; 2) set common goals and work together to achieve the goals; and 3) provide joint solutions that improve patient outcomes. The success of IPECP is anchored on the effectiveness of individual team members and their collective capacities (Meleis, 2016). Hence, health professions students must actively interact with peers by getting involved in interprofessional co-curricular and extracurricular activities.

One example of an extracurricular activity is the Institute for Healthcare Improvement (IHI) Open School chapters at US university campuses and other countries. The IHI Open School chapter is an interprofessional student organization committed to improving healthcare quality. In this organization, health professions students work with peers and faculty advisors across the health professions on health-related student-driven projects and may present their projects at IHI conferences. Students in this IHI club learn specialized skills in team building and organizing for change that may empower them to become performance improvement leaders in team-based environments.

Given the advancement of IPECP and interprofessional collaborative research at US universities and health systems, complementary efforts to improve the K-12 curricula are needed such that K-12 students begin to develop team characteristics prior to attending college. To guide K-12 students towards learning team characteristics, pedagogical approaches that highlight the essential roles of the community, peers, families, and teachers as part of a child's social development (Powers & de Waters, 2004; Papatheodorou & Moyles, 2008) must be strongly emphasized in K-12 curricula. Students who learn the basics of teamwork prior to college may be better prepared for the post-secondary IPECP curricula.

Students trained using interprofessional models of research are more likely to become interprofessional team members (IOM, 2001). Models used in IPE broadly could be adapted to fit interprofessional collaborative research training specifically. Collaboration is a long-term process and requires investment. Therefore, the organizational cultures and leadership across stakeholder groups have to invest and commit to formational relationships, nurturing it both in principle and in resources (Green & Johnson, 2015). This includes providing necessary training for faculty involved; making the necessary changes in content and conduct of health research training to pre- and postdoctoral fellows. These investments and commitments will lead to a cadre of interprofessional collaborative practice-ready researchers who will work with not only one another but also patient populations served (WHO, 2010; Bridges et al., 2011).

FUTURE RESEARCH DIRECTIONS

Few available studies show promise that interprofessional health care teams can make significant and meaningful contributions to improvement of patient and population health outcomes and to the redesign of the US health care delivery system (Lutfiyya, Brandt, & Cerra, 2016; Lutfiyya et al., 2019; Nelson-Brantley & Warshawsky, 2018). However, there is need for more evidence that explicitly map IPE and CP training to the outcomes of improved population health, reduced healthcare costs, and are patient health-related; and better linkage between health professions education or training and practice (Gilbert, 2013; Lutfiyya et al., 2016; Lutfiyya et al., 2019). Compared to IPECP broadly, interprofessional collaborative research training lags behind in its implementation; and as such, there is a paucity of evaluation research. Future research directions may focus on several questions: (1) what are the specific training requirements and competencies for interprofessional collaborative research training for students and faculty educators alike (Bridges et al., 2011; Lutfiyya et al., 2016; Paradis, & Whitehead, 2018)? (2) What are requisite curricular mechanisms (i.e., logistics and scheduling, program content, compulsory attendance, shared objectives, learning principles, and contextual learning), [WHO, 2010]? (3) How should health profession teams be constituted to achieve desired health-related outcomes (Lutfiyya et al., 2016)? (4) What is the effect of interprofessional collaborative research training on practice and outcomes of improved population health and reduced health care costs; and how to measure these outcomes (Lutfiyya et al., 2016)?

CONCLUSION

There is a paucity of IPE activities for health professions students training for research. IPE activities need to be threaded across all dimensions of research training for undergraduate and graduate or pre- and post-doctoral students at all educational levels in order to develop a collaborative practice-ready biomedical and biobehavioral research workforce. We need interprofessional collaborative research workforce to jointly create and disseminate new knowledge to health professionals in order to provide the highest quality of patient care to improve patient-level and population-level health outcomes. Hence, an urgent need for increased IPECP scientific conferences across the US to: build capacity for all stakeholders (students, educators, clinicians, patients, families, communities, and researchers) and disseminate models of excellence that 1) improve access to care, 2) decrease costs, and 3) improve quality of care.

Healthcare reform will be accelerated once the inseparable link between interprofessional education, interprofessional collaborative practice, and research is adequately addressed by all stakeholders. New or redesigned models of care will lose value without a workforce that is versatile in knowledge and skills that would effectively coordinate the implementation of the models. Regardless of the model of care, the US is long overdue for a coordinated health care system in which IPECP is adequately implemented among educators, practitioners, researchers, and policy-makers at all levels of the health system. Finally, to achieve a sustainable healthcare reform, the educational, social, and health systems must establish a shared goal that recognizes patients, families, and communities as partners in the delivery of care.

REFERENCES

Alexandraki, I., Hernandez, C., Torre, D., Chretien, K., Hernandez, C. A., Torre, D. M., & Chretien, K. C. (2017). Interprofessional Education in the Internal Medicine Clerkship Post-LCME Standard Issuance: Results of a National Survey. *Journal of General Internal Medicine*, *32*(8), 871–876. doi:10.1007/s11606-017-4004-3 PubMed

Alper, E., Rosenberg, E. I., O'Brien, K. E., Fischer, M., & Durning, S. J. (2009). Patient safety education at US and Canadian medical schools: Results from the 2006 Clerkship Directors in Internal Medicine survey. *Academic Medicine*, *84*(12), 1672–1676. doi:10.1097/ACM.0b013e3181bf98a4 PubMed

Altpeter, T., Luckhardt, K., Lewis, J. N., Harken, A. H., & Polk, H. C. Jr. (2007). Expanded surgical time out: A key to real-time data collection and quality improvement. *Journal of the American College of Surgeons*, *204*(4), 527–532. doi:10.1016/j.jamcollsurg.2007.01.009 PubMed

American Association of Colleges of Nursing Essentials of Baccalaureate Education for and interprofessional education: An emerging concept. (2008). Journal of interprofessional care, 19(sup1), 8-20. Retrieved from http://www.aacnnursing.org/portals/42/publications/baccessentials08.pdf

Andel, C., Davidow, S. L., Hollander, M., & Moreno, D. A. (2012). The economics of health care quality and medical errors. *Journal of Health Care Finance*, *39*(1), 39. PubMed

Berwick, D. M., Nolan, T. W., & Whittington, J. (2008). The triple aim: Care, health, and cost. *Health Affairs*, *27*(3), 759–769. doi:10.1377/hlthaff.27.3.759 PubMed

Bridges, D. R., Davidson, R. A., Odegard, S., Maki, I. V., & Tomkowiak, J. (2011). Interprofessional collaboration: Three best practice models of interprofessional education. *Medical Education Online*, *1*(0). doi: PubMed doi:10.3402/meo.v16i0.6035

Clarke, J. L., Bourn, S., Skoufalos, A., Beck, E. H., & Castillo, D. J. (2016). An innovative approach to health care delivery for patients with chronic conditions. *Population Health Management, 20*(1), 23–30. doi:10.1089/pop.2016.0076 PubMed

Cox, M., Cuff, P., Brandt, B., Reeves, S., & Zierler, B. (2016). Measuring the impact of interprofessional education on collaborative practice and patient outcomes. Journal of Interprofessional Care, 30(1), 1–3. https://doi-org.proxynw.uits.iu.edu/10.3109/13561820.2015.1111052

Creighton University. (2017). News Center: University Campus of CHI Health-Creighton University Medical Center opens new era for health care. Retrieved from https://www.creighton.edu/publicrelations/newscenter/news/2017/january2017/january52017/chicumcnr010517/

D'Amour D, & Oandasan I. (2005). Interprofessionality as the field of interprofessional practice and interprofessional education: An emerging concept. Journal of Interprofessional Care, 19(sup1), 8-20.

Earnest, M., & Brandt, B. (2014). Aligning practice redesign and interprofessional education to advance triple aim outcomes. *Journal of Interprofessional Care, 28*(6), 497–500. doi:10.3109/13561820.2014.933650 PubMed

Emanuel, E. J., & Orszag, P. R. (2010). Health care reform and cost control. *The New England Journal of Medicine, 363*(7), 601–603. doi:10.1056/NEJMp1006571 PubMed

Gilbert, J. H. (2013). Interprofessional education, learning, practice and care. Journal of Interprofessional Care, 27(4), 283–285. https://doi-org.proxynw.uits.iu.edu/10.3109/13561820.2012.755807

Gilligan, C., Outram, S., & Levett-Jones, T. (2014). Recommendations from recent graduates in medicine, nursing and pharmacy on improving interprofessional education in university programs: A qualitative study. *BMC Medical Education*, (1). doi:10.1186/1472-6920-14-52

Gordon, M. A., Lasater, K., Brunett, P., & Dieckmann, N. F. (2015). Interprofessional Education Finding a Place to Start. Nurse Educator, 40(5), 249–253. 00000000000164 doi:10.1097/NNE.00

Green, B. N., & Johnson, C. (2015). Interprofessional collaboration in research, education, and clinical practice: Working together for a better future. Journal of Chiropractic Education, 29(1), 1-10. doi:10.7899ljce-14-36

Guck, T. P., Potthoff, M. R., Walters, R. W., Doll, J., Greene, M. A., & DeFreece, T. (2019). Improved outcomes associated with interprofessional collaborative practice. *Annals of Family Medicine, 17*(Suppl 1), S82–S82. doi:10.1370/afm.2428 PubMed

Hall, L. W., & Zierler, B. K. (2015). Interprofessional Education and Practice Guide No. 1: Developing faculty to effectively facilitate interprofessional education. Journal of Interprofessional Care, 29(1), 3–7. https://doi-org.proxynw.uits.iu.edu/10.3109/13561820.2014.937483

Hall, P. (2005). Interprofessional teamwork: Professional cultures as barriers. Journal of Interprofessional care, 19(sup1), 188-196.

Hardin L., & Spykerman, K. (2017). Competing health care systems and complex patients: An inter-professional collaboration to improve outcomes and reduce health care costs. Journal of Interprofessional Education & Practice, (7), 5-10.

Institute of Medicine. (2001). *Committee on Quality of Health Care in America. Crossing the quality chasm: A new health system for the 21st century.* National Academies Press.

Institute of Medicine. (2015). *Measuring the Impact of Interprofessional Education on Collaborative Practice and Patient Outcomes.* National Academies Press.

James, J. T. (2013). A new, evidence-based estimate of patient harms associated with hospital care. *Journal of Patient Safety, 9*(3), 122–128. doi:10.1097/PTS.0b013e3182948a69 PubMed

Khan, C. T., Louie, A. K., Reicherter, D., & Roberts, L. W. (2016). What Is the Role of Academic Departments of Psychiatry in Advancing Global Mental Health? *Academic Psychiatry, 40*(4), 672–678. doi:10.1007/s40596-016-0497-z PubMed

Kirsh, S. B., Schaub, K., & Aron, D. C. (2009). Shared Medical Appointments: A Potential Venue for Education in Interprofessional Care. Quality Management in Health Care, 18(3), 217–224. https://doi-org.proxynw.uits.iu.edu/10.1097/QMH.0b013e3181aea27d

Lakhani, J., Benzies, K., & Hayden, K. A. (2012). Attributes of Interdisciplinary Research Teams: A Comprehensive Review of the Literature. *Clinical and Investigative Medicine. Medecine Clinique et Experimentale, 35*(5), E260–E265. doi:10.25011/cim.v35i5.18698

Levett-Jones, T., Burdett, T., Chow, Y. L., Jönsson, L., Lasater, K., Mathews, L. R., ... Wihlborg, J. (2018). Case Studies of Interprofessional Education Initiatives from Five Countries. *Journal of Nursing Scholarship*, *50*(3), 324–332. doi:10.1111/jnu.12384 PubMed

Little, M. M., St Hill, C., Ware, K. B., Swanoski, M. T., Chapman, S. A., Lutfiyya, M. N., & Cerra, F. (2017). Team science as interprofessional collaborative research practice: A systematic review of the science of team science literature. *Journal of Investigative Medicine: The Official Publication of The American Federation for Clinical Research*, *65*(1), 15–22. doi:10.1136/jim-2016-000216 PubMed

Lutfiyya, M. M., Chang, L. F., McGrath, C., Dana, C., & Lipsky, M. S. (2019). The state of the science of interprofessional collaborative practice: A scoping review of the patient health-related outcomes-based literature published between 2010 and 2018. *PLoS One*, *14*(6), 1–18. doi:10.1371/journal.pone.0218578 PubMed

Lutfiyya, M. N., Brandt, B., Delaney, C., Pechacek, J., & Cerra, F. (2016). Setting a research agenda for interprofessional education and collaborative practice in the context of United States health system reform. *Journal of Interprofessional Care*, *30*(1), 7–14. doi:10.3109/13561820.2015.1040875 PubMed

Lutfiyya, M. W., Brandt, B. F., & Cerra, F. (2016). Reflections from the intersection of health professions education and clinical practice: The state of the science of interprofessional education and collaborative practice. *Academic Medicine*, *91*(6), 766–771. doi:10.1097/ACM.0000000000001139 PubMed

Makary, M. A., & Daniel, M. (2016). Medical error--the third leading cause of death in the US. *British Medical Journal*, *1*, ●●●. Retrieved from http://search.ebscohost.com/login.aspx?direct=true&db=edb&AN=115194747&site=eds-live PubMed

Meleis, A. I. (2016). Interprofessional education: A summary of reports and barriers to recommendations. *Journal of Nursing Scholarship*, *48*(1), 106–112. doi:10.1111/jnu.12184 PubMed

Nagarajan, R., Kalinka, A. T., & Hogan, W. R. (2013). Evidence of community structure in biomedical research grant collaborations. *Journal of Biomedical Informatics*, *46*(1), 40–46. doi:10.1016/j.jbi.2012.08.002 PubMed

National Institutes of Health. (n.d.). Research training and career development. Retrieved from https://researchtraining.nih.gov/programs/fellowships

Nelson-Brantley, H. V., & Warshawsky, e. (2018). Interprofessional education: Advancing team science to create collaborative safety cultures. The Journal of Nursing Administration, 48(5), 235–237. doi:10.1097/NNA.0000000000000607 PubMed

Papatheodorou, T., & Moyles, J. R. (Eds.). (2008). Learning together in the early years: Exploring relational pedagogy. Routledge. Paradis. E., & Whitehead, C. R. (208). Beyond the lamppost: A proposal for a fourth wave of education for collaboration. *Academic Medicine, 93*(10), 1457–1463.

Patient Safety Movement. (n.d.). Resources for Policy Makers. Retrieved from https://patientsafetymovement.org/advocacy/policy-makers/resources-for-policy-makers/

Powers, S. E., & de Waters, J. (2004). Creating project-based learning experiences for university-k-12 partnerships. 34th Annual Frontiers in Education, 2004, F3D–18.

Reeves, S., Pelone, F., Harrison, R., Goldman, J., & Zwarenstein, M. (2017). Interprofessional collaboration to improve professional practice and healthcare outcomes. *Cochrane Database of Systematic Reviews, 6*(6), CD000072. doi:10.1002/14651858.CD000072.pub3

Reeves, S., Perrier, L., Goldman, J., Freeth, D., & Zwarenstein, M. (2013). Interprofessional education: Effects on professional practice and healthcare outcomes (update). *Cochrane Database of Systematic Reviews*, (3): CD002213. doi:10.1002/14651858.CD002213.pub3

Retchin, S. M. (2008). A conceptual framework for interprofessional and co-managed care. *Academic Medicine, 83*(10), 929–933. doi:10.1097/ACM.0b013e3181850b4b PubMed

Rivers, R. M., Swain, D., & Nixon, W. R. (2003). Using aviation safety measures to enhance patient outcomes. *AORN Journal, 77*(1), 158–162. doi:10.1016/S0001-2092(06)61385-9 PubMed

Robertson, J. J., & Long, B. (2018). Suffering in silence: Medical error and its impact on health care providers. *The Journal of Emergency Medicine, 54*(4), 402–409. doi:10.1016/j.jemermed.2017.12.001 PubMed

Rogers, G. D., Thistlethwaite, J. E., Anderson, E. S., Abrandt Dahlgren, M., Grymonpre, R. E., Moran, M., & Samarasekera, D. D. (2017). International consensus statement on the assessment of interprofessional learning outcomes. *Medical Teacher, 39*(4), 347–359. doi:10.1080/0142159X.2017.1270441 PubMed

Rozensky, R. H., & Janicke, D. M. (2012). Commentary: Healthcare reform and psychology's workforce: Preparing for the future of pediatric psychology. *Journal of Pediatric Psychology, 37*(4), 359–368. doi:10.1093/jpepsy/jsr111 PubMed

Schuetz, B., Mann, E., & Everett, W. (2010). Educating Health Professionals Collaboratively For Team-Based Primary Care. *Health Affairs*, *29*(8), 1476–1480. doi:10.1377/hlthaff.2010.0052 PubMed

Southerland, J. H., Webster-Cyriaque, J., Bednarsh, H., & Mouton, C. P. (2016). Interprofessional collaborative practice models in chronic disease management. Dental Clinics, 60(4), 789–809. doi: PubMed doi:10.1016/j.cden.2016.05.001

Starmer, A. J., Spector, N. D., Srivastava, R., West, D. C., Rosenbluth, G., Allen, A. D., ... Lipsitz, S. R. (2014). Changes in medical errors after implementation of a handoff program. *The New England Journal of Medicine*, *371*(19), 1803–1812. doi:10.1056/NEJMsa1405556 PubMed

Thom, K. A., Heil, E. L., Croft, L. D., Duffy, A., Morgan, D. J., & Johantgen, M. (2016). Advancing interprofessional patient safety education for medical, nursing, and pharmacy learners during clinical rotations. *Journal of Interprofessional Care*, *30*(6), 819–822. doi:10.1080/13561820.2016.1215972 PubMed

Thomas, E. J., Sherwood, G. D., & Helmreich, R. L. (2003). Lessons from aviation: Teamwork to improve patient safety. *Nursing Economics*, *21*(5), 241. PubMed

Tracy, C. S., Bell, S. H., Nickell, L. A., Charles, J., & Upshur, E. G. (2013). Innovative Model of interprofessional primary care for elderly patients with complex health care needs. *Canadian Family Physician Medecin de Famille Canadien*, *59*(3), e148–e155. PubMed

Vanderbilt University. (2019). About the Program. Retrieved from https://medschool.vanderbilt.edu/vpil/about-the-program/

Vanderbilt University. (2019). Vanderbilt Program in Interprofessional Learning: About the Program. Retrieved from https://medschool.vanderbilt.edu/vpil/

Veterans Health Administration Patient Aligned Care Team. (2019). Retrieved from https://www.pcpcc.org/initiative/veterans-health-administration-patient-aligned-care-team-pact

Wachter, R. M., & Gupta, K. (2019). *Understanding Patient Safety* (3rd ed.)., Retrieved from https://accessmedicine-mhmedical-com.ezproxy.rosalindfranklin.edu/book.aspx? bookid=2203

Wagner, E. H. (1998). Chronic disease management: What will it take to improve care for chronic illness? *Effective Clinical Practice*, *1*(1), 2–4. PubMed

Wakefield, M. (2000). To err is human: An Institute of Medicine report. *Professional Psychology, Research and Practice*, *31*(3), 243–244. doi:10.1037/h0092814

World Health Organization. (2010). The WHO Framework for Action. *Journal of Interprofessional Care, 24*(5), 475–478. doi:10.3109/13561820.2010.504134 PubMed

Zwarenstein, M., Goldman, J., & Reeves, S. (2009). Interprofessional collaboration: Effects of practice-based interventions on professional practice and healthcare outcomes. *Cochrane Database of Systematic Reviews.* https://doi-org.proxynw.uits. iu.edu/10.1002/14651858.CD000072

ADDITIONAL READING

Alexandraki, I., Hernandez, C., Torre, D., Chretien, K., Hernandez, C. A., Torre, D. M., & Chretien, K. C. (2017). Interprofessional education in the internal medicine clerkship post-LCME standard issuance: Results of a national survey. *Journal of General Internal Medicine, 32*(8), 871–876. doi:10.1007/s11606-017-4004-3 PubMed

Danielson, J., & Willgerodt, M. (2018). Building a theoretically grounded curricular framework for successful interprofessional education. *American Journal of Pharmaceutical Education, 82*(10), 1133–1139. PubMed

Gonzalo, J. D., Haidet, P., Papp, K. K., Wolpaw, D. R., Moser, E., Wittenstein, R. D., & Wolpaw, T. (2017). Educating for the 21st-century health care system: An interdependent framework of basic, clinical, and systems sciences. *Academic Medicine, 92*(1), 35–39. doi:10.1097/ACM.0000000000000951 PubMed

Kim, J., Lowe, M., Srinivasan, V., Gairy, P., & Sinclair, L. (2010). *Enhancing capacity for interprofessional collaboration: A resource to support program planning.* Toronto: Toronto Rehabilitation Institute.

Maeno, T., Haruta, J., Takayashiki, A., Yoshimoto, H., Goto, R., & Maeno, T. (2019). Interprofessional education in medical schools in Japan. *PLoS One, 14*(1), 1–10. doi:10.1371/journal.pone.0210912 PubMed

Resnick, J. C. (2011). Increasing opportunity through interdisciplinary research: Climbing down and shattering a tower of babel. *Frontiers in Psychiatry, 2.* doi:10.3389/ fpsyt.2011.00020 PubMed

Sinclair, L., Lowe, M., Paulenko, T., & Walczak, A. (2007). *Facilitating interprofessional clinical learning: Interprofessional education placements and other opportunities.* Toronto: University of Toronto, Office of Interprofessional Education.

Zorek, J., & Raehl, C. (2013). Interprofessional education accreditation standards in the USA: A comparative analysis. *Journal of Interprofessional Care, 27*(2), 123–130. doi:10.3109/13561820.2012.718295 PubMed

KEY TERMS AND DEFINITIONS

Chronic Disease/Chronic Condition: A health condition that has one or more of the following characteristics: permanent; leaves lingering disability; non-reversible pathological condition.

Collaboration: Collaboration implies two or more individuals working together for a desired outcome or goal. For this chapter, that goal is oriented toward improved patient health outcomes through a team-based approach to care.

Collaborative Research Practice: Occurs when researchers from more than one health-related profession engage in scientific inquiry to jointly create and disseminate new knowledge to clinical and research health professionals in order to provide the highest quality of patient care to improve population health outcomes.

Complex Chronic Disease/Complex Chronic Condition: Refers to a health condition that has one or more chronic diseases and one or more of the following characteristics: permanent; leaves lingering disability; non-reversible pathological condition; co-exists with a psychological illness.

Health Professions Students: Health professions students are learners from healthcare disciplines (e.g., dentistry, nursing, nutrition, medicine, pharmacy, physical therapy, radiology, health information management, and social work).

Interdisciplinary Research: Research that cuts across the disciplines and fosters the integration of ideas.

Interprofessional and Interdisciplinary Research Collaboration: Occurs when researchers from more than one profession or discipline work together to achieve the common goal of producing new scientific.

Interprofessional Collaborative Practice: Occurs when multiple health workers from different professional backgrounds work together with patients, families, caregivers and communities to deliver the highest quality of care.

Interprofessional Education: Occurs when students from two or more professions learn about, from and with each other to enable effective collaboration and improve health outcomes. Once students understand how to work interprofessionally, they are ready to enter the workplace as a member of the collaborative practice team.

Simulation: A pedagogical approach tailored to realistic scenarios in a safe, controlled environment for learners to demonstrate their knowledge and practice the learned skills without consequences of their actions.

Chapter 10
Overview of Professionalism Competence:
Bringing Balance to the Medical Education Continuum

Barry A. Doublestein
Regent University, USA

Walter T. Lee
Duke University Medical School, USA

Richard M. Pfohl
Leadership Peaks, LLC, USA

ABSTRACT

Lately, the term 'high-value care' has become a popular mantra among healthcare leaders and policymakers. These people claim that changes are necessary in healthcare to reduce costs, minimize overuse, and optimize outcomes. While few can argue that changes are needed in these areas, there is disagreement as to how to make the largest impact. The authors agree with those who believe that the greatest potential for success is found in professionalism improvements, not through payment or policy reforms. While medical education prides itself on producing highly competent and technically proficient physicians, it has generally neglected professionalism development considering these skills something to be acquired outside of formal medical education. The authors consider recent efforts to define professionalism competency and offer a useful model that brings parity to physician training. If professionalism is the bedrock of high-value care, the time has come to provide physicians with the skills to excel.

DOI: 10.4018/978-1-7998-2949-2.ch010

INTRODUCTION

Healthcare is an economic system which is engaged in a constant balancing act of providing care to people while making sure that reimbursements are sufficient to support the continuation of the infrastructure used to provide that care. By its nature, it depends upon profit in order to reinvest into research and development which brings about new technologies that make the care more efficient and effective. There is often friction between those that are concerned over the economic viability of the infrastructure through which patients receive care and those that carry out the processes that actually bring about the best health outcomes for their patients. While these providers are cognizant of the costs most of the time, they are often willing to do everything possible to bring about health and wellness as their primary purpose even when those costs are very high.

While the healthcare infrastructure is important to the delivery of care, it does not, on its own, provide value, for it only produces value when someone uses it to treat people. Jac Fitz-enz in his book, *The ROI of Human Capital: Measuring the Economic Value of Employee Performance*, says that people alone generate value. *People are the only element with the inherent power to generate value. All other variables—cash and its cousin credit, materials, plant and equipment, and energy—offer nothing but inert potentials. By their nature, they add nothing, and they cannot add anything until some human being, be it the lowest-level laborer, the most ingenious professional, or the loftiest executive, leverages that potential by putting it into play.* (Fitz-enz, 2000, p. xii). If it is people who put the potential into play, they alone, are the factor that determines the value of the patient/provider encounter. They also hold the power to stifle or damage value if they fail to *put the potential into play*.

Putting the potential into play, is fundamentally about being competent in the use of the 'tools-of-the-trade,' which are the technical skills used to provide care during the patient encounter. However, it is also about how those skills are carried out as the provider engages with patients and their families, peers, and fellow healthcare team members; something that is often overlooked or undervalued. These skills have often been called 'soft skills (McClelland, 1973; Goleman, 2013; Murphy, Putter, Johnson, 2014),' but use of the term offers up connotations of being somewhat subservient, or less important, than the technical skills. Nothing could be further from the truth; these skills are at least equally as important as the technical skills, and may even be more important as they relate to a 'value-added' experience for the patient.

Lately, the term, 'high-value care,' has become a popular mantra among healthcare leaders and health-policy makers. Those that use the term claim that changes are necessary to reduce costs, minimize overuse, and optimize outcomes throughout the US healthcare system (Marcotte, Moriates, Wolfson, Frankel, 2019). Marcotte, et al, however, claim that professionalism, not payment or policy reform, offers the greatest potential for improving healthcare outcomes. The authors of this chapter agree whole-heartedly with them that *professionalism is the bedrock of high-value care*. Therefore, the aim of this chapter, and its follow-up found in Chapter 11, is to offer a challenge to the medical education community to elevate the importance of these non-technical skills in the training of physicians, for it is here where the greatest potential for improvement of health outcomes is made.

Since the authors of this chapter believe that the term 'soft skills' inadequately describes the scope of their use, they propose the term, 'professionalism competence,' as an apt descriptor to cover these non-technical skills. Instead of ignoring or relegating professionalism competence to secondary status, its importance must be recognized and promoted throughout the medical education continuum, finally bringing long-overdue balance to training.

Unfortunately, the current medical education system is more focused on providing rising-physicians with the 'skills of the trade' (Cooke, Irby, O'Brien, 2010) than how those skills are used to provide value to the patient, their families, and fellow healthcare team members.

With medical knowledge growing at such a rapid pace (Glasziou, 2008), many medical school deans are flummoxed with how to integrate this rapid knowledge expansion into the medical school curriculum, which is focused on basic-science and clinical didactics, while balancing the expansion of clinical 'skills of the trade', all within a fixed period; four years of undergraduate medical education (UME). Lest the reader think that this problem is isolated to the UME portion of the medical education continuum, it simply is compounded during graduate medical education (GME) when the resident is expected to learn the lion's share of the 'skills of the trade' of their specialty.

From the outside looking in, one might think that implementing professionalism competency skill development in in both UME and GME might be a simple task, but it is more complicated than just adding new elements into the ongoing curriculum. The authors, in their expansive medical education experience, have had countless discussions with medical educators who confirm this conundrum. There is little time to teach everything that needs to be confronted in both the UME and GME environments from a technical perspective, let alone the professionalism competency skills expected as a pre-requisite to entry, even if they are rudimentary in practice. Byyny, Papadakis, and Paauw speak to this problem in their book: *Medical Professionalism: Best Practices* (2015). While medical schools would like to select students, who demonstrate competence in professional values and ethics, they depend more on academic performance for admission because they lack the tools that would help them in assessing competence. Competence models, however, have shown that academic success has little to do with predicting job performance success (Mount, 2005), rather non-academic abilities typically outweigh cognitive talents in the makeup of outstanding leaders (Goleman, 2013). In fact, Goleman states: *Academic intelligence has little to do with emotional life* (1995, p. 33). In a study done by the Hay Group, leaders who showed strengths in eight or more of their non-cognitive competencies (think: professionalism competence) created highly-energizing, top-performing climates (Hay Group, 2011; Goleman, 1998; Goleman, 2013). Unfortunately, leaders in this category are quite rare in that only 19% of studied executives attained this level.

For a number of reasons, medical education leaders expect that those entering their schools as physicians-in-training, or as residents, already demonstrate competency as it relates to these skills. Unfortunately, very few, as the Hay Study finds fall into this category. So, it makes sense to push the acquisition of these professionalism competence skills to the pre-medical school level, where prospective physicians are introduced to the skills required of practicing physicians.

This leaves a glaring question to be answered: is it possible to effectively translate professionalism competence knowledge into a practical development program that brings about change resulting in highly skilled, and technically and professionally competent practitioners? The answer to the question is a resounding, yes, but it requires the same level of commitment that has been given to technical-skill development for the past century of medical education's history. Some might argue that psychosocial development is fixed once one attains adulthood and any attempt to modify it is a losing endeavor and a waste of time. Fortunately, there is hope, for these skills can be taught and acquired and must be recognized as of equal importance in the medical education process (Goleman, 1995; Doublestein, Lee, Pfohl, 2015).

If, the US healthcare system hopes to achieve 'high-value care,' it must collectively demand that those entering the practice of medicine demonstrate outstanding professionalism competence. But, in order for that to happen, it bears repeating that the medical education community must elevate and promote the role of professionalism competency training throughout the medical education continuum. As Chip and Dan Heath suggest in their 2010 New York Times Bestseller, *Switch: How to Change Things When Change is Hard,* in order to bring about change, someone needs to act differently. If collective healthcare hopes to move into the new paradigm of 'high-value care,' the time has come to 'act differently' by ushering in this needed professionalism reform. But before any type of reform is discussed more completely, it is necessary to first provide an overview of the concept of professionalism in medical education, and second, to provide a more complete definition of professionalism competence.

CONSIDERING ELEMENTS RELATED TO 'SOFT SKILLS'

As stated earlier, the term, '*soft skills*' has been used in the past (McClelland, 1973; Goleman, 2013) to define these value-added skills, yet none offers an overarching and complete definition that satisfies the varied nature of the healthcare environment. They do, however, provide elements that play a part in what the authors call professionalism competence. Therefore, it would be prudent to consider how the literature and different industries define these skills, in part. A more complete and overarching definition follows, but one can see that the variety of elements makes any meaningful consensus difficult. Following are various elements:

1) Managing self, communicating, supporting, motivating, managing conflict (Pichler, Beenen, 2014; Beenen, Pichler, Davoudpour, 2018);

2) Sensitivity to others' needs, flexibility, perceptiveness, instilling trust in others, consistency across interactions, accountability, effective communication (Hogan, Lock, 1995);

3) Self-awareness, listening, helping, facilitating, asserting, influencing, negotiating, working with groups, and managing relationships (Hayes, 2002);

4) The five skills of communication: listening, oral, written, assertive, nonverbal (Klein, DeRouin, Salas, 2006);

5) The seven skills of relationship building: cooperation/coordination, trust, intercultural sensitivity, service orientation, self-presentation, social influence, conflict resolution/negotiation (Klein, DeRouin, Salas, 2006);

6) Communication and interpersonal skills (Murphy, Putter, Johnson, 2014);

7) Emotional Intelligence (Goleman, 1995); Goleman defines it as: *abilities such as being able to motivate oneself and persist in the face of frustrations; to control impulse and delay gratification; to regulate one's moods and keep distress from swamping the ability to think: to empathize and to hope* (p.34). In other words, emotional intelligence is a set of emotional and social skills that influence the way one perceives and expresses themselves, develops and maintains social relationships, copes with challenges, and uses emotional information in an effective and meaningful way. It has also been defined as the ability to understand and manage one's own emotions and those of the people around them (Doublestein, Pfohl, 2013).

8) Goleman further defined the four domains of emotional intelligence: self-awareness, self-management, social awareness, and relationship management. Within these four domains, he found twelve competencies (learned and learnable) that allow for outstanding performance at work or as a leader. These are: emotional self-awareness, emotional self-control, adaptability, achievement orientation, positive outlook, empathy, organizational awareness, influence,

coach and mentor, conflict management, teamwork, inspirational leadership (Goleman, Boyatzis, 2017);

9) The American Board of Internal Medicine (ABIM) went one step further in their *ABIM Physician Charter* by defining professionalism through a series of fundamental principles:

    a.   Primacy of patient welfare

    b.   Patient autonomy

    c.   Social justice

10) It went on to define nine professional responsibilities expected of physicians:

    a.   Professional competence – through a commitment to lifelong learning the medical knowledge and clinical and team skills necessary for the provision of quality care through demonstrated competency.

    b.   Honesty with patients

    c.   Confidentiality

    d.   Maintaining appropriate relations with patients

    e.   Improving quality of care

    f.   Improving access to care

    g.   A just distribution of finite resources

    h.   Scientific knowledge

    i.   Maintaining trust by managing conflicts of interest (ABIM Foundation, 2005);

11) While Abraham Flexner, the author of the much-heralded report on the condition of medical education in the US and Canada, did not specifically deal with the '*soft-skills*' of physician education, he did, however, deal with what he called: professional formation (1910). The term referred to establishment of a set of standards expected of practicing physicians. In a sense, it deals with the traits, trappings, and traditions of physician-hood. Although it was not his intention to tackle problems beyond a few decades after the publication of his report (Ludmerer, 1999), his original recommendations became the standard for medical education at least until the centennial follow-up report was published in 2010. This follow-up report spoke of the need for clear demonstration of competence in *personal characteristics to ensure lifelong commitment to the aspirational goals of excellence, accountability, humanism, altruism, and continued progress toward expertise after completion of training* (Cooke, Irby, O'Brien, 2010, p. 146).

While this is not an exhaustive list of elements of '*soft skills*, each aid in understanding the broad scope of what is expected of high-performing physician leaders. One thing that is clear about attempting to define professionalism in medicine is that there is a considerable difference of opinion across the literature, as to its scope. There appears to be a divide over whether it should be viewed as a set of attributes or an overarching ethos that grounds the practice of medicine (Birden, Glass, Wilson, Harrison, Usherwood, Nass, 2014). The ABIM report (2005) underscores this point in that it focuses on professional responsibilities required of competent physicians, rather than a set of skills or characteristics.

Many seem to agree that the focus of any conversations about professionalism in medicine is best reflected in the term professional identity formation (Weld, 2015; Cooke, Irby, O'Brien, 2010). Weld (2015) believes that the end of professional identity formation is the creation of a humanistic, ethically vigilant, reflective, socially responsive and responsible, resilient health care professional. While the authors of this chapter would not disagree with Weld, for they believe competent physicians should hold the characteristics of which he speaks as ultimate expressions of their formation. However, professionalism competency is more than acquiring and practicing the traits, trappings, and traditions of being a physician. Rather, the authors believe that professionalism is a set of high performing actions practiced with skill as one engages with patients, peers, and members of the healthcare team. People operating in accordance with these high performing actions reflect the various characteristics to which Weld refers. The authors are focused on developing the skills that, when practiced consistently, result in highly competent humanistic, ethically vigilant, reflective, socially responsive and responsible, resilient physicians.

AN OVERARCHING DEFINITION OF PROFESSIONALISM COMPETENCE

Professionalism competence defines the non-technical skills necessary for maximizing patient care in the 21st Century. It is comprised of a series of elements centered around the amended Miller's Prism of Clinical Competence (Cruess, Cruess, Steinert, 2016) in which the ultimate goal of clinical competence is to attain the '*Is*' level. The ultimate end of medical education competence is not accomplished by one merely moving through Miller's four-steps to clinical competence: *Knows* (knowledge); *Knows How* (Competence); *Shows How* (Performance); and *Does* (Action). Rather the ultimate goal of medical education is for the physician to *Be* a physician – that is to consistently demonstrate the attitudes, values, and behaviors expected of one who has come to think, act, and feel like a physician (Cruess, Cruess, Steinert, 2016).

The authors of this chapter began discussions in early 2012 about putting together a model of professionalism competence that would provide a useable framework from which to assess and guide any specific physician-in-training. The substance of the Professionalism Intelligence Model (PIM) is found in the following two phrases: *Behaviors are conditioned by how one thinks and feels and guided by a certain set of virtues* (Doublestein, Lee, Pfohl, 2015); and, *Every physician is a leader* (as in self-leadership, leadership in the patient relationship, team leadership, and vocational or avocational leadership) (Doublestein, Pfohl, 2013). Professionalism competence is about striving for balance across three intelligences: cognitive (CI), emotional (EI), and leadership (LI), while being guided by a certain set of virtues.

The first component of the model deals with Cognitive Intelligence (CI) *How One Thinks.* One should not make the mistake of believing that CI is the same thing as IQ. On one hand, IQ is a measure of an individual's personal information bank which includes their memory, vocabulary, and visual-motor coordination (Stein, Book, 2003). On the other hand, CI is about how one handles or expresses that personal information as they go about their daily lives (Doublestein, Pfohl, 2013).

While there are more elements that encompass CI, the authors suggest that every physician should demonstrate a high level of cognition skill in at least the following five areas:

1. Focused Thinking – This competency deals with the question: *To what level am I able to block out distractions in order to think clearly?* Focused thinking, however, is not always about blocking out certain things that one might consider distractions, rather it is also about being able to determine if these seemingly identified distractions really are distractions or not; simultaneously processing in a way that is focused on the matter at hand.

2. Problem Solving – Deals with the question: *To what level am I able to break problems into elements and find a solution?* Problem-solving consists of five components: 1) the ability to dissect a problem into workable parts; 2) the ability to form questions from the workable parts; 3) the ability to identify causation; 4) the ability to seek and gather complete and accurate information; and, 5) the willingness to seek counsel.

3. Critical Thinking – Deals with the question: *To what level am I able to make clear and reasoned judgments?* Critical-thinking is an intellectually-disciplined process of actively and skillfully: 1) conceptualizing – forming an idea or a picture of something – making it possible to understand; 2) applying – putting two or more disparate pieces of information together in a way that makes it possible to understand; 3) analyzing – looking at data from various perspectives; not just from one view that might be based in self-bias; 4) synthesizing – taking these differing viewpoints and combining them to form a new thought or a new direction; and 5) evaluating data – asking if the information gleaned or generated fits the situation at hand. In summation, critical thinking is an intellectually-disciplined process which requires purposeful and genuine attention to intellectual pursuits.

4. <u>Decision-Making</u> – Deals with the question; *To what level can I make good decisions based upon known facts?* Decision-making involves certain fundamental elements, when combined that result in a process that consistently offers the participant with good results. The elements are recognizing: 1) that a decision must be made; 2) that information surrounding the problem must be gathered in a way that defines the problem correctly; 3) the need to take the gathered information and appraise or weigh its importance in bringing about a preferred future; 4) the motivations behind a particular decision; 5) the correct solution from the many options, for with the right information and the right motives, one can determine the best option; and, 6) that one must act – they cannot afford to sit back and hope that the problem goes away; they must be decisive.

5. <u>Explanation</u> – Deals with the question: *To what level can I offer a logical and well-thought out explanation of my actions?* This involves the ability to explain one's thoughts clearly and be able to understand the causes, context, and consequences of those thoughts while interacting with others. It is insufficient in itself to explain oneself clearly, rather it is about gaining a more complete understanding of the results of one's actions; which requires being continuously attuned to how someone else feels.

While an important part of one's success, both Goleman (1995) and McClelland (1973) have advocated that success in whatever a person does is not predicted by that person's IQ, or CI alone; rather successful leaders demonstrate a high level of emotional intelligence (EI) as well, underscoring that balance across various intelligences is necessary for success. Most see the value in a physician demonstrating expertise in these CI areas as they engage with patients and fellow-team members, but expertise here alone does not guarantee a successful engagement. Some readers will confirm in their own personal experience that a smart physician does not necessarily equate to one who demonstrates 'excellent bedside manner.

The second component of the PIM model deals with Emotional Intelligence (EI) *How One Feels.* Through extensive research, Goleman found that emotional competencies are twice as important in contributing to excellence as compared to pure intellect (1998). Goleman (1995) defines the essence of emotional intelligence as being aware of one's self and of others and being able to manage one's inner world and relationships with others.

While Goleman (1995) purports that EI has 12 domains, the authors suggest that every physician should, at least, demonstrate a high level of skill in the following five competencies:

1. Self-awareness – The ability to be aware of one's own deficiencies or shortcomings. High-performing leaders are aware of their limits so that they know where they need to improve or find someone with the skills, they may be lacking to work with them (Goleman, 1998). This factor is found to be the most important of all EI competencies (Goleman, 2013). It deals with the question: *To what extent do I understand my own self?* If one cannot understand their own self, how can they hope to understand others?

2. Self-regulation – Deals with the question: *To what level do I regulate my emotions?* It involves the ability of one to act consistently in their long-term best interest which is in accordance with their deepest values. This requires that a person develop a set of standards (values) by which they will operate on a day-to-day basis. These standards or values in essence establish the boundaries in which one will interact; being careful to not operate outside their standards. Self-regulation is the process of keeping one's actions within a defined set of parameters. The key here is found in the word: values, for it establishes the guidelines for action.

3. Interpersonal relationships – Deals with the question: *To what level do I interact with others?* It is about successfully developing and keeping enduring relationships with others. It includes: 1) being able to get along with others; 2) focusing on others and their needs over one's own; 3) attracting people with an engaging personality that is not mean-spirited or selfish; 4) being loyal to someone even in difficult times or when it might be inconvenient or financially not rewarding – it is about persevering in faith in others; and, 5) valuing the confidences of others.

4. Empathy – Deals with the question: *How strong is my empathy for others and their plights?* It is about understanding or feeling what another being is experiencing from that person's frame of reference. It is about placing oneself in another's position, or discerning what they are thinking or feeling. It is comprised of: 1) an ability to see the world from another's perspective; 2) having a desire to help others; 3) having concern over another's present condition; and, 4) willfully putting another person ahead of themselves.

5. Motivation – Deals with the questions: *To what level am I motivated to do my job? Am I committed?* It is about understanding the motivations behind one's service. Patients will follow a physician who demonstrates that their genuine motivation stems from serving them, as is the focus of servant-leadership theory (Greenleaf, 2002).

While these skills are valuable when engaging patients and fellow-team members, expertise in these areas without the added CI skills, in part, does not guarantee successful engagement, as well.

The third component of the model is Leadership Intelligence (LI) *How One Acts.* Jim Kouzes and Barry Posner (2010) in the early 1980s began searching out the characteristics of admired leaders. They sought to know what successful leaders do to *...inspire people to do things differently, to struggle against uncertain odds, and to persevere toward a misty image of a better future* (p.1). Their research over the last three decades across cultures, sex, and age groups, have found five practices (behaviors or acts) that leaders employ to make extraordinary things happen as they engage with others (Kouzes, Posner, 2012). Since the PIM is based upon the belief that all physicians are leaders, successful leaders should practice:

1. Embodiment – Modeling the behaviors expected of others. This competency deals with the question: *To what level do I model behaviors expected of others?* Few people will follow someone who is unwilling to do the things they expect of others. As an example, patients are less willing to comply with an obese physician's directives than one who is not (Phul, Gold, Leudicke, DePierre, 2013). Patients don't necessarily want to follow what one says, rather they want to follow their example.

2. Inspiration – Inspiring others to attain the best that they can be and encouraging them with a vision of what could be. This deals with the question: *To what level do I inspire others to be the best they can be?*

3. Excellence – Aspiring to achieve the best in everything they do. This also includes an element of dedication to a process of self-betterment. This deals with the question: *To what level am I committed to seeking excellence in all that I do?* A person dedicated to excellence is dissatisfied with the status quo, so they seek ways to improve.

4. Empowerment – Providing opportunities for others to act in ways that release them to be what they are intended to be, not merely replicas of the leader. These people are provided a goal for which to aspire while being freed to act in a personalized way, using the skills, talents, and personality they have to accomplish the shared goals or vision of the leader and the organization. This deals with the question: *To what level do I empower others to be and seek their best?*

5. Recognition – Recognizing people for their work or accomplishments. This deals with the question: *To what level do I recognize others and their accomplishments?*

While these skills are extremely valuable, they alone in themselves, do not guarantee success; but must be combined with one's high-performing cognitive and emotional intelligence characteristics in a way that finds balance such that the sum is greater than its individual parts.

The PIM has, at its center, the concept of the three intelligences being guided by a set of virtues. These are the guiding principles by which the person or that organization operates. Without a certain set of clearly-defined virtues, no one can be held accountable for how a specific physician *thinks (CI), feels (EI), or acts (LI)* (Cruess, Cruess, Steinert, 2016).

SUMMARY

While not an exhaustive study of professionalism, the authors have provided a fairly accurate overview of current thinking as it relates to the subject. First of all, few can argue that there is balance across the medical education continuum of focus on technical and professionalism competency skills. The authors believe that this imbalance is not caused by some sinister conspiracy of neglect, but rather related to a need to focus on integrating rapid technological advancements into an ever-expanding curriculum.

Second, if Marcotte, Moriates, Wolfson, and Frankel (2019) are correct in their claim that professionalism, not payment or policy reform, offers the greatest potential for improving healthcare outcomes, failing to consider its importance in patient care is the ultimate form of malpractice. Medical education leadership can no longer neglect finding ways to integrate professionalism competency education into physician development.

Third, because the subject of professionalism competence, as a vital component of physician development, is a relatively new concept, it may seem premature to settle on one unifying model or definition that settles the argument. The authors, however, believe that their model of professionalism competence offers a practical framework around which action can be taken immediately to deal with the rebalancing of medical education's focus on skill development.

In this chapter, the authors provided their Professionalism Intelligence Model as one way to define professionalism competence. This model deals directly with the skills that the competent physician demonstrates as they attain the ultimate goal of medical education; that is to consistently demonstrate the attitudes, values, and behaviors expected of one who has come to think, act, and feel like a physician (Cruess, Cruess, Steinert, 2016).

In Chapter 11, the authors take the concept of professionalism competence further as they discuss the most significant barrier to professionalism competency development in the medical education continuum, the benefits to implementing professionalism competency training, a short case study on a successful professionalism competency-based program, and provide a few recommendations to bring about reform.

REFERENCES

ABIM Foundation. (2005). *Medical Professionalism in the New Millennium: A Physician Charter.* American Board of Internal Medicine Foundation. Available from: https://abimfoundation.org/wp-content/uploads/2015/12/Medical-Professionalism-in-the-New-Millenium-A-Physician-Charter.pdf. Accessed: August, 2019.

Beenen, G., Pichler, S., & Davoudpour, S. (2018). Interpersonal Skills in MBA Admission: How Are They Conceptualized and Assessed? *Journal of Management Education, 42*(1), 34–54. doi:10.1177/1052562917703743

Birden, H., Glass, N., Wilson, I., Harrison, M., Usherwood, T., & Nass, T. (2014). Defining professionalism in medical education: A systematic review. *Medical Teacher, 36*(1), 47–61. doi:10.3109/0142159X.2014.850154 PMID:24252073

Byyny, R., Papadakis, M., & Paauw, D. (Eds.). (2015). *Medical Professionalism: Best Practices.* Menlo Park, CA: Alpha Omega Alpha Honor Medical Society.

Cooke, M., Irby, D. M., & O'Brien, B. C. (2010). *Educating Physicians: A Call for Reform of Medical School and Residency. The Carnegie Foundation for the Advancement of Teaching.* San Francisco, CA: Jossey-Bass.

Cruess, R., Cruess, S., & Steinert, Y. (2016). Amending Miller's Pyramid to Include Professional Identity Formation. *Academic Medicine, 91*(2), 180–185. doi:10.1097/ACM.0000000000000913 PMID:26332429

Doublestein, B., Lee, W., & Pfohl, R. (2015). Healthcare 2050: Anticipatory Leadership. In *Critical Challenges, Key Contexts, and Emerging Trends.* Emerald.

Doublestein, B., & Pfohl, R. (2013). *Leadership Lived Out: Training Exemplary Resident Leaders.* Faculty Planning Meeting (July 13). Department of Otolaryngology: Head & Neck Surgery, Duke Medical School.

Fitz-enz, J. (2000). *The ROI of Human Capital: Measuring the Economic Value of Employee Performance.* New York, NY: AMACOM.

Flexner, A. (1910). *Medical Education in the United States and Canada.* New York, NY: The Carnegie Foundation for the Advancement of Teaching.

Glasziou, P. (2008). Evidence based medicine and the medical curriculum. *BMJ (Clinical Research Ed.), 337.* PMID:18815165

Goleman, D. (1995). *Emotional Intelligence: Why It Can Matter More Than IQ.* New York, NY: Bantam Books.

Goleman, D. (1998). *Working with Emotional Intelligence*. New York, NY: Bantam Books.

Goleman, D. (2013). *Focus: The Hidden Driver of Excellence*. New York, NY: Harper.

Goleman, D., & Boyatzis, R. (2017). Emotional Intelligence Has 12 Elements. Which Do You Need to Work On? *Harvard Business Review*. Available from: https://hbr.org/2017/02/emotional-intelligence-has-12-elements-which-do-you-need-to-work-on

Greenleaf, R. (2002). *Servant Leadership: A Journey into the Nature of Legitimate Power and Greatness 25th Anniversary Edition*. Paulist Press.

Hay Group. (2011). *Emotional and social competency inventory (ESCI): A user guide for accredited practitioners*. Available from: http://eiconsortium.org/pdf/ESCI_user_guide.pdf

Hayes, J. (2002). *Interpersonal skills at work* (2nd ed.). New York, NY: Routledge. doi:10.4324/9780203465783

Heath, C., & Heath, D. (2010). *Switch: How to Change Things When Change is Hard*. New York, NY: Broadway Books.

Hogan, J., & Lock, J. (1995, May). *A taxonomy of interpersonal skills for business interactions*. Paper presented at the 10th Annual Conference of the Society for Industrial and Organizational Psychology, Orlando, FL.

Klein, C., DeRouin, R., & Salas, E. (2006). Uncovering workplace interpersonal skills: A review, framework, and research agenda. *International Review of Industrial and Organizational Psychology, 21*, 80–126.

Kouzes, J., & Posner, B. (2010). *The Truth About Leadership: The No-fads Heart-of-the-Matter Facts You Need to Know*. San Francisco, CA: Jossey-Bass.

Kouzes, J., & Posner, B. (2012). *The Leadership Challenge: How to Make Extraordinary Things Happen in Organizations* (5th ed.). San Francisco, CA: Jossey-Bass.

Ludmerer, K. M. (1999). *Time to Heal: American Medical Education from the Turn of the Century to the Era of Managed Care*. New York, NY: Oxford University Press.

Marcotte, L., Moriates, C., Wolfson, D., & Frankel, R. (2019). Professionalism as the Bedrock of High-Value Care. *Academic Medicine*. Available from: https://journals.lww.com/academicmedicine/Abstract/publishahead/Professionalism_as_the_Bedrock_of_High_Value_Care.97538.aspx

McClelland, D. C. (1973, January). Testing for Competence Rather Than for 'Intelligence.' *The American Psychologist, 28*(1), 1–14. doi:10.1037/h0034092 PMID:4684069

Mount, G. (2005). The Role of Emotional Intelligence in Developing International Business Capability: EI Provides Traction. In *Linking Emotional Intelligence and Performance at Work.* Mahwah, NJ: Lawrence Erlbaum.

Murphy, S. E., Putter, S., & Johnson, S. (2014). Soft skills training: Best practices in industry and higher education. In R. E. Riggio & S. J. Tan (Eds.), *Leader interpersonal and influence skills: The soft skills of leadership* (pp. 276–310). New York, NY: Taylor & Francis.

Pichler, S., & Beenen, G. (2014). Toward the development of a model and a measure of managerial interpersonal skills. In R. E. Riggio & S. J. Tan (Eds.), *Leader interpersonal and influence skills: The soft skills of leadership* (pp. 11–30). New York, NY: Taylor & Francis.

Puhl, R., Gold, J., Luedicke, J., & DePierre, J. (2013). The effect of physicians' body weight on patient attitudes: implications for physician selection, trust and adherence to medical advice. *International Journal of Obesity, 37*(11), 1415-21.

Stein, S., & Book, H. (2003). *The EQ Edge: Emotional Intelligence and Your Success.* Toronto, Canada: Multi-Health Systems.

Weld, H. (2015, June). Professional Identity (Trans)Formation in Medical Education. *Academic Medicine, 90*(6), 701–706. doi:10.1097/ACM.0000000000000731 PMID:25881651

ADDITIONAL READING

Cooke, M., Irby, D. M., & O'Brien, B. C. (2010). *Educating Physicians: A Call for Reform of Medical School and Residency. The Carnegie Foundation for the Advancement of Teaching.* San Francisco, CA: Jossey-Bass.

Goleman, D. (2006). Social Intelligence: The New Science of Human Relationships. New York. NY: Bantam.

Kouzes, J., & Posner, B. (2012). *The Leadership Challenge: How to Make Extraordinary Things Happen in Organizations* (5th ed.). San Francisco, CA: Jossey-Bass.

Quinn, R. (2000). *Change the World: How Ordinary People Can Accomplish Extraordinary Results*. San Francisco, CA: Jossey-Bass.

Schein, E. (1992). *Organizational Culture and Leadership* (2nd ed.). San Francisco, CA: Jossey-Bass.

KEY TERMS AND DEFINITIONS

Clinical Competence: The end result of clinical medical education in which the physician *becomes* a physician – where they consistently demonstrate the attitudes, values, and behaviors expected of one who has come to think, act, and feel like a physician (Cruess, Cruess, & Steinert, 2016).

Cognitive Intelligence (CI): CI, is one equally important element of the Professionalism Intelligence Model. It is focused on how one *Thinks as a physician.* While IQ is a measure of an individual's personal information bank which includes their memory, vocabulary, and visual-motor coordination (Stein & Book, 2003) CI is about how one handles or expresses that personal information as they go about their daily lives (Doublestein & Pfohl, 2013).

Emotional Intelligence (EI): EI is one equally important element of the Professionalism Intelligence Model. It is focused on how one *feels as a physician.* EI is being aware of one's self and of others and being able to manage one's inner world and relationships with others (Goleman, 1995).

High-Value Care: Healthcare to patients which is cost-conscience, coordinated, and highly-efficient resulting in optimized outcomes. This type of care is focused on best practices from a technical and delivery perspective. Some believe high-value care is advanced through payment or policy reform. While important, its greatest opportunity for reform comes through professionalism advancements (Marcotte, Moriates, Wolfson, & Frankel, 2019). Professionalism is the bedrock of high-value care.

Leadership Intelligence (LI): LI is one equally important element of the Professionalism Intelligence Model. It is focused on how one *Acts as a physician.* LI consists of practices (behaviors or acts) that leaders employ to make extraordinary things happen as they engage with others (Kouzes & Posner, 2012).

Professional Competence: The term used to define the skills necessary to deliver high-value care. Professionalism competence is a set of high performing non-technical actions practiced with skill as one engages with patients, peers, and members of the healthcare team. People operating in accordance with these high-performing actions result in highly competent humanistic, ethically vigilant, reflective, socially responsive and responsible, resilient physicians (Weld, 2015). These skills transcend the traits, trappings, and traditions of being a physician.

Chapter 11
Professionalism Competence:
Its Role in Bringing About High-Value Care – A Case Study

Barry A. Doublestein
Regent University, USA

Walter T. Lee
Duke University Medical School, USA

Richard M. Pfohl
Leadership Peaks, LLC, USA

ABSTRACT

The existing medical education paradigm is not structured in a way that prepares future physicians with knowledge or the skill set to excel in professionalism. The authors provide information in the form of a case study of a professionalism competency development program that was undertaken in the Duke University Medical School Division of Head and Neck Surgery and Communications Sciences, barriers found that impede development, and offer five reforms that are necessary in order to bring about the movement toward high-value care. The authors propose to 1) prioritize professionalism competency training in medical education, 2) make curricular revisions to promote professionalism competency training across the continuum, 3) revise selection criteria for entrance to the profession that deals with basic professionalism skills, 4) institute new prerequisite requirements for entrance to the profession centered on professionalism competency, and 5) require professionalism competency training as part of certification and re-certification processes.

DOI: 10.4018/978-1-7998-2949-2.ch011

INTRODUCTION

As the authors discussed in Chapter 10, medical education has arrived at a critical stage in which circumstances are demanding reform in how future physicians and residents are trained. Rising costs, an aging patient population, physician shortages, and reliance on an outdated education paradigm are some of the things that are structurally standing in the way of *high-value care* outcomes. As Marcotte, Moriates, Wolfson, and Frankel (2019) suggest, *high-value care* will not find its greatest potential through policy or payment reforms, but through professionalism reform. The existing medical education paradigm is not structured in a way that prepares future physicians with knowledge or the skill set to excel in professionalism. This chapter intends to provide information in the form of a case study of a professionalism competency development program that was undertaken in the Duke University Medical School – Division of Head and Neck Surgery and Communication Sciences (Duke – HNSCS) called: Leadership Lived Out® (LLO®), barriers found that impede development, and five reforms that the authors believe are necessary in order to bring about the movement toward *high-value care*.

In 2013, the authors of this chapter began a program designed to improve professionalism competence in the Duke University Medical School – Division of Head and Neck Surgery and Communication Sciences. The program concept began as a proactive endeavor to bring about a division-wide commitment to excellence in patient care.

The first step in creating the program was to identify a set of virtues that the division agreed would guide those involved in patient care. They chose: integrity, initiative, self-discipline, responsibility (later changed to: compassion), and accountability (Lee, 2013). In a sense, all thoughts, actions, engagements, and decisions are judged, or guided through these shared virtues. Without these fundamental virtues guiding behavior, it would be impossible to grow or learn as individuals or as an organization. These shared virtues provide a definable set of standards that in essence are the worldview from and through which all interact and are held accountable.

So, Duke – HNSCS values: integrity, initiative, self-discipline, compassion, and accountability, while another institution or department might value: honesty, competence, respect, grace, or justice. What matters most is that there is an established set of virtues moderating or guiding action and setting the standards for professionalism competence. The purpose of these virtues is to set a standard of greatness, a goal for all to achieve which results in better people, teams and organizations. With these virtues as guiding principles driving how one thinks, feels or acts, others are able to determine through observation whether one is truly thinking, feeling, or acting from an intrinsic perspective or from one imposed (or expected) by others. The underlying motivation matters for intrinsic-based actions outlast those which are extrinsically imposed (Pink, 2011). So, by identifying Duke – HNSCS virtues, the authors were able to establish the foundational principles against which all division employees' behaviors could be evaluated.

The LLO® program offered the authors an excellent opportunity to practically apply the concept that *behaviors are conditioned by how one thinks and feels and guided by a certain set of virtues* (Doublestein, Lee, Pfohl, 2015), the substance of the Professionalism Intelligence Model (PIM) which is described more fully in Chapter 10. Once basic foundational virtues were identified, the next step in the process was to find a way to assess each program participant's professional competence as it relates to the major cognitive, emotional, and leadership intelligence scales and their respective sub-scales. To accomplish this, the authors developed the Professionalism Quotient Inventory (PQ-i), with its two component parts; the PQ-i – Self and the PQ-i – 360. The PQ-i – Self establishes how one assesses their actions across the five subscales of each of the Cognitive, Emotional, and Leadership Intelligences. The PQ-i – 360 provides feedback from individuals to whom the participant looks for leadership, are among their peers, and those to whom the participant provides leadership. Data from the two parts are comingled to provide a report that focuses on the participant's areas of agreement and gaps (as to how they and others see them). The open-ended section of the PQ-i – 360 offers excellent insights that help to bring clarity about what the raters observe about the participant's cognitive, emotional and leadership intelligences. One strength of the PQ-i assessment tool is that it provides a unique snapshot specifically tailored to a particular participant.

Once the report is produced, participants meet with a coach to: 1) discuss report findings, 2) help guide the participant to discovering strategies that would overcome the identified gaps or reinforce the agreements; and, 3) to debrief regarding the success of the strategies and find ways to modify them if necessary. This phase of the program is individually applied (for no two people experience the same level of professionalism competence).

The LLO® program led to the formation of the process of professionalism competency development which yielded a series of steps through which one must go in order to advance in competence. There are no shortcuts in that each step leads to the next, in a cyclical progression, gaining more expertise as they continually progress. The professionalism competence cycle contains the following steps:

1) <u>Self-assessment</u> – This step equates to Miller's first stage of clinical competence – *Knows* (Miller, 1990). It is here that one begins to understand how they and others see them across the three intelligences and their corresponding sub-scales.

2) <u>Self-awareness</u> – This step is extremely important for it is here that one begins to take knowledge and accept it as reality. It equates to Miller's second stage of clinical competence – *Knows How* (Miller, 1990). These first two stages are about discovery.

3) <u>Self-analysis</u> – This step is where one accepts or approves of provided gaps and agreements discovered during the self-assessment process. This is the end stage of single-loop learning (Argyris, 1977) in which the learned information will not bring about change unless it is applied. It is here where one must make a willful decision to apply the knowledge gained to lead to betterment. This step equates to Miller's third stage of clinical competence – *Shows How* (Miller, 1990). Famed psychologist, Carl Rogers, underscores the value of this stage to bring about change when he said: *We cannot change, we cannot move away from what we are, until we thoroughly accept what we are. Then change seems to come about almost unnoticed* (1961, p. 1).

4) <u>Self-improvement strategy</u> – This step is where one considers the development of strategies to either reinforce agreements or improve gaps uncovered during the discovery process. If the goal is to advance in professionalism competence, one must develop and practice actions that will move them from complaisance to excellence. This stage equates to Miller's final stage of clinical competence – *Does* (Miller, 1990).

5) <u>Evaluation</u> – This step is where one considers whether their improvement strategies have brought about professionalism improvement. If successful, one will consider ways to continuously improve on those strategies, ultimately leading to overall professionalism growth. If not successful, one would identify new ways to bring about the needed improvement. This stage equates to Cruess, et al's final stage of Miller's model of clinical competence (amended) – *Is* (Cruess, Cruess, Steinert, 2016). Those dedicated to betterment are constantly considering how they can improve as they move along in practice.

The latter two steps in the professionalism competence cycle are part of the double-loop learning proposed by Argyris (1977). The things learned here are run back through the cycle for further refinement and improvement.

The best leaders are learners (Kouzes, Posner, 2010). As such, the process of professionalism competency development requires that people within the organization are committed to learning. It is important for the medical educator to remember that one purpose of medical education is to take people from novice to expert (Miller, 1990). The process of moving people along this continuum is often fueled by failure, the very thing that physicians hope never happens. But it is often inevitable, and as such, it is important to process every failure, large or small, in a way that maximizes learning opportunities (Edmondson, 2012). Organizations or institutions that maximize learning opportunities are those that leverage their failures and seek the best in their people and processes (Senge, 1990).

And, learning institutions are 'safe' places where psychological safety is practiced (Edmondson, 2012). Leape, Shore, Dienstag, Mayer, Edgman-Levitan, Meyer, and Healy (2012) speak to the dangers associated with psychologically-unsafe cultures in medicine. Patient safety is negatively impacted when widespread disrespect for patients, peers and fellow-team members is found across the culture. Disrespect has no place in the medical education continuum and is clearly an enemy to *high-value care* and professionalism competence. Unfortunately, disrespect can be found in even the best organizations; something that cannot and should not be tolerated at all.

In summary, the PIM is about an individual seeking balance across how their three intelligences (cognitive, emotional, and leadership) form them as individuals for success. There is one remaining factor, however, that one must also consider when attempting to define professionalism competence. While the PIM is about personal competence, one must also consider that people do not act in a vacuum for every engagement is social. One might be moving along the novice-to-expert continuum gaining the hoped-for movement toward personal excellence, yet still fail in engagements with patients, peers, and fellow-team members. This happens because people must also have a separate set of skills that aid them as they engage one another in the social construct. Therefore, it is important to place the PIM in the social economy for it does not reside in isolation. Unless an individual understands that every interaction takes place in a social construct that requires individuals to be operating at a high-performing level, seeking professionalism competency is a hollow endeavor. Daniel Goleman calls these social skills, Social Intelligence (2006). He says that every interaction has an emotional subtext in that whatever one is doing as they engage with others; they are able to *make each other feel a little better, or even a lot better, or a little worse—or a lot worse* (Goleman, 2006, p.14).

So, it is most important for the reader to understand that having high-value technical skills and professionalism competence alone (outside of the social construct) is well and good, however, better is practice of those traits skillfully and properly as one engages with another.

Social Intelligence used to be folded into the Emotional Intelligence construct, but Goleman (2006) found that in the human aptitude for relationship there are two distinct categories relating to social engagement: 1) Social awareness, and 2) Social facility.

Social awareness refers to a variety of abilities that run from being able to instantaneously sense another's inner state, to understanding their feelings and thoughts, and finally to understanding complicated social situations. Goleman identifies four categories of awareness: 1) *primal empathy* – which is about feeling with others by sensing non-verbal emotional signals; 2) *attunement* – which is about listening with full receptivity by attuning oneself to another; 3) *empathic accuracy* – which is about understanding another's thoughts, feelings, and intentions; and, 4) *social cognition* – which is about knowing how the social world works.

Social facility builds upon social awareness to allow smooth and effective interactions. It is not sufficient in itself to be able to simply sense how others feel, or know what they intend, rather, social facility involves: 1) synchrony – interacting with others smoothly at the nonverbal level; 2) *self-presentation* – presenting oneself effectively as they engage with others; 3) *influence* – being able to shape outcomes of social interactions; and, 4) *concern* – caring about others' needs and taking actions that demonstrate concern.

The key point here is to remember that professionalism competence is about practicing balance across the three intelligences *while* engaging with others, whether they are patients, peers, or fellow-healthcare team members. If one fails to practice professionalism competence in social interactions, they fail to bring about *high-value care*.

BARRIER TO PROFESSIONALISM COMPETENCE

In the early stages of the LLO® professionalism competency program, the authors discovered that success was predicated on each participant's level of commitment to self-betterment. Some involved in the program saw it as one more item to check off their list of 'items required for graduation.' Some took the attitude of 'I'll do whatever you want me to do, just tell me what I need to do.' This clearly is not the end goal of professionalism competency, for it gives the impression that the end-stage of Miller's Prism of Clinical Competence, the Action stage: *Does* demonstrates their competence; negating the importance of why they are performing their actions, whether they come from personal commitment to excellence or from some outside set of rules or expectations. Professionalism competence is something that is expected to flow from an intrinsic desire to *Be* – that is to think, feel, and act as a physician (Cruess, Cruess, Steinert, 2016; Doublestein, Lee, Pfohl, 2015).

The major barrier to professionalism competency efforts is found in this willful commitment by each individual to self-betterment. Unfortunately, very few people are committed to this process. If one were to use goal-setting as a benchmark to determine commitment to self-betterment, only 30% of people set goals, with only 20% of them accomplishing them, resulting in a mere 6 in 100 achieving them (Vermeeren, 2007). In another study, Schwantes (2016) reports similar findings in that only 8 in 100 achieve their goals.

Argyris and Schon (1974) argue that everyone has an *espoused theory* (as to how they claim to behave) and a *theory in action* (as to how they actually behave). They contend that most are unaware of this discrepancy and that this personal condition has a collective outcome that complicates matters. It results in miscommunication, self-fulfilling prophecies, and escalating errors. These people fizzle out before they achieve their personal or collective potential. Argyris later contends that there is a universal pattern in professional life, a set of values, around which people tend to organize their lives:

1) To remain in control;
2) To win;
3) To suppress negative feelings; and,
4) To pursue rational objectives (Argyris, 1991).

Anything that suggests failure throughout this pattern, is seen as a threat and is avoided as all costs, just when transformation is about to happen – they fail to transform. As medical educators, it is imperative to fully understand why so few desire the transformation necessary to bring professionalism competence to the practice of medicine on a daily basis.

Robert Fritz (1989) offers one possible reason why so few want to transform. He says that people make three types of choices as they engage on a day-to-day basis; fundamental, primary, and secondary. He describes the difference between making the primary choice of becoming a physician (being married, or making a religious choice), and making the fundamental choice of living by the principles of that choice; that is living one's life, filtering all decisions or actions, through the lens of the worldview governing the decision (fundamental choice). Some like the thought of being a physician (altruism, lifestyle, career challenge, financial reward), yet follow a path that often opposes the very nature of the idealized physician character. This is often perpetuated throughout the medical education continuum through socialization by means of the *hidden curriculum* (Mahood, 2011; Haferty, 1998).

The *hidden curriculum* is more of a socialization process than it is a transmission of knowledge or skills (Mahood, 2011). In essence, it is about the transmission of norms and values that undermine the formal message. It is devious for it is taught and perpetuated implicitly by example. While medical students and residents are often taught that empathy for patients and their conditions are paramount in providing excellent care, they are often called out for being unprofessional when displaying emotions as they empathize. This process is akin to what happens when children watch their parents' actions as opposed to what they say.

Lest the reader minimize the impact of the *hidden curriculum* in professionalism competence they need to consider that there are serious ramifications associated with its practice:

1) It causes students (residents included) to move from being open-minded to closed-minded;
2) They move from being intellectually curious to narrowly focused on facts;
3) They move from empathy to emotional detachment;
4) They move from idealism to cynicism;
5) They move from civility and caring to arrogance and irritability; and
6) It causes an erosion of ethics (Mahood, 2011).

Feundtner, Christakis, and Christakis (1994) found that 62% of medical students had done unethical behaviors because of the pressures exerted through the *hidden curriculum*. Some of these behaviors are: pretending to examine patients or making up vitals, ignoring contamination, obtaining informed consent without knowledge of the procedure, withholding results from patients, and doing unnecessary procedures for experience.

Unless professionalism competence is reinforced at all levels of the medical education continuum, including at the *hidden curriculum* level, *high-value care* will never be attainable. There is no middle ground, one is either transformed at the fundamental level, or not.

BENEFITS OF PROFESSIONALISM COMPETENCY TRAINING

One cannot ignore the benefits of professionalism competency training to the practice of medicine as physicians begin to put the 'potential into play (Fitz-enz, 2000)' that results in a new culture of *high-value care*. This does not take place by accident, rather it requires a true commitment to excellence beyond just the technical-skill training processes of the past. For when this new culture begins to take hold, the change for which many have longed comes as an unstoppable avalanche. Professionalism competency positively impacts patient safety (Leape, Shore, Dienstag, Mayer, Edgman-Levitan, Meyer, Healy, 2012), patient satisfaction (Lee, 2004), more productive teams (Lencioni, 2012), well-rounded and balanced physicians between technical and professionalism competency skills (Doublestein, Lee, Pfohl, 2015), and transformed physicians and cultures (Doublestein, Lee, Pfohl, 2015). It also deals with unprofessional attitudes or instances immediately rather than 'kicking the proverbial can down the road' hoping that someone else will confront professionalism lapses (Papadakis, Teherani, Banach, Knettler, Rattner, Stern, 2005).

If professionalism competency is the bedrock of *high-value care* (Marcotte, Moriates, Wolfson, Frankel, 2019), its practice will bring about a second revolution on par with the impact of Abraham Flexner's report (1910) as it changed the fundamental nature of medical education, and therefore, the practice of medicine.

INTEGRATING PROFESSIONALISM COMPETENCY INTO THE MEDICAL EDUCATION CONTINUUM

A workable solution to bringing about this necessary professionalism competency reform would be for collective medical education to agree to pursue the following recommendations:

1) *Prioritize professionalism competency training* – The first step in the process of reform is to agree that the time has come to elevate the role of professionalism competency in the practice of medicine. Cooke, Irby, and O'Brien (2010) call out for an expansion on Flexner's original recommendation on professional formation. They suggest the five following actions:

   a. Offering formal ethics instruction;
   b. Confronting the underlying messages expressed in the hidden curriculum and find ways to align espoused values with actual clinical practice;
   c. Promoting more role-modeling experiences between faculty and students that offer accountability for holding them to high moral standards;
   d. A high commitment to excellence and continuous improvement; and,
   e. Developing feedback and opportunities for reflection and assessment of professionalism in the context of longitudinal mentoring and advising.

   These recommendations deal with issues equally as important as technical skill development. In fact, each have elements associated with leadership training; something that Cooke, Irby, and O'Brien suggest is an underdeveloped skill and needs attention (2010).

2) *Make curricular revisions to promote professionalism competency training* – As discussed in Chapter 10, many medical school deans are flummoxed with how to integrate more into a process that is already at maximum overload. While this appears to be true, professionalism competency training can easily be integrated across the medical education continuum if it is prioritized as a skill to be developed. It can be integrated across all clinical rotations and be made an integral part of the clinical evaluation process. Making curricular changes in this way elevates professionalism competency just as technical

240

skill revisions are made from time to time, resulting in new standards of care. Another component of this recommendation is to actively integrate highly-professional role models throughout the medical education continuum (Kenny, Mann, MacLeod, 2003).

3) *Change selection criteria for entrance to the profession* – As stated earlier in this chapter, the present selection process for entry into UME and GME is heavily weighted toward academic credentials. Byyny, Papadakis, and Paauw (2015) suggest that this is because many believe that there are few tools available through which professionalism competency can be assessed. Assessment tools can be developed, like the PQ-i – Self and 360 that adequately provide admission committees with a glimpse into an applicant's level of professionalism competence prior to admission. As discussed earlier, professionalism competency, like other technical skills, fall along the medical education continuum and some enter the system as a novice, while others are more advanced. Knowing where the applicant falls in specific aspects of professionalism competence aids the educator in where to place emphasis for each to move along the continuum toward expert.

4) *Institute new prerequisite requirements for entrance to the profession* – Papadakis, Teherani, Banach, Knettler, Rattner, and Stern (2005) found a correlation between professionalism lapses in medical school and residency with state medical board actions later in practice. They suggested that earlier intervention in the medical education continuum would reduce incidence of action later in practice. The authors of this chapter suggest that introduction to professionalism competency training is best handled at the pre-medical level of education. It is generally here where prospective students begin the process of preparing for the rigorous challenge of medical school from an academic perspective, so it makes sense that during this time, the prospective student is introduced to professionalism competency expectations as well. To aid pre-medical programs with this new prerequisite, a standardized program of instruction, similar to the LLO®, would be provided for students in an online format that centers on the goals and objectives of professionalism in medicine.

5) *Require professionalism competency training as part of certification and re-certification processes* – While professionalism competency training is interwoven into the pre-medical, UME, and GME structure, it should also be a requirement for certification and re-certification through continuing medical education programs. Once professionalism competency training is brought to equal status with technical skills training throughout medical education, ease of integration into future practice standards is uncomplicated.

Making these reforms will change the very nature and culture of physician engagement across the practice of medicine, ushering in a new level of *high-value care*, previously unseen. While to some, these reforms may seem unattainable because of lack of consensus of definition, steps must be taken now that will begin the process of change, for if action is delayed, future generations will accuse this one of 'kicking the can down the road, hoping for someone to do something differently.' There is no excuse for inaction.

SUMMARY

If professionalism is the bedrock of *high-value care*, as purported by Marcotte, et al (2019), healthcare leadership must find ways to help providers *put the potential into play*, by educating them and holding them accountable for demonstrating those practices that elevate professionalism as they engage with patients, peers, and fellow team members. Unfortunately, the existing medical education paradigm is not structured in a way that prepares future physicians with knowledge or the skill set to excel in professionalism. The authors of this chapter, in an effort to proactively offer a response to this systemic problem in medical education, initiated a professionalism competency development program (Leadership Lived Out®) in the Duke University Medical School – Division of Head and Neck Surgery and Communication Sciences, which offered a mechanism through which personal growth could be nurtured. They built the program around the concept that *behaviors are conditioned by one's cognitive and emotional intelligences and guided by a certain set of virtues,* and the belief that the end goal of medical education is to create physicians who are able to *think, feel and act like physicians should* in a way that is not imposed externally, but flows from an intrinsic desire to be the best they can be. This is attained when one strikes a balance between their cognitive, emotional, and leadership intelligences, while engaging with others, with skill, in a social construct. Professionalism competency is predicated upon acquiring the knowledge and skills associated with these intelligences and taking steps to commit to their practice in everyday life, both personally and vocationally. The acquisition of these skills is incumbent on a physician's willful decision to engage in daily self-betterment practices.

The authors propose five reforms to be implemented in the medical education continuum that would usher in a revolution in *high-value care*, unparalleled in recent history. The five reforms are: 1) prioritize professionalism competency training; 2) make curricular revisions to promote professionalism competency training; 3) change selection criteria for entrance to the profession; 4) institute new prerequisite requirements for entrance to the profession; and, 5) require professionalism competency training as part of certification and re-certification processes.

Little could be more important in healthcare reform than to prioritize professionalism competency training as the substance that releases people to generate *high-value care*. The time to act is now.

REFERENCES

Argyris, C. (1977). Double Loop Learning in Organizations. *Harvard Business Review*. Available from: https://hbr.org/1977/09/double-loop-learning-in-organizations

Argyris, C. (1991, May). Teaching Smart People How to Learn. *Harvard Business Review*, 99–109.

Argyris, C., & Schon, D. (1974). *Theory in practice: Increasing professional effectiveness*. San Francisco, CA: Jossey-Bass.

Byyny, R., Papadakis, M., & Paauw, D. (Eds.). (2015). *Medical Professionalism: Best Practices*. Menlo Park, CA: Alpha Omega Alpha Honor Medical Society.

Cooke, M., Irby, D. M., & O'Brien, B. C. (2010). *Educating Physicians: A Call for Reform of Medical School and Residency. The Carnegie Foundation for the Advancement of Teaching*. San Francisco, CA: Jossey-Bass.

Cruess, R., Cruess, S., & Steinert, Y. (2016). Amending Miller's Pyramid to Include Professional Identity Formation. *Academic Medicine*, *91*(2), 180–185. doi:10.1097/ACM.0000000000000913 PMID:26332429

Doublestein, B., Lee, W., & Pfohl, R. (2015). Healthcare 2050: Anticipatory Leadership. In *Critical Challenges, Key Contexts, and Emerging Trends*. Emerald.

Edmondson, A. (2012). *Teaming: How Organizations Learn, Innovate, and Compete in the Knowledge Economy*. San Francisco, CA: Jossey-Bass.

Feudtner, C., Christakis, D., & Christakis, N. (1994). Do clinical clerks suffer ethical erosion? Students' perceptions of their ethical environment and personal development. *Academic Medicine*, *69*(8), 670–679. doi:10.1097/00001888-199408000-00017 PMID:8054117

Fitz-enz, J. (2000). *The ROI of Human Capital: Measuring the Economic Value of Employee Performance*. New York, NY: AMACOM.

Flexner, A. (1910). *Medical Education in the United States and Canada*. New York, NY: The Carnegie Foundation for the Advancement of Teaching.

Fritz, R. (1989). *The Path of Least Resistance: Learning to Become the Creative Force in Your Own Life*. New York, NY: Fawcett.

Goleman, D. (2006). *Social Intelligence: The New Science of Human Relationships*. New York, NY: Bantam Books.

Haferty, F. (1998). Beyond curriculum reform: Confronting medicine's hidden curriculum. *Academic Medicine*, *73*(4), 403–407. doi:10.1097/00001888-199804000-00013 PMID:9580717

Kenny, N., Mann, K., & MacLeod, H. (2003). Role modeling in physicians' professional formation: Reconsidering an essential but untapped educational strategy. *Academic Medicine*, *78*(11), 1076–1083. PMID:14660418

Kouzes, J., & Posner, B. (2010). *The Truth About Leadership: The No-fads Heart-of-the-Matter Facts You Need to Know*. San Francisco, CA: Jossey-Bass.

Leape, L., Shore, M., Dienstag, J., Mayer, R., Edgman-Levitan, S., Meyer, G., & Healy, G. (2012). A culture of respect, part 1: The nature and causes of disrespectful behavior by physicians. *Academic Medicine, 87*(7), 845-852.

Lee, F. (2004). *If Disney Ran Your Hospital: 9 1/2 Things You Would Do Differently*. Second River Healthcare.

Lee, W. (2013). Measuring the immeasurable core competency of professionalism. *JAMA Otolaryngology-Head & Neck Surgery*, *139*(1), 12–13. doi:10.1001/jamaoto.2013.1071 PMID:23329086

Lencioni, P. (2012). *The Advantage: Why Organizational Health Trumps Everything Else in Business*. San Francisco, CA: Jossey-Bass.

Mahood, S. (2011). Medical education: Beware the hidden curriculum. *Canadian Family Physician Médecin de Famille Canadien*, *57*(9), 983–985. PMID:21918135

Marcotte, L., Moriates, C., Wolfson, D., & Frankel, R. (2019). Professionalism as the Bedrock of High-Value Care. *Academic Medicine*. Available from: https://journals.lww.com/academicmedicine/Abstract/publishahead/Professionalism_as_the_Bedrock_of_High_Value_Care.97538.aspx

Miller, G. E. (1990). The Assessment of Clinical Skills/Competence/Performance. *Academic Medicine*, *65*(9), 63–67. doi:10.1097/00001888-199009000-00045 PMID:2400509

Papadakis, M., Teherani, A., Banach, M., Knettler, T., Rattner, S., Stern, D., ... Hodgson, C. S. (2005). Disciplinary action by medical boards and prior behavior in medical school. *The New England Journal of Medicine, 353*(25), 2673–2682. doi:10.1056/NEJMsa052596 PMID:16371633

Pink, D. (2011). *Drive: The Surprising Truth About What Motivates Us*. Riverhead Books.

Rogers, C. (1961). *On Becoming a Person: A Therapist's View of Psychotherapy*. Houghton Mifflin.

Schwantes, M. (2016). Science Says 92 Percent of People Don't Achieve Their Goals. Here's How the Other 8 Percent Do. *Inc.* Available from: https://www.inc.com/marcel-schwantes/science-says-92-percent-of-people-dont-achieve-goals-heres-how-the-other-8-perce.html

Senge, P. (1990). *The Fifth Discipline: The Art & Practice of the Learning Organization*. New York, NY: Doubleday Currency.

Vermeeren, D. (2007). *365 Lessons from Amazing Success*. Business Boost SUCCESS.

ADDITIONAL READING

Argyris, C., & Schon, D. (1974). *Theory in practice: Increasing professional effectiveness*. San Francisco, CA: Jossey-Bass.

Cooke, M., Irby, D. M., & O'Brien, B. C. (2010). *Educating Physicians: A Call for Reform of Medical School and Residency. The Carnegie Foundation for the Advancement of Teaching*. San Francisco, CA: Jossey-Bass.

Cruess, R., Cruess, S., & Steinert, Y. (2016). Amending Miller's Pyramid to Include Professional Identity Formation. *Academic Medicine, 91*(2), 180–185. doi:10.1097/ACM.0000000000000913 PMID:26332429

Edmondson, A. (2012). *Teaming: How Organizations Learn, Innovate, and Compete in the Knowledge Economy*. San Francisco, CA: Jossey-Bass.

Fritz, R. (1989). *The Path of Least Resistance: Learning to Become the Creative Force in Your Own Life*. New York, NY: Fawcett.

Lee, W. (2013). Measuring the immeasurable core competency of professionalism. *JAMA Otolaryngology-Head & Neck Surgery, 139*(1), 12–13. doi:10.1001/jamaoto.2013.1071 PMID:23329086

KEY TERMS AND DEFINITIONS

Hidden Curriculum: The hidden curriculum is a socialization process that transmits norms and values that undermine the formal message taught during the medical education continuum. The hidden curriculum disrupts training in that its message (as it is practiced by others in authority) implies that what is formally taught as best practices is less important than what is practiced. It causes students (residents included) to move from being open-minded to closed-minded; move from being intellectually curious to narrowly focused on facts; from empathy to emotional detachment; from idealism to cynicism; from civility and caring to arrogance and irritability; and, an erosion of ethics (Mahood, 2011).

Leadership Lived Out® (LLO®): Leadership Lived Out® is a program developed in the Duke University Medical School – Division of Head and Neck Surgery and Communication Sciences to improve professionalism competence as members engage with patients and fellow team members. The program began as a proactive endeavor to bring about a division-wide commitment to excellence in patient care. The LLO® program is based on the concept that *behaviors are conditioned by how one thinks and feels and guided by a certain set of virtues* (Doublestein, Lee, & Pfohl, 2015).

Learning Opportunities: The process of professionalism competency development requires that people within the organization are committed to learning. One purpose of medical education is to take people from novice to expert (Miller, 1990). The process of moving people along this continuum is often fueled by failure, the very thing that physicians hope never happens. But it is often inevitable, and as such, it is important to process every failure, large or small, in a way that maximizes learning opportunities (Edmondson, 2012). Organizations or institutions that maximize learning opportunities are those that leverage their failures and seek the best in their people and processes (Senge, 1990).

Professional Competence: The term used to define the skills necessary to deliver *high-value care*. Professionalism competence is a set of high-performing, non-technical actions practiced with skill as one engages with patients, peers, and members of the healthcare team. People operating in accordance with these high-performing actions result in highly-competent humanistic, ethically vigilant, reflective, socially responsive and responsible, resilient physicians (Weld, 2015). These skills transcend the traits, trappings, and traditions of being a physician.

Professional Competency Cycle: The professionalism competency cycle is a learning process which moves people from novice to expert status. While the term 'expert' is an ever-changing target, the cyclical process provides structure to the learning process. The cycle consists of self-assessment, self-awareness, self-analysis, self-improvement strategy development, and evaluation. The first three steps are about discovery, with the final two about active application and learning.

Shared Virtues: They are the fundamental guiding principles that support all thoughts, actions, engagements, and decisions through which team members are judged or guided as they go about their patient care activities. Without these fundamental virtues guiding behavior, it would be impossible to grow or learn as individuals or as an organization. These shared virtues provide a definable set of standards that in essence are the worldview from and through which everyone interacts and is held accountable.

Social Economy: Every interaction with patients or team members occurs in a social construct. One might be gaining excellent personal professionalism competence yet fail to achieve desired *high-value care* outcomes. The practitioner must gain understanding and competence of social intelligence skills in order to fully gain high-performing status. Professionalism competence is fully achieved when practiced in the social construct.

Social Intelligence: Social Intelligence refers to one's human aptitude for relationship. It is comprised of two distinct categories relating to social engagement: social awareness, and social facility (Goleman, 2006). Social awareness refers to a variety of abilities that run from being able to instantaneously sense another's inner state, to understanding their feelings and thoughts, and finally to understanding complicated social situations. Social facility builds upon social awareness to allow smooth and effective interactions and it involves: 1) *synchrony* – interacting with others smoothly at the nonverbal level; 2) *self-presentation* – presenting oneself effectively as they engage with others; 3) *influence* – being able to shape outcomes of social interactions; and, 4) *concern* – caring about others' needs and taking actions that demonstrate concern (Goleman, 2006).

Compilation of References

10. Paths to Innovation in Health Care Delivery. (2019, October). *NEJM Catalyst*. Retrieved from https://cdn2.hubspot.net/hubfs/558940/Event_October_2019/Landing/10-Paths-to-Innovation-in-Health-Care-Delivery.pdf

ABIM Foundation. (2005). *Medical Professionalism in the New Millennium: A Physician Charter*. American Board of Internal Medicine Foundation. Available from: https://abimfoundation.org/wp-content/uploads/2015/12/Medical-Professionalism-in-the-New-Millenium-A-Physician-Charter.pdf. Accessed: August, 2019.

Accident Compensation Corporation of New Zealand. (2016). *ACC Privacy Maturity Plan 2016/17*. Retrieved from https://www.acc.co.nz/

ADM Biopolis core expertise is finding, designing and developing microorganisms for industrial and health-related purposes. To develop ground-breaking products, our R&D is based on a series of harmonized, interconnected research platforms. (n.d.). Retrieved from http://biopolis.es/

Aggelidis, V. P., & Chatzoglou, P. D. (2009). Using a modified technology acceptance model in hospitals. *International Journal of Medical Informatics*, *78*(2), 115–126. doi:10.1016/j.ijmedinf.2008.06.006 PMID:18675583

Ahmed, E., Evans, T. G., Standing, H., & Mahmud, S. (2013). Harnessing pluralism for better health in Bangladesh. *Lancet*, *382*(9906), 1746–1755. doi:10.1016/S0140-6736(13)62147-9 PMID:24268003

AICPA/CICA Privacy Maturity Model. (2011). Retrieved from https://iapp.org/media/pdf/resource_center/aicpa_cica_privacy_maturity_model_final-2011.pdf

Ajjan, H., & Hartshorne, R. (2008). Investigating faculty decisions to adopt Web 2.0 technologies: Theory and empirical tests. *The Internet and Higher Education*, *11*(2), 71–80. doi:10.1016/j.iheduc.2008.05.002

Akter, M. S., Upal, M., & Hani, U. (2008). Service quality perception and satisfaction: A study over sub-urban public hospitals in Bangladesh. *Journal of Services Research*, 125.

Akter, S., D'Ambra, J., & Ray, P. (2011). Trustworthiness in mHealth information services: An assessment of a hierarchical model with mediating and moderating effects using partial least squares (PLS). *Journal of the Association for Information Science and Technology*, *62*(1), 100–116.

Alaboudi, A., Atkins, A., Sharp, B., Balkhair, A., Alzahrani, M., & Sunbul, T. (2016). Barriers and challenges in adopting Saudi telemedicine network: The perceptions of decision makers of healthcare facilities in Saudi Arabia. *Journal of Infection and Public Health, 9*(6), 725–733. doi:10.1016/j.jiph.2016.09.001 PMID:27649882

Alexandraki, I., Hernandez, C., Torre, D., Chretien, K., Hernandez, C. A., Torre, D. M., & Chretien, K. C. (2017). Interprofessional Education in the Internal Medicine Clerkship Post-LCME Standard Issuance: Results of a National Survey. *Journal of General Internal Medicine, 32*(8), 871–876. doi:10.1007/s11606-017-4004-3 PubMed

Alper, E., Rosenberg, E. I., O'Brien, K. E., Fischer, M., & Durning, S. J. (2009). Patient safety education at US and Canadian medical schools: Results from the 2006 Clerkship Directors in Internal Medicine survey. *Academic Medicine, 84*(12), 1672–1676. doi:10.1097/ACM.0b013e3181bf98a4 PubMed

Altpeter, T., Luckhardt, K., Lewis, J. N., Harken, A. H., & Polk, H. C. Jr. (2007). Expanded surgical time out: A key to real-time data collection and quality improvement. *Journal of the American College of Surgeons, 204*(4), 527–532. doi:10.1016/j.jamcollsurg.2007.01.009 PubMed

Amadeo, K. (2019, August 22). *4 Reasons Why We Need Healthcare Reform.* Retrieved from https://www.thebalance.com/why-reform-health-care-3305749

America Next. (2014). *The freedom and empowerment plan: The prescription for conservative consumer-focused health reform.* Alexandria, VA: America Next.

American Association of Colleges of Nursing Essentials of Baccalaureate Education for and interprofessional education: An emerging concept. (2008). Journal of interprofessional care, 19(sup1), 8-20. Retrieved from http://www.aacnnursing.org/portals/42/publications/baccessentials08.pdf

Andaleeb, S. S., Siddiqui, N., & Khandakar, S. (2007). Patient satisfaction with health services in Bangladesh. *Health Policy and Planning, 22*(4), 263–273. doi:10.1093/heapol/czm017 PMID:17545252

Andel, C., Davidow, S. L., Hollander, M., & Moreno, D. A. (2012). The economics of health care quality and medical errors. *Journal of Health Care Finance, 39*(1), 39. PubMed

Appari, A., & Johnson, M. E. (2010). Information security and privacy in healthcare: current state of research. *International Journal of Internet and Enterprise Management, 6*(4), 279-314.

Aranda-Jan, C. B., Mohutsiwa-Dibe, N., & Loukanova, S. (2014). Systematic review on what works, what does not work and why of implementation of mobile health (mHealth) projects in Africa. *BMC Public Health, 14*(1), 188. doi:10.1186/1471-2458-14-188 PMID:24555733

Argyris, C. (1977). Double Loop Learning in Organizations. *Harvard Business Review.* Available from: https://hbr.org/1977/09/double-loop-learning-in-organizations

Argyris, C. (1991, May). Teaching Smart People How to Learn. *Harvard Business Review,* 99–109.

Argyris, C., & Schon, D. (1974). *Theory in practice: Increasing professional effectiveness.* San Francisco, CA: Jossey-Bass.

Arrow, K. J. (1963). Uncertainty and the Welfare Economics of Medical Care. *The American Economic Review, 53*(5), 941–973.

Arthur, W., & Day, E. A. (2011). Assessment centers. In S. Zedock (Ed.), APA Handbook of Industrial and Organizational Psychology (vol. 2). Washington, DC: American Psychological Association. doi:10.1037/12170-007

Ashford, S. J., & Detert, J. (2015). Get the boss to buy-in. *Harvard Business Review, 93*(1/2), 72–79.

Aubrey, A. (2017, May 8). *Fresh Food By Prescription: This Health Care Firm Is Trimming Costs - And Waistlines.* Retrieved from https://www.npr.org/sections/thesalt/2017/05/08/526952657/fresh-food-by-prescription-this-health-care-firm-is-trimming-costs-and-waistline

Bagayoko, C. O., Traoré, D., Thevoz, L., Diabaté, S., Pecoul, D., Niang, M., ... Geissbuhler, A. (2014). Medical and economic benefits of telehealth in low-and middle-income countries: Results of a study in four district hospitals in Mali. *BMC Health Services Research, 14*(1), S9. doi:10.1186/1472-6963-14-S1-S9 PMID:25080312

Bain, D. M. (2006). *The Influences on Physician Attitudes Toward the Use of Telemedicine for the Delivery of Patient Care.* ProQuest.

Baker, D. P., Horvath, L., Campion, M. A., Offermann, L., & Salas, E. (2005). The ALL Teamwork Framework. In T. S. Murray, Y. Clermont, & M. Binkley (Eds.), *International Adult Literacy Survey, Measuring Adult Literacy and Life Skills: New Frameworks for Assessment.* Ottawa: Ministry of Industry.

Bales, R. F. (1950). A set of categories for the analysis of small group interaction. *American Sociological Review, 15*(2), 257–263. doi:10.2307/2086790

Bartrom, S., & Stanton, T. (2011). High performance work systems: The gap between policy and practice in healthcare reform. *Journal of Health Organization and Management, 25*(3), 281–297. doi:10.1108/14777261111143536 PMID:21845983

Bashshur, R. L. (1995). On the definition and evaluation of telemedicine. *Telemedicine Journal, 1*(1), 19–30. doi:10.1089/tmj.1.1995.1.19 PMID:10165319

Bashshur, R. L., Howell, J. D., Krupinski, E. A., Harms, K. M., Bashshur, N., & Doarn, C. R. (2016). The empirical foundations of telemedicine interventions in primary care. *Telemedicine Journal and e-Health, 22*(5), 342–375. doi:10.1089/tmj.2016.0045 PMID:27128779

Bashshur, R. L., Reardon, T. G., & Shannon, G. W. (2000). Telemedicine: A new health care delivery system. *Annual Review of Public Health, 21*(1), 613–637. doi:10.1146/annurev.publhealth.21.1.613 PMID:10884967

Bashshur, R., Shannon, G., Krupinski, E., & Grigsby, J. (2011). The Taxonomy of Telemedicine. *Telemedicine Journal and e-Health, 17*(6), 484–494. doi:10.1089/tmj.2011.0103 PMID:21718114

Bayer. (2018). *Finding a cure for cancer – is big data the solution?* Retrieved from https://www.canwelivebetter.bayer.com/innovation/finding-cure-cancer-big-data-solution#the-data-mountain

Becker's Hospital Review. (2015, December 7). *The corner office: Dr. David Feinberg on raising the patient experience to a whole new level.* Retrieved from https://www.beckershospitalreview.com/hospital-management-administration/the-corner-office-dr-david-feinberg-on-raising-the-patient-experience-to-a-whole-new-level.html

Beenen, G., Pichler, S., & Davoudpour, S. (2018). Interpersonal Skills in MBA Admission: How Are They Conceptualized and Assessed? *Journal of Management Education, 42*(1), 34–54. doi:10.1177/1052562917703743

BenMessaoud, C., Kharrazi, H., & MacDorman, K. F. (2011). Facilitators and barriers to adopting robotic-assisted surgery: Contextualizing the unified theory of acceptance and use of technology. *PLoS One, 6*(1), e16395. doi:10.1371/journal.pone.0016395 PMID:21283719

Berry, L. L. (2019). Service innovation is urgent in healthcare. *AMS Review*, 1-15.

Berry, L., & Beckham, D. (2014). Team-based care at Mayo Clinic: A Model for ACOs. *Journal of Healthcare Management, 59*(1), 9–13. doi:10.1097/00115514-201401000-00003 PMID:24611420

Berry, L., & Seltman, K. (2008). *Management lessons from Mayo Clinic.* New York, NY: McGraw Hill.

Berwick, D. M., Nolan, T. W., & Whittington, J. (2008). The triple aim: Care, health, and cost. *Health Affairs, 27*(3), 759–769. doi:10.1377/hlthaff.27.3.759 PubMed

Bessard, P. (2008, December 22). Challenges of Mixed Economy Solutions in Healthcare: The Examples of Switzerland and Singapore. *Economic Affairs, 28*(4), 16–21. doi:10.1111/j.1468-0270.2008.00863.x

Betz, E. (2018). Advantages and limitations of the direct primary care model. *MGMA STAT.* Retrieved from https://www.mgma.com/data/data-stories/advantages-and-limitations-of-the-direct-primary-c

Birden, H., Glass, N., Wilson, I., Harrison, M., Usherwood, T., & Nass, T. (2014). Defining professionalism in medical education: A systematic review. *Medical Teacher, 36*(1), 47–61. doi:10.3109/0142159X.2014.850154 PMID:24252073

Bodenheimer, T., & Sinsky, C. (2014). From triple to quadruple aim: Care of the patient requires care of the provider. *Annals of Family Medicine, 12*(8), 573–576. doi:10.1370/afm.1713 PMID:25384822

Bomey, N. (2018, Feb. 25). How Amazon, JPMorgan, Berkshire could transform American healthcare. *USA Today (Online).* Retrieved from https://www.usatoday.com/story/money/2018/02/25/amazon-jpmorgan-berkshire-health-care/350625002

Boonstra, A., & Broekhuis, M. (2010). Barriers to the acceptance of electronic medical records by physicians from systematic review to taxonomy and interventions. *BMC Health Services Research, 10*(1), 231. doi:10.1186/1472-6963-10-231 PMID:20691097

Bray, D. W., Campbell, R. J., & Grant, D. L. (1979). *Formative years in business: A long-term AT&T study of managerial lives*. R.E. Krieger Publishing Co.

Bridges, D. R., Davidson, R. A., Odegard, S., Maki, I. V., & Tomkowiak, J. (2011). Interprofessional collaboration: Three best practice models of interprofessional education. *Medical Education Online, 1*(0). doi: PubMed doi:10.3402/meo.v16i0.6035

Bureau of Labor Statistics. (2019). *Employment, Hours, and Earnings from the Current Employment Statistics survey*. Author.

Byyny, R., Papadakis, M., & Paauw, D. (Eds.). (2015). *Medical Professionalism: Best Practices*. Menlo Park, CA: Alpha Omega Alpha Honor Medical Society.

Cancer Data and Statistics. (2019, July 9). Retrieved from https://www.cdc.gov/cancer/dcpc/data

Cannon-Bowers, J. A., Tannenbaum, S. I., Salas, E., & Volpe, C. E. (1995). Defining competencies and establishing team training requirements. In R. Guzzo & E. Salas (Eds.), *Team effectiveness and decision making in organizations* (pp. 333–380). San Francisco: Jossey Bass.

Cardon, J., & Hendel, I. (2001). Asymmetric Information in Health Insurance: Evidence from the National Medical Expenditure Survey. *The Rand Journal of Economics, 32*(3), 408–427. doi:10.2307/2696362 PMID:11800005

Carlson, R. (2015, March 1). Direct primary care practice model drops insurance and gains providers and consumers. *Physician Leadership Journal*. Retrieved from https://www.thefreelibrary.com/Direct+primary+care+practice+model+drops+insurance+and+gains...-a0409422676

Casey, B. R., Chisholm-Burns, M., Passiment, M., Wagner, R., & Riordan, L. (n.d.). *Weiss KB for the NCICLE Quality Improvement: Focus on Health Care Disparities Work Group*. The role of the clinical learning environment in preparing new clinicians to engage in quality improvement efforts to eliminate health care disparities. Retrieved from http://ncicle.org

CBS. (2019). *Carol's second act*. Retrieved from https://www.cbs.com/shows/carols-second act/about/

Celdrán, A. H., Pérez, M. G., Clemente, F. J. G., & Pérez, G. M. (2018). Sustainable securing of Medical Cyber-Physical Systems for the healthcare of the future. *Sustainable Computing: Informatics and Systems*.

Centers for Medicare & Medicaid Services. (2018). *National Health Accounts Historical: NHE Tables*. Author.

Centers for Medicare & Medicaid Services. (2018). *National Health Accounts Historical: NHE Tables*. Retrieved from https://www.cms.gov/research-statistics-data-and-systems/statistics

Centers for Medicare and Medicaid. (2019). *Medicare shared savings program.* Retrieved from https://www.cms.gov/Medicare/Medicare-Fee-for-Service-Payment/sharedsavingsprogram/index.html

Chandler, C. I. R., Chonya, S., Mtei, F., Reyburn, H., & Whitty, C. J. M. (2009). Motivation, money and respect: A mixed-method study of Tanzanian non-physician clinicians. *Social Science & Medicine, 68*(11), 2078–2088. doi:10.1016/j.socscimed.2009.03.007 PMID:19328607

Chang, H. (2015). Evaluation framework for telemedicine using the logical framework approach and a fishbone diagram. *Healthcare Informatics Research, 21*(4), 230–238. doi:10.4258/hir.2015.21.4.230 PMID:26618028

Chen, L., & Troy, T. (2017, February 2). *Trump wants health 'insurance for everybody.' Here's how the GOP can make it happen.* Retrieved from https://www.washingtonpost.com/opinions/trump-wants-health-insurance-for-everybody-heres-how-the-gop-can-make-it-happen/2017/02/02/284e51b0-e4f1-11e6-a547-5fb9411d332c_story.html

Chen, G., Donahue, L. M., & Klimoski, R. J. (2004). Training undergraduates to work in organizational teams. *Academy of Management Learning & Education, 3*(1), 27–40. doi:10.5465/amle.2004.12436817

Chen, L. (2018, December). Getting Ready for Health Reform 2020: Republicans' Options before Improving upon the State Innovation Approach. *Health Affairs, 37*(12), 2076–2083. doi:10.1377/hlthaff.2018.05119 PMID:30444425

Cheong, L. (2004). *Medical savings accounts in Singapore: The impact of Medisave and income on healthcare expenditure.* Stanford, CA: Center for Primary Care and Outcomes Research, Stanford University.

Christensen, C. (1997). *Disruptive Innovation.* Retrieved from https://www.christenseninstitute.org/disruptive-innovations/

Christensen, C. (2018). *Christensen Institute: Healthcare.* Retrieved from https://www.christenseninstitute.org/results/?_sft_topics=healthcare

Christensen, J. (2018, June 4). *Same cancer, worse results and twice the cost in the US. CNN.* Retrieved from https://www.cnn.com/2018/06/01/health/us-canada-health-care-spending-study/index.html

Clapesattle, H. (1941). *The doctors Mayo.* Minneapolis, MN: University of Minnesota Press.

Clarke, J. L., Bourn, S., Skoufalos, A., Beck, E. H., & Castillo, D. J. (2016). An innovative approach to health care delivery for patients with chronic conditions. *Population Health Management, 20*(1), 23–30. doi:10.1089/pop.2016.0076 PubMed

Classen, D. C., Resar, R., Griffin, F., Federico, F., Frankel, T., Kimmel, N., ... James, B. C. (2011). "Global trigger tool" shows that adverse events in hospitals may be ten times greater than previously measured. *Health Affairs, 30*(4), 581–589. doi:10.1377/hlthaff.2011.0190 PMID:21471476

Comstock, J. (2019, September 24). *Amazon launches Amazon Care, a telemedicine-driven care offering for Seattle employees.* Retrieved from https://www.mobihealthnews.com/news/nortamerica/amazon-launches-amazon-

Consumer Reports. (2013, May). *Safety still lags in ILS hospitals.* Retrieved from http://www.consumerreports.org/cro/magazine/2013/05/safety-still-lags-in-u-s-hospiitals/index.htm

Contributor, Q. (2013, February 7). *Where Do the Millions of Cancer Research Dollars Go Every Year?* Retrieved from https://slate.com/human-interest/2013/02/where-do-the-millions-of-cancer-research-dollars-go-every-year.html

Cooke, M., Irby, D. M., & O'Brien, B. C. (2010). *Educating Physicians: A Call for Reform of Medical School and Residency. The Carnegie Foundation for the Advancement of Teaching.* San Francisco, CA: Jossey-Bass.

Coopers, P. W. (2013*). Socio-economic impact of mHealth.* An assessment report for the European Union.

Copeland, B. Bill, & US Life Sciences & Health Care. (2018, January 18). *Top 10 health care innovations: Deloitte US.* Retrieved from https://www2.deloitte.com/us/en/pages/life-sciences-and-health-care/articles/top-10-health-care-innovations.html

Costigan, R. D., & Donahue, L. (2009). Developing the great eight competencies with leaderless group discussion. *Journal of Management Education, 33*(5), 596–616. doi:10.1177/1052562908318328

Cox, M., Cuff, P., Brandt, B., Reeves, S., & Zierler, B. (2016). Measuring the impact of interprofessional education on collaborative practice and patient outcomes. Journal of Interprofessional Care, 30(1), 1–3. https://doi-org.proxynw.uits.iu.edu/10.3109/13561820.2015.1111052

Creighton University. (2017). News Center: University Campus of CHI Health-Creighton University Medical Center opens new era for health care. Retrieved from https://www.creighton.edu/publicrelations/newscenter/news/2017/january2017/january52017/chicumcnr010517/

Cresswell, K., & Sheikh, A. (2013). Organizational issues in the implementation and adoption of health information technology innovations: An interpretative review. *International Journal of Medical Informatics, 82*(5), e73–e86. doi:10.1016/j.ijmedinf.2012.10.007 PMID:23146626

Cruess, R., Cruess, S., & Steinert, Y. (2016). Amending Miller's Pyramid to Include Professional Identity Formation. *Academic Medicine, 91*(2), 180–185. doi:10.1097/ACM.0000000000000913 PMID:26332429

Cuomo, M. I. (2012, October 2). *Are We Wasting Billions Seeking a Cure for Cancer?* Retrieved from https://www.thedailybeast.com/are-we-wasting-billions-seeking-a-cure-for-cancer

Cuomo, M. I. (2013). *World without cancer: the making of a new cure and the real promise of prevention.* New York: Rodale.

Cutler, D. M., & Reber, S. J. (1998). The Trade-Off Between Competition and Adverse Selection. *The Quarterly Journal of Economics, 113*(2), 433–466. doi:10.1162/003355398555649

Cutler, D. M., Rosen, A. B., & Vijan, S. (2006). The Value of Medical Spending in the United States, 1960–2000. *The New England Journal of Medicine, 355*(9), 920–927. doi:10.1056/ NEJMsa054744 PMID:16943404

Cutts, H. (2017). *An Investigation of Circumstances Affecting Consumer Behavioral Intentions to Use Telemedicine Technology: An Interpretative Phenomenological Study.* Northcentral University.

D'Amour D, & Oandasan I. (2005). Interprofessionality as the field of interprofessional practice and interprofessional education: An emerging concept. Journal of Interprofessional Care, 19(sup1), 8-20.

Dávalos, M. E., French, M. T., Burdick, A. E., & Simmons, S. C. (2009). Economic evaluation of telemedicine: Review of the literature and research guidelines for benefit–cost analysis. *Telemedicine Journal and e-Health, 15*(10), 933–948.

Davis, P. (2018, December 5). *A new theory of cancer.* Retrieved from https://www.themonthly. com.au/issue/2018/november/1540990800/paul-davies/new-theory-cancer

Davis, S. M, & Gourdji, J. (n.d.). *Making the Healthcare Shift: The Transformation to Consumer-Centricity.* New York, NY: James Morgan Publishing.

Davis, S., & Gourdji, J. (2019). *Making the healthcare shift: The transformation to consumer-centricity.* New York: Morgan James Publishing.

Deber, R., Hollander, M. J., & Jacobs, P. (2008). Models of funding and reimbursement in health care: A conceptual framework. *Canadian Public Administration, 51*(3), 381–405. doi:10.1111/ j.1754-7121.2008.00030.x

Demaerschalk, B. M., Berg, J., Chong, B. W., Gross, H., Nystrom, K., Adeoye, O., ... Whitchurch, S. (2017). American telemedicine association: Telestroke guidelines. *Telemedicine Journal and e-Health, 23*(5), 376–389. doi:10.1089/tmj.2017.0006 PMID:28384077

Dolgin, E. (2018). Cancer's cost conundrum. *Nature, 555*(7695). doi: 10.1038-d41486-018-02483-3

Donovan, F. (2018, August 22). *Judge Gives Final OK to $115M Anthem Data Breach Settlement.* Retrieved from https://healthitsecurity.com/news/judge-gives-final-ok-to-115m-anthem-data-breach-settlement

Doswell, W. M., Braxter, B., Dabbs, A. D., Nilsen, W., & Klem, M. L. (2013). mHealth: Technology for nursing practice, education, and research. *Journal of Nursing Education and Practice, 3*(10), 99. doi:10.5430/jnep.v3n10p99

Doublestein, B., & Pfohl, R. (2013). *Leadership Lived Out: Training Exemplary Resident Leaders.* Faculty Planning Meeting (July 13). Department of Otolaryngology: Head & Neck Surgery, Duke Medical School.

Doublestein, B., Lee, W., & Pfohl, R. (2015). Healthcare 2050: Anticipatory Leadership. In *Critical Challenges, Key Contexts, and Emerging Trends.* Emerald.

Draycott, T., Sibanda, T., & Owen, L. (2009). Does training in obstetric emergencies improve neonatal outcome? *BJOG*, *112*, 177–182. PMID:16411995

Dünnebeil, S., Sunyaev, A., Blohm, I., Leimeister, J. M., & Krcmar, H. (2012). Determinants of physicians' technology acceptance for e-health in ambulatory care. *International Journal of Medical Informatics*, *81*(11), 746–760. doi:10.1016/j.ijmedinf.2012.02.002 PMID:22397989

Dutot, V., Bergeron, F., Rozhkova, K., & Moreau, N. (2019). Factors Affecting the Adoption of Connected Objects in e-Health: A Mixed Methods Approach. *Systèmes d'Information et Management*, *23*(4), 3.

Earnest, M., & Brandt, B. (2014). Aligning practice redesign and interprofessional education to advance triple aim outcomes. *Journal of Interprofessional Care*, *28*(6), 497–500. doi:10.3109/13561820.2014.933650 PubMed

Edmondson, A. (2012). *Teaming: How Organizations Learn, Innovate, and Compete in the Knowledge Economy*. San Francisco, CA: Jossey-Bass.

Ellis, R. P., & McGuire, T. G. (1993). Supply-side and demand-side cost sharing in health care. *The Journal of Economic Perspectives*, *7*(4), 135–151. doi:10.1257/jep.7.4.135 PMID:10130330

Emanuel, E. J., & Orszag, P. R. (2010). Health care reform and cost control. *The New England Journal of Medicine*, *363*(7), 601–603. doi:10.1056/NEJMp1006571 PubMed

Ervin, J. N., Kahn, J. M., Cohen, T. R., & Weingart, L. R. (2018). Teamwork in the intensive care unit. *The American Psychologist*, *73*(4), 468–477. doi:10.1037/amp0000247 PMID:29792461

Esmaeilzadeh, P. (2019). The effects of public concern for information privacy on the adoption of Health Information Exchanges (HIEs) by healthcare entities. *Health Communication*, *34*(10), 1202–1211. doi:10.1080/10410236.2018.1471336 PMID:29737872

Evans, P. R. (2015). *An exploration of the perceptions of a US Midwest acute care hospital organization regarding the adoption and acceptance of telemedicine*. Capella University.

Everett, B. (2019, July 15). Republicans ready to dive off a cliff on Obamacare. *Politico*. Retrieved from https://a.msn.com/r/2/AAEj9o3?m=en-us&referrerID=InAppShare

Fanta, G. B., Pretorius, L., & Erasmus, L. (2015). An evaluation of eHealth systems implementation frameworks for sustainability in resource constrained environments: A literature review. *IAMOT 2015 Conference Proceedings*.

Farr, C. (2019, March 13). Cardiologist Eric Topol explains how artificial intelligence can make doctors more humane. *Health Tech Matters*. Retrieved from https://www.cnbc.com/2019/03/13/eric-topol-interview-with-christina-farr-on-ai-and-doctors.html

Farr, C. (2019, March 14). Everything we know about Haven, the Amazon joint venture to revamp healthcare. *Health Tech Matters*. Retrieved from https://www.cnbc.com/2019/03/13/what-is-haven-amazon-jpmorgan-berkshire-revamp-health-care.html

Faulkner, G., Dale, L. P., & Lau, E. (2019). Examining the use of loyalty point incentives to encourage health and fitness centre participation. *Preventive Medicine Reports, 14*, 100831. doi:10.1016/j.pmedr.2019.100831 PMID:30886815

Feke, T. (2015). *Medicare*. New York: Alpha, a member of Penguin Group USA Inc.

Feldstein, M. (1973). The Welfare Loss of Excess Health Insurance. *Journal of Political Economy, 81*(2), 251–280. doi:10.1086/260027

Feudtner, C., Christakis, D., & Christakis, N. (1994). Do clinical clerks suffer ethical erosion? Students' perceptions of their ethical environment and personal development. *Academic Medicine, 69*(8), 670–679. doi:10.1097/00001888-199408000-00017 PMID:8054117

Fickenscher, K., & Bakerman, M. (2011). Change management in health care IT. *Physician Executive, 37*(2), 64–67. PMID:21465898

Financial Burden of Cancer Care. (2019, February). National Cancer Institute. Retrieved from https://progressreport.cancer.gov/after/economic_burden

Fiscella, K., & McDaniel, S. H. (2018). The complexity, diversity, and science of primary care teams. *The American Psychologist, 73*(4), 451–467. doi:10.1037/amp0000244 PMID:29792460

Fitz-enz, J. (2000). *The ROI of Human Capital: Measuring the Economic Value of Employee Performance*. New York, NY: AMACOM.

Flexner, A. (1910). *Medical Education in the United States and Canada*. New York, NY: The Carnegie Foundation for the Advancement of Teaching.

Folland, S., Goodman, A. C., & Stano, M. (2013). *The economics of health and health care* (7th ed.). Boston: Pearson.

Fontenot, S. F. (2013). The affordable care act and electronic health care records. *Physician Executive, 39*(6), 72–76. PMID:24354149

Ford, J., & Ford, L. (2009). Decoding resistance to change. *Harvard Business Review*, 99–103.

Franco, L. M., Bennett, S., & Kanfer, R. (2002). Health sector reform and public sector health worker motivation: A conceptual framework. *Social Science & Medicine, 54*(8), 1255–1266. doi:10.1016/S0277-9536(01)00094-6 PMID:11989961

Fritz, R. (1989). *The Path of Least Resistance: Learning to Become the Creative Force in Your Own Life*. New York, NY: Fawcett.

Gallegos, A. (2019). Direct primary care: What makes a practice successful? *Family Practice News, 49*(7), 1–23.

Gandhi, V., & Jalali, R. (2017, January 15). *A Conference of New Ideas in Cancer-Challenging Dogmas*. Retrieved from https://www.ncbi.nlm.nih.gov/pubmed/28062401

Gatenby, R. (2009). A chance of strategy in the way on cancer. *Nature, 459*.

Gatewood, R. D., Feild, H. S., & Barrick, M. R. (2016). *Human Resource Selection* (8th ed.). Boston: Cengage Learning.

Gaynor, M., & Vogt, W. B. (2000). Antitrust and competition in health care markets. In A. Culyer & J. Newhouse (Eds.), *Handbook of Health Economics* (pp. 1405–1487). New York: Elsevier Science, North-Holland.

Geeta, S. M., & Barad, T. (2016, November 18). *Challenging cancer dogma in Mumbai*. Retrieved from https://cancerworld.net/cutting-edge/challenging-cancer-dogma-in-mumbai/

Gilbert,J.H.(2013).Interprofessionaleducation,learning,practiceandcare.JournalofInterprofessional Care, 27(4), 283–285. https://doi-org.proxynw.uits.iu.edu/10.3109/13561820.2012.755807

Gilligan, C., Outram, S., & Levett-Jones, T. (2014). Recommendations from recent graduates in medicine, nursing and pharmacy on improving interprofessional education in university programs: A qualitative study. *BMC Medical Education*, (1). doi:10.1186/1472-6920-14-52

Ginsburg, P. B. (2012). Fee-For-Service Will Remain A Feature Of Major Payment Reforms, Requiring More Changes In Medicare Physician Payment. *Health Affairs*, 31(9), 1977–1983. doi:10.1377/hlthaff.2012.0350 PMID:22949446

Glasziou, P. (2008). Evidence based medicine and the medical curriculum. *BMJ (Clinical Research Ed.)*, 337. PMID:18815165

Goleman, D., & Boyatzis, R. (2017). Emotional Intelligence Has 12 Elements. Which Do You Need to Work On? *Harvard Business Review*. Available from: https://hbr.org/2017/02/emotional-intelligence-has-12-elements-which-do-you-need-to-work-on

Goleman, D. (1995). *Emotional Intelligence: Why It Can Matter More Than IQ*. New York, NY: Bantam Books.

Goleman, D. (1998). *Working with Emotional Intelligence*. New York, NY: Bantam Books.

Goleman, D. (2006). *Social Intelligence: The New Science of Human Relationships*. New York, NY: Bantam Books.

Goleman, D. (2013). *Focus: The Hidden Driver of Excellence*. New York, NY: Harper.

Gordon, M. A., Lasater, K., Brunett, P., & Dieckmann, N. F. (2015). Interprofessional Education Finding a Place to Start. Nurse Educator, 40(5), 249–253. 00000000000164 doi:10.1097/NNE.00

Gottlieb, J., & Shephard, M. (2018, September 6). How large a burden are administrative costs in healthcare? *Econofact*. Retrieved from https://econofact.org/how-large-a-burden-are-administrative-costs-in-health-care

Gourdji, J., & Davis, S. (2019). *Making the Healthcare Shift: The Transformation to Consumer-Centricity*. New York: Morgan James.

Green, B. N., & Johnson, C. (2015). Interprofessional collaboration in research, education, and clinical practice: Working together for a better future. Journal of Chiropractic Education, 29(1), 1-10. doi:10.7899ljce-14-36

Greenleaf, R. (2002). *Servant Leadership: A Journey into the Nature of Legitimate Power and Greatness 25th Anniversary Edition*. Paulist Press.

Grossman, M. (1972). On the Concept of Health Capital and the Demand for Health. *Journal of Political Economy, 80*(2), 223–255. doi:10.1086/259880

Guck, T. P., Potthoff, M. R., Walters, R. W., Doll, J., Greene, M. A., & DeFreece, T. (2019). Improved outcomes associated with interprofessional collaborative practice. *Annals of Family Medicine, 17*(Suppl 1), S82–S82. doi:10.1370/afm.2428 PubMed

Gustke, S. S., Balch, D. C., West, V. L., & Rogers, L. O. (2000). Patient satisfaction with telemedicine. *Telemedicine Journal, 6*(1), 5–13. doi:10.1089/107830200311806

Haferty, F. (1998). Beyond curriculum reform: Confronting medicine's hidden curriculum. *Academic Medicine, 73*(4), 403–407. doi:10.1097/00001888-199804000-00013 PMID:9580717

Hagar, S. (2017, Feb. 5). Health share ministries offer alternatives to ACA. *TCA Regional News*.

Hage, E., Roo, J. P., van Offenbeek, M. A., & Boonstra, A. (2013). Implementation factors and their effect on e-Health service adoption in rural communities: A systematic literature review. *BMC Health Services Research, 13*(1), 19. doi:10.1186/1472-6963-13-19 PMID:23311452

Hagist, C., & Kotliko, L. J. (2006). *Who's Going Broke? Comparing Healthcare Costs in ten OECD Countries*. NBER Working Paper 11833.

Hale, T. M., & Kvedar, J. C. (2014). Privacy and security concerns in telehealth. *The Virtual Mentor, 16*(12), 981. PMID:25493367

Hall, L. W., & Zierler, B. K. (2015). Interprofessional Education and Practice Guide No. 1: Developing faculty to effectively facilitate interprofessional education. Journal of Interprofessional Care, 29(1), 3–7. https://doi-org.proxynw.uits.iu.edu/10.3109/13561820.2014.937483

Hall, P. (2005). Interprofessional teamwork: Professional cultures as barriers. Journal of Interprofessional care, 19(sup1), 188-196.

Hardin L., & Spykerman, K. (2017). Competing health care systems and complex patients: An inter-professional collaboration to improve outcomes and reduce health care costs. Journal of Interprofessional Education & Practice, (7), 5-10.

Hay Group. (2011). *Emotional and social competency inventory (ESCI): A user guide for accredited practitioners*. Available from: http://eiconsortium.org/pdf/ESCI_user_guide.pdf

Hayes, J. (2002). *Interpersonal skills at work* (2nd ed.). New York, NY: Routledge. doi:10.4324/9780203465783

Health Professions Accreditors Collaborative. (2019). *Guidance on developing quality interprofessional education for the health professions.* Chicago, IL: Health Professions Accreditors Collaborative.

HealthMarkets. (2019, October 1). *Healthcare Reform News Updates. CMS announces 10-state pilot wellness program for ACA marketplace.* Retrieved from https://www.healthmarkets.com/resources/health-insurance/trumpcare-news-updates/

Heath, C., & Heath, D. (2010). *Switch: How to Change Things When Change is Hard.* New York, NY: Broadway Books.

Henderson, J., & Cavalancia, N. (2019) Insider Threat Program Maturity Model. *Techvangelism & Insider Threat Defense.* Retrieved from https://www.veriato.com/docs/default-source/collateral-assets/insider-threat-maturity-report.pdf

Hill, M. H., & Doddato, T. (2002). Relationships among patient satisfaction, intent to return, and intent to recommend services provided by an academic nursing center. *Journal of Cultural Diversity, 9*(4), 108–112. PMID:12674887

Himmelstein, D. (2014, Sept. 8). A Comparison of hospital administrative costs in eight nations: US costs exceed other nations by far. *The Commonwealth Fund.* Retrieved from https://www.commonwealthfund.org/publications/journal-article/2014/sep/comparison-hospital-administrative-costs-eight-nations-us

HIPAA Journal. (2018). *What Happens if UPi Break HIPAA Rules.* Retrieved from https://www.hipaajournal.com/what-happens-if-you-break-hipaa-rules/

HIPAA Journal. (2019). *The Most Common HIPAA Violations You Should Be Aware Of.* Retrieved from https://www.hipaajournal.com/common-hipaa-violations/

Historical. (2019, December 17). *Centers for Medicare & Medicaid Services.* Retrieved from https://www.cms.gov/Research-Statistics-Data-and-Systems/Statistics-Trends-and-Reports/NationalHealthExpendData/NationalHealthAccountsHistorical

Hobson, C. J., Strupeck, D., Griffin, A., Szostek, J., & Rominger, A. S. (2014). Teaching MBA students teamwork and team leadership skills: An empirical evaluation of a classroom educational program. *American Journal of Business Education, 7*(3), 191–212. doi:10.19030/ajbe.v7i3.8629

Hobson, C. J., Strupeck, D., Griffin, A., Szostek, J., Selladurai, R., & Rominger, A. (2013). Facilitating and documenting behavioral improvements in business student teamwork skills. *Business Education Innovation Journal, 5*(1), 83–95.

Hogan, J., & Lock, J. (1995, May). *A taxonomy of interpersonal skills for business interactions.* Paper presented at the 10th Annual Conference of the Society for Industrial and Organizational Psychology, Orlando, FL.

Holden, R. J., & Karsh, B.-T. (2010). The technology acceptance model: Its past and its future in health care. *Journal of Biomedical Informatics, 43*(1), 159–172. doi:10.1016/j.jbi.2009.07.002 PMID:19615467

Hoque, B., Bao, Y., & Sorwar, G. (2017). Investigating factors influencing the adoption of e-Health in developing countries: A patient's perspective. *Informatics for Health & Social Care, 42*(1), 1–17. doi:10.3109/17538157.2015.1075541 PMID:26865037

Hoque, M. R., Mazmum, M., & Bao, Y. (2014). e-Health in Bangladesh: Current status, challenges, and future direction. *Int Tech Manag Rev, 4*(2), 87–96. doi:10.2991/itmr.2014.4.2.3

Hossain, A., Quaresma, R., & Rahman, H. (2019). Investigating factors influencing the physicians' adoption of electronic health record (EHR) in healthcare system of Bangladesh: An empirical study. *International Journal of Information Management, 44*, 76–87. doi:10.1016/j.ijinfomgt.2018.09.016

How many people in the world die from cancer? (n.d.). Retrieved from https://ourworldindata.org/how-many-people-in-the-world-die-from-cancer

Hsia, T.-L., Chiang, A.-J., Wu, J.-H., Teng, N. N., & Rubin, A. D. (2019). What Drives E-Health Usage? Integrated Institutional Forces and Top Management Perspectives. *Computers in Human Behavior, 97*, 260–270. doi:10.1016/j.chb.2019.01.010

Hsu, J. (2019, July 31). *Artificial intelligence could improve healthcare for all-unless it doesn't.* Retrieved from https://www.fastcompany.com/90384481/artificial-intelligence-could-improve-health-care-for-all-unless-it-doesnt

Huckabee, M. (2019, August 17). *Free healthcare for everyone! Bad idea!* Retrieved from https://www.youtube.com/watch?v=4IacUBgGz7w

Huckabee, M. (2019, October 5). *Is John K. Delaney too moderate for the democratic elections? Find out!* Retrieved from https://www.facebook.com/HuckabeeOnTBN/videos/2485494795013107/

Huckabee, M. (n.d.). *Free healthcare for everyone! Bad idea!* Retrieved from https://www.youtube.com/watch?v=4IacUBgGz7w

Hulet, M. (2012). *Privacy Risk Assessments. Nov. 2012 Perkins and Company.* Retrieved from: http://perkinsaccounting.com/wp-content/uploads/ISACA-Privacy-Risk-Assessmentv7.pdf

Institute of Medicine. (2001). *Committee on Quality of Health Care in America. Crossing the quality chasm: A new health system for the 21st century.* National Academies Press.

Institute of Medicine. (2015). *Measuring the Impact of Interprofessional Education on Collaborative Practice and Patient Outcomes.* National Academies Press.

Institute of Medicine. (2015). *Measuring the impact of interprofessional education on collaborative practice and patient outcomes.* Washington, DC: National Academies Press.

International Association of Privacy Professionals. (2019). *Overview of Privacy Maturity Models,* Retrieved from https://iapp.org/resources/tools/

Interprofessional Education Collaborative Expert Panel. (2011). *Core competencies for interprofessional collaborative practice: Report of an expert panel.* Washington, DC: Interprofessional Education Collaborative.

James, J. T. (2013). A new, evidence-based estimate of patient harms associated with hospital care. *Journal of Patient Safety*, *9*(3), 122–128. doi:10.1097/PTS.0b013e3182948a69 PubMed

Jayasuriya, R., Jayasinghe, U. W., & Wang, Q. (2014). Health worker performance in rural health organizations in low- and middle-income countries: Do organizational factors predict non-task performance? *Social Science & Medicine*, *113*, 1–4. doi:10.1016/j.socscimed.2014.04.042 PMID:24820407

Jennett, H., Hall, L. A., Hailey, D., Ohinmaa, A., Anderson, C., Thomas, R., ... Scott, R. E. (2003). The socio-economic impact of telehealth: A systematic review. *Journal of Telemedicine and Telecare*, *9*(6), 311–320. doi:10.1258/135763303771005207 PMID:14680514

Jennett, S., Scott, R. E., Affleck Hall, L., Hailey, D., Ohinmaa, A., Anderson, C., ... Lorenzetti, D. (2004). Policy implications associated with the socioeconomic and health system impact of telehealth: A case study from Canada. *Telemedicine Journal and e-Health*, *10*(1), 77–83. doi:10.1089/153056204773644616 PMID:15104919

Jha, A. (2017, September 20). *What Does an Ideal Healthcare System Look Like?* Retrieved from https://thehealthcareblog.com/blog/2017/09/20/what-does-an-ideal-healthcare-system-look-like/

Joos, O., Silva, R., Amouzou, A., Moulton, L. H., Perin, J., Bryce, J., & Mullany, L. C. (2016). Evaluation of a mHealth data quality intervention to improve documentation of pregnancy outcomes by health surveillance assistants in Malawi: A cluster randomized trial. *PLoS One*, *11*(1), e0145238. doi:10.1371/journal.pone.0145238 PMID:26731401

Jost, T. J., & Pollock, H. (2016). Making Healthcare Truly Affordable after Healthcare Reform. *The Journal of Law, Medicine & Ethics*, *44*(4), 546–554. doi:10.1177/1073110516684785 PMID:28661251

Kash, B. A., Spaulding, A., Johnson, C. E., & Gamm, L. (2014, January/February). Success Factors for Strategic Change Initiatives: A Qualitative Study. *Journal of Healthcare Management*, *59*(1), 65–82. doi:10.1097/00115514-201401000-00011 PMID:24611428

Kenny, N., Mann, K., & MacLeod, H. (2003). Role modeling in physicians' professional formation: Reconsidering an essential but untapped educational strategy. *Academic Medicine*, *78*(11), 1076–1083. PMID:14660418

Kerber, K., & Buono, A. (2005, Fall). Rethinking organizational change: Reframing the Challenge of Change Management. *Organization Development Journal*, *23*, 3.Kotter, J. P. (2007). Leading Change: Why Transformation Efforts Fail. *Harvard Business Review*, *85*(1), 96–103.

Kessler, G. (2019, September 24). Biden's bungled attack on medicare-for-all. *The Washington Post*. Retrieved from https://www.washingtonpost.com/politics/2019/09/24/bidens-bungled-attack-medicare-for-all/

Khan, C. T., Louie, A. K., Reicherter, D., & Roberts, L. W. (2016). What Is the Role of Academic Departments of Psychiatry in Advancing Global Mental Health? *Academic Psychiatry*, *40*(4), 672–678. doi:10.1007/s40596-016-0497-z PubMed

Khan, S. Z., Shahid, Z., Hedstrom, K., & Andersson, A. (2012). Hopes and fears in implementation of electronic health records in Bangladesh. *The Electronic Journal on Information Systems in Developing Countries*, *54*(1), 1–18. doi:10.1002/j.1681-4835.2012.tb00387.x

Kiberu, V. M., Mars, M., & Scott, R. E. (2017). Barriers and opportunities to implementation of sustainable e-Health programmes in Uganda: A literature review. *African Journal of Primary Health Care & Family Medicine*, *9*(1). doi:10.4102/phcfm.v9i1.1277 PMID:28582996

Kiberu, V. M., Scott, R. E., & Mars, M. (2019). Assessing core, e-learning, clinical and technology readiness to integrate telemedicine at public health facilities in Uganda: A health facility–based survey. *BMC Health Services Research*, *19*(1), 266. doi:10.118612913-019-4057-6 PMID:31035976

Kifle, M., Mbarika, V. W., Tsuma, C., Wilkerson, D., & Tan, J. (2008). A telemedicine transfer model for Sub-Saharan Africa. *Hawaii International Conference on System Sciences, Proceedings of the 41st Annual*. 10.1109/HICSS.2008.41

Kiley, J. (2018, October 3). *60% in US say health care coverage is government's responsibility*. Retrieved from https://www.pewresearch.org/fact-tank/2018/10/03/most-continue-to-say-ensuring-health-care-coverage-is-governments-responsibility/

Kim, E., Gellis, Z. D., Bradway, C., & Kenaley, B. (2018). Key determinants to using telehealth technology to serve medically ill and depressed homebound older adults. *Journal of Gerontological Social Work*, 1–24. doi:10.1080/01634372.2018.1499575 PMID:30040598

King, D. A. (2018, February). *Using technology to drive behavioural change in healthcare*. Retrieved from https://www.warc.com/content/article/bestprac/using_technology_to_drive_behavioural_change_in_healthcare/120037?utm_source=DailyNews&utm_medium=email&

King, R., Rose, R., Merritt, M., & Okray, J. (2014). *The ABCs of ACOs : a practical handbook on accountable care organizations*. Chicago, IL: ABA, Health Law Section.

Kirsh, S. B., Schaub, K., & Aron, D. C. (2009). Shared Medical Appointments: A Potential Venue for Education in Interprofessional Care. Quality Management in Health Care, 18(3), 217–224. https://doi-org.proxynw.uits.iu.edu/10.1097/QMH.0b013e3181aea27d

Klein, C., DeRouin, R., & Salas, E. (2006). Uncovering workplace interpersonal skills: A review, framework, and research agenda. *International Review of Industrial and Organizational Psychology*, *21*, 80–126.

Klingberg, A., Sawe, H. R., Hammar, U., Wallis, L. A., & Hasselberg, M. (2019). mHealth for burn injury consultations in a low-resource setting: An acceptability study among health care providers. *Telemedicine Journal and e-Health*, tmj.2019.0048. doi:10.1089/tmj.2019.0048 PMID:31161967

Koenig, M. A. (2019). *Telemedicine in the ICU*. Springer. doi:10.1007/978-3-030-11569-2

Koetsier, J. (2018, April 5). *Why every Amazon meeting has atleast one empty chair?* Retrieved from https://www.inc.com/john-koetsier/why-every-amazon-meeting-has-at-least-one-empty-chair.html

Koné Péfoyo, A. J., & Wodchis, W. P. (2013). Organizational performance impacting patient satisfaction in Ontario hospitals: A multilevel analysis. *BMC Research Notes*, *6*(1), 509–509. doi:10.1186/1756-0500-6-509 PMID:24304888

Korner, M., Lippenberger, C., Becker, S., Reichler, L., Müller, C., Zimmermann, L., ... Baumeister, H. (2016). Knowledge integration, teamwork, and performance in healthcare. *Journal of Health Organization and Management*, *30*(2), 227–243. doi:10.1108/JHOM-12-2014-0217 PMID:27052623

Kotter, J. P., & Schlesinger, L. A. (2008). Choosing Strategies for Change. *Harvard Business Review*, *86*(7/8), 130–139. PMID:10240501

Kouzes, J., & Posner, B. (2010). *The Truth About Leadership: The No-fads Heart-of-the-Matter Facts You Need to Know*. San Francisco, CA: Jossey-Bass.

Kouzes, J., & Posner, B. (2012). *The Leadership Challenge: How to Make Extraordinary Things Happen in Organizations* (5th ed.). San Francisco, CA: Jossey-Bass.

Krämer, J., & Schreyögg, J. (2019). Demand-side determinants of rising hospital admissions in Germany: The role of ageing. *The European Journal of Health Economics*, 1–14. PMID:30739296

Kruse, C. S., Atkins, J. M., Baker, T. D., Gonzales, E. N., Paul, J. L., & Brooks, M. (2018). Factors influencing the adoption of telemedicine for treatment of military veterans with post-traumatic stress disorder. *Journal of Rehabilitation Medicine*, *50*(5), 385–392. doi:10.2340/16501977-2302 PMID:29700551

Lagarde, M., Huicho, L., & Papanicolas, I. (2019). Motivating provision of high quality care: It is not all about the money. *BMJ (Clinical Research Ed.)*, *366*, l5210. doi:10.1136/bmj.l5210 PMID:31548200

Lakhani, J., Benzies, K., & Hayden, K. A. (2012). Attributes of Interdisciplinary Research Teams: A Comprehensive Review of the Literature. *Clinical and Investigative Medicine. Medecine Clinique et Experimentale*, *35*(5), E260–E265. doi:10.25011/cim.v35i5.18698

Lapointe, L., Lamothe, L., & Fortin, J. (2006). The Dynamics of IT Adoption in a Major Change Process in Healthcare Delivery. In T. Spil & R. Schuring (Eds.), *E-Health Systems Diffusion and Use: The Innovation, the User and the Use IT Model* (pp. 107–127). Hershey, PA: IGI Global. doi:10.4018/978-1-59140-423-1.ch007

Leaming, L. E. (2007). *Barriers to physician adoption of telemedicine and best practices for overcoming these barriers*. Medical University of South Carolina.

Leape, L., Shore, M., Dienstag, J., Mayer, R., Edgman-Levitan, S., Meyer, G., & Healy, G. (2012). A culture of respect, part 1: The nature and causes of disrespectful behavior by physicians. *Academic Medicine*, *87*(7), 845-852.

Lee, F. (2004). *If Disney Ran Your Hospital: 9 1/2 Things You Would Do Differently.* Second River Healthcare.

Lee, J. Y., & Lee, S. W. H. (2018). Telemedicine Cost–Effectiveness for Diabetes Management: A Systematic Review. *Diabetes Technology & Therapeutics.*

Lee, W. (2013). Measuring the immeasurable core competency of professionalism. *JAMA Otolaryngology-Head & Neck Surgery, 139*(1), 12–13. doi:10.1001/jamaoto.2013.1071 PMID:23329086

Lencioni, P. (2012). *The Advantage: Why Organizational Health Trumps Everything Else in Business.* San Francisco, CA: Jossey-Bass.

Leonard, M., & Frankel, A. (2011). Role of effective teamwork and communication in delivering safe, high-quality care. *The Mount Sinai Journal of Medicine, New York, 78*(6), 820–826. doi:10.1002/msj.20295 PMID:22069205

Levett-Jones, T., Burdett, T., Chow, Y. L., Jönsson, L., Lasater, K., Mathews, L. R., ... Wihlborg, J. (2018). Case Studies of Interprofessional Education Initiatives from Five Countries. *Journal of Nursing Scholarship, 50*(3), 324–332. doi:10.1111/jnu.12384 PubMed

Lewis, S., Synowiec, C., Lagomarsino, G., & Schweitzer, J. (2012). E-health in low-and middle-income countries: Findings from the Center for Health Market Innovations. *Bulletin of the World Health Organization, 90*(5), 332–340. doi:10.2471/BLT.11.099820 PMID:22589566

Li, Y., Li, Y., Deng, Z., & Zhu, Z. (2018). *A Collaborative Telemedicine Platform Focusing on Paranasal Sinus Segmentation.* Paper presented at the International Conference on Intelligent Interactive Multimedia Systems and Services.

Lincoff, N. (2015, June 30). *The future of healthcare could be in concierge medicine.* Retrieved from https://www.healthline.com/health-news/the-future-of-healthcare-could-be-in-concierge-medicine-063015

Little, M. M., St Hill, C., Ware, K. B., Swanoski, M. T., Chapman, S. A., Lutfiyya, M. N., & Cerra, F. (2017). Team science as interprofessional collaborative research practice: A systematic review of the science of team science literature. *Journal of Investigative Medicine: The Official Publication of The American Federation for Clinical Research, 65*(1), 15–22. doi:10.1136/jim-2016-000216 PubMed

Lohr, K., Brook, R., Kamberg, C., Goldberg, G., Leibowitz, A., Keesey, J., ... Newhouse, J. (1986). Use of Medical Care in the Rand Health Insurance Experiment: Diagnosis- and Service-Specific Analyses in a Randomized Controlled Trial. *Medical Care, 24*(9). PMID:3093785

Ludmerer, K. M. (1999). *Time to Heal: American Medical Education from the Turn of the Century to the Era of Managed Care.* New York, NY: Oxford University Press.

Lu, J., Yu, C.-S., & Liu, C. (2005). Facilitating conditions, wireless trust and adoption intention. *Journal of Computer Information Systems, 46*(1), 17–24.

Lundy, J. (2018, June 5). Sharing health costs with faith: Ministries offer coverage, savings as an alternative to traditional insurance. *TCA Regional News.*

Lutfiyya, M. M., Chang, L. F., McGrath, C., Dana, C., & Lipsky, M. S. (2019). The state of the science of interprofessional collaborative practice: A scoping review of the patient health-related outcomes-based literature published between 2010 and 2018. *PLoS One, 14*(6), 1–18. doi:10.1371/journal.pone.0218578 PubMed

Lutfiyya, M. N., Brandt, B., Delaney, C., Pechacek, J., & Cerra, F. (2016). Setting a research agenda for interprofessional education and collaborative practice in the context of United States health system reform. *Journal of Interprofessional Care, 30*(1), 7–14. doi:10.3109/13561820.2015.1040875 PubMed

Lutfiyya, M. W., Brandt, B. F., & Cerra, F. (2016). Reflections from the intersection of health professions education and clinical practice: The state of the science of interprofessional education and collaborative practice. *Academic Medicine, 91*(6), 766–771. doi:10.1097/ACM.0000000000001139 PubMed

Macy, J., Jr. Foundation. (2013). Transforming patient care: Aligning interprofessional education with clinical practice redesign. New York, NY: Author.

Mahood, S. (2011). Medical education: Beware the hidden curriculum. *Canadian Family Physician Médecin de Famille Canadien, 57*(9), 983–985. PMID:21918135

Makary, M. A., & Daniel, M. (2016). Medical error--the third leading cause of death in the US. *British Medical Journal, 1*, ●●●. Retrieved from http://search.ebscohost.com/login.aspx?direct=true&db=edb&AN=115194747&site=eds-live PubMed

Manning, W. G., & Susan Marquis, M. (1996). Health Insurance: The Tradeoff Between Risk Pooling and Moral Hazard. *Journal of Health Economics, 15*(5), 609–639. doi:10.1016/S0167-6296(96)00497-3 PMID:10164045

Marcotte, L., Moriates, C., Wolfson, D., & Frankel, R. (2019). Professionalism as the Bedrock of High-Value Care. *Academic Medicine.* Available from: https://journals.lww.com/academicmedicine/Abstract/publishahead/Professionalism_as_the_Bedrock_of_High_Value_Care.97538.aspx

Martin, A. B., Probst, J. C., Shah, K., Chen, Z., & Garr, D. (2012). Differences in readiness between rural hospitals and primary care providers for telemedicine adoption and implementation: Findings from a statewide telemedicine survey. *The Journal of Rural Health, 28*(1), 8–15. doi:10.1111/j.1748-0361.2011.00369.x PMID:22236310

McCarthy, A. (2013, October 5). Obamacare's unconstitutional origins. *National Review.* Retrieved from https://www.nationalreview.com/2013/10/obamacares-unconstitutional-origins-andrew-c-mccarthy/

McCarthy, J. (2018, December 7). Most Americans rate still rate their healthcare quality quite positively. *Well-Being*. Retrieved from https://news.gallup.com/poll/245195/americans-rate-healthcare-quite-positively.aspx

McCarthy, N. (2019, August 8). How U.S. Healthcare Spending Per Capita Compares With Other Countries [Infographic]. *Forbes*. Retrieved from https://www.forbes.com/sites/niallmccarthy/2019/08/08/how-us-healthcare-spending-per-capita-compares-with-other-countries-infographic/#37dfa6fd575d

McClelland, D. C. (1973, January). Testing for Competence Rather Than for 'Intelligence.' *The American Psychologist*, *28*(1), 1–14. doi:10.1037/h0034092 PMID:4684069

Medicopedia. (n.d.). Retrieved from https://medicopedia.co/

Meleis, A. I. (2016). Interprofessional education: A summary of reports and barriers to recommendations. *Journal of Nursing Scholarship*, *48*(1), 106–112. doi:10.1111/jnu.12184 PubMed

Mello, M., Chandra, A., Gawande, A., & Studdert, D. (2010). National costs of the medical liability system. *Health Affairs*. Retrieved from https://www.healthaffairs.org/doi/10.1377/hlthaff.2009.0807

Menvielle, L., Audrain-Pontevia, A.-F., & Menvielle, W. (2017). *The digitization of healthcare: New challenges and opportunities*. Springer. doi:10.1057/978-1-349-95173-4

Mgawadere, F., Smith, H., Asfaw, A., Lambert, J., & van den Broek, N. (2019). "There is no time for knowing each other": Quality of care during childbirth in a low resource setting. *Midwifery*, *75*, 33–40. doi:10.1016/j.midw.2019.04.006 PMID:30986692

Miller & Grant. (2004, May 31). *The Role of Public Health Improvements in Health Advances: The 20th Century United States*. Academic Press.

Miller, E. (2010). *Telemedicine and the provider-patient relationship: What we know so far*. Report prepared for the Nuffield Council's Working Party on Medical Profiling and Online Medicine.

Miller, G. E. (1990). The Assessment of Clinical Skills/Competence/Performance. *Academic Medicine*, *65*(9), 63–67. doi:10.1097/00001888-199009000-00045 PMID:2400509

Millman, M. (1993). *18 Institute of Medicine Committee on Monitoring Access to Personal Healthcare Services. In Access to Healthcare in America*. Washington, DC: National Academics Press.

Modi, P. K., Portney, D., Hollenbeck, B. K., & Ellimoottil, C. (2018). Engaging telehealth to drive value-based urology. *Current Opinion in Urology*, *28*(4), 342–347. PMID:29697472

Moon, M. (2001). Medicare. *The New England Journal of Medicine*, *344*(12), 928–931. doi:10.1056/NEJM200103223441211 PMID:11259729

Mount, G. (2005). The Role of Emotional Intelligence in Developing International Business Capability: EI Provides Traction. In *Linking Emotional Intelligence and Performance at Work*. Mahwah, NJ: Lawrence Erlbaum.

Mukherjee, N., & Sexton, J. (2008). Impact of preoperative briefings on operating room delays. *Archives of Surgery*, *143*(11), 1068–1072. doi:10.1001/archsurg.143.11.1068 PMID:19015465

Mukherjee, S. (2012). *The emperor of all maladies a biography of cancer*. Detroit, MI: Gale, Cengage Learning. doi:10.5005/jp-journals-10028-1025

Mun, Y. Y., Jackson, J. D., Park, J. S., & Probst, J. C. (2006). Understanding information technology acceptance by individual professionals: Toward an integrative view. *Information & Management*, *43*(3), 350–363. doi:10.1016/j.im.2005.08.006

Murphy, K. M., & Topel, R. H. (2006). The Value of Health and Longevity. *Journal of Political Economy*, *114*(October), 871–904. doi:10.1086/508033

Murphy, S. E., Putter, S., & Johnson, S. (2014). Soft skills training: Best practices in industry and higher education. In R. E. Riggio & S. J. Tan (Eds.), *Leader interpersonal and influence skills: The soft skills of leadership* (pp. 276–310). New York, NY: Taylor & Francis.

Nagarajan, R., Kalinka, A. T., & Hogan, W. R. (2013). Evidence of community structure in biomedical research grant collaborations. *Journal of Biomedical Informatics*, *46*(1), 40–46. doi:10.1016/j.jbi.2012.08.002 PubMed

Nardi, M. D., French, E., Jones, J. B., & Mccauley, J. (2016). Medical Spending of the US Elderly. *Fiscal Studies*, *37*(3-4), 717–747. doi:10.1111/j.1475-5890.2016.12106 PMID:31404348

Narine, L., & Persaud, D. D. (2003). Gaining and maintaining commitment to large-scale change in healthcare organizations. *Health Services Management*, *16*(3), 179–187. doi:10.1258/095148403322167933 PMID:12908992

National Center for Health Statistics. (2018). Health, United States, 2017: With Special Feature on Mortality. Hyattsville, MD: Author.

National Institutes of Health. (n.d.). Research training and career development. Retrieved from https://researchtraining.nih.gov/programs/fellowships

Neily, J., Mills, P., & Young-Xu, Y. (2010). Impact of a comprehensive patient safety strategy on obstetric adverse events. *Journal of the American Medical Association*, *304*, 1693–1700. doi:10.1001/jama.2010.1506 PMID:20959579

Nelson-Brantley, H. V., & Warshawsky, e. (2018). Interprofessional education: Advancing team science to create collaborative safety cultures. The Journal of Nursing Administration, 48(5), 235–237. doi:10.1097/NNA.0000000000000607 PubMed

Newhouse, J. P. (2002). Why Is There A Quality Chasm? *Health Affairs*, *21*(4), 13–25. doi:10.1377/hlthaff.21.4.13 PMID:12117124

OECD. (2017). *Health at a Glance 2017: OECD Indicators*. Paris: OECD Publishing.

OECD. (2019). *Health at a Glance 2019: OECD Indicators*. Paris: OECD Publishing; doi:10.1787/4dd50c09-

Office for Civil Rights. (2015, November 6). *Methods for De-identification of PHI*. Retrieved from https://www.hhs.gov/hipaa/for-professionals/privacy/special-topics/de-identification/index.html

Office of the Management and Budget. (2018). *Budget of the US Government: FY 2019*. Washington, DC: Government Publishing Office. Available from: https://www.govinfo.gov/content/pkg/BUDGET-2019-BUD/pdf/BUDGET-2019-BUD.pdf

Olsen, J. A., Smith, R. D., & Harris, A. (1999, April). *Economic Theory and the Monetary Valuation of Health Care: An Overview of the Issues as Applied to the Economic Evaluation of Health Care Programs*. Centre for Health Program Evaluation: Working Paper No. 82.

OpenStax CNX. (2016). *8.4 Efficiency in Perfectly Competitive Markets*. Retrieved from http://cnx.org/contents/69619d2b-68f0-44b0-b074-a9b2bf90b2c6@11.330

Or, C. K., Karsh, B.-T., Severtson, D. J., Burke, L. J., Brown, R. L., & Brennan, P. F. (2011). Factors affecting home care patients' acceptance of a web-based interactive self-management technology. *Journal of the American Medical Informatics Association, 18*(1), 51–59. doi:10.1136/jamia.2010.007336 PMID:21131605

Organization, W. H. (1998). A Health Telematics Policy in Support of WHO'S Health-For-All Strategy for Global Development: Report of the WHO Group Consultation on Health Telematics 11-16 December, Geneva, 1997. World Health Organization.

Oriade, A., & Schofield, P. (2019). An examination of the role of service quality and perceived value in visitor attraction experience. *Journal of Destination Marketing & Management, 11*, 1–9. doi:10.1016/j.jdmm.2018.10.002

Panner, M. (2019, March 25). *Cancer Treatment Costs Imperil Patients*. Forbes. Retrieved from https://www.forbes.com/sites/forbestechcouncil/2019/03/25/cancer-treatment-costs-imperil-patients/#1e91a53f2b6f

Papadakis, M., Teherani, A., Banach, M., Knettler, T., Rattner, S., Stern, D., ... Hodgson, C. S. (2005). Disciplinary action by medical boards and prior behavior in medical school. *The New England Journal of Medicine, 353*(25), 2673–2682. doi:10.1056/NEJMsa052596 PMID:16371633

Papanicolas, I., Woskie, L. R., & Jha, A. K. (2018). Health care spending in the United States and other high-income countries. *Journal of the American Medical Association, 319*(10), 1024–1039. doi:10.1001/jama.2018.1150 PMID:29536101

Papatheodorou, T., & Moyles, J. R. (Eds.). (2008). Learning together in the early years: Exploring relational pedagogy. Routledge. Paradis. E., & Whitehead, C. R. (208). Beyond the lamppost: A proposal for a fourth wave of education for collaboration. *Academic Medicine, 93*(10), 1457–1463.

PAR-19-101: Physical Sciences-Oncology Network (PS-ON): Physical Sciences-Oncology Projects (PS-OP) (U01 Clinical Trial Optional). (n.d.). Retrieved from https://grants.nih.gov/grants/guide/pa-files/PAR-19-101.html

Patient Safety Movement. (n.d.). Resources for Policy Makers. Retrieved from https://patientsafetymovement.org/advocacy/policy-makers/resources-for-policy-makers/

Pauly, M. V., & Satterthwaite, M. A. (1981). The Pricing of Primary Care Physicians' Services: A Test of the Role of Consumer Information. *The Bell Journal of Economics, 12*(2), 488–506. doi:10.2307/3003568

Pettker, C., Thung, S., & Norwit. (2009). Impact of a comprehensive patient safety strategy on obstetric adverse events. *American Journal of Obstetrics Gynecology, 200*, 492e1-492e8.

Phelps, C. E. (2012). *Health Economics* (5th ed.). Pearson.

Physical Sciences in Oncology. (2018). Retrieved from https://physics.cancer.gov/

Pichler, S., & Beenen, G. (2014). Toward the development of a model and a measure of managerial interpersonal skills. In R. E. Riggio & S. J. Tan (Eds.), *Leader interpersonal and influence skills: The soft skills of leadership* (pp. 11–30). New York, NY: Taylor & Francis.

Pink, D. (2011). *Drive: The Surprising Truth About What Motivates Us*. Riverhead Books.

Powers, S. E., & de Waters, J. (2004). Creating project-based learning experiences for university-k-12 partnerships. 34th Annual Frontiers in Education, 2004, F3D–18.

Principles for Health Care Payment Reform to Improve Cancer Care Quality. (n.d.). Retrieved from https://www.canceradvocacy.org/cancer-policy/principles-for-health-care-payment-reform-to-improve-cancer-care-quality/

Promoting a More Balanced Approach to Cancer Prevention and Treatment. (n.d.). Retrieved from https://www.ascopost.com/issues/december-15-2012/promoting-a-more-balanced-approach-to-cancer-prevention-and-treatment/

Puhl, R., Gold, J., Luedicke, J., & DePierre, J. (2013). The effect of physicians' body weight on patient attitudes: implications for physician selection, trust and adherence to medical advice. *International Journal of Obesity, 37*(11), 1415-21.

Rajaram, R., & Bilimoria, K. Y. (2015). Medicare. *Journal of the American Medical Association, 314*(4), 420. doi:10.1001/jama.2015.8049 PMID:26219069

Rajteric, I. H. (2010). Overview of business intelligence maturity models. *Journal of Contemporary Management Issues, 15*(1), 47–67.

Reeves, S., Pelone, F., Harrison, R., Goldman, J., & Zwarenstein, M. (2017). Interprofessional collaboration to improve professional practice and healthcare outcomes. *Cochrane Database of Systematic Reviews, 6*(6), CD000072. doi:10.1002/14651858.CD000072.pub3

Reeves, S., Perrier, L., Goldman, J., Freeth, D., & Zwarenstein, M. (2013). Interprofessional education: Effects on professional practice and healthcare outcomes (update). *Cochrane Database of Systematic Reviews*, (3): CD002213. doi:10.1002/14651858.CD002213.pub3

Retchin, S. M. (2008). A conceptual framework for interprofessional and co-managed care. *Academic Medicine*, *83*(10), 929–933. doi:10.1097/ACM.0b013e3181850b4b PubMed

Rho, M. J., Choi, I., & Lee, J. (2014). Predictive factors of telemedicine service acceptance and behavioral intention of physicians. *International Journal of Medical Informatics*, *83*(8), 559–571. doi:10.1016/j.ijmedinf.2014.05.005 PMID:24961820

Richard, M. (1996). NHS waiting lists have been a boon for private medicine in the UK. *Canadian Medical Association Journal*, *154*(3), 378–381. PMID:8564909

Rittenhouse, D., Shortell, S., & Fisher, E. (2009). Primary Care and Accountable Care— Two Essential Elements of Delivery-System Reform. *The New England Journal of Medicine*, *361*(24), 2301–2303. doi:10.1056/NEJMp0909327 PMID:19864649

Rivers, R. M., Swain, D., & Nixon, W. R. (2003). Using aviation safety measures to enhance patient outcomes. *AORN Journal*, *77*(1), 158–162. doi:10.1016/S0001-2092(06)61385-9 PubMed

Roberto, M. A., & Levesque, L. C. (2005). The art of making change initiatives stick. *MIT Sloan Management Review*, *46*(4), 53.

Robertson, J. J., & Long, B. (2018). Suffering in silence: Medical error and its impact on health care providers. *The Journal of Emergency Medicine*, *54*(4), 402–409. doi:10.1016/j.jemermed.2017.12.001 PubMed

Rogers, C. (1961). *On Becoming a Person: A Therapist's View of Psychotherapy*. Houghton Mifflin.

Rogers, G. D., Thistlethwaite, J. E., Anderson, E. S., Abrandt Dahlgren, M., Grymonpre, R. E., Moran, M., & Samarasekera, D. D. (2017). International consensus statement on the assessment of interprofessional learning outcomes. *Medical Teacher*, *39*(4), 347–359. doi:10.1080/014215 9X.2017.1270441 PubMed

Rose, M., & Ritchie, H. (2015, July 3). *Cancer.* Retrieved from https://ourworldindata.org/cancer

Rosen, M. A., DiazGranados, D., Dietz, A. S., Benishek, L. E., Thompson, D., Pronovost, P. J., & Weaver, S. J. (2018). Teamwork in healthcare: Key discoveries enabling safer, high-quality care. *The American Psychologist*, *73*(4), 433–450. doi:10.1037/amp0000298 PMID:29792459

Rosenthal, E. (2018). *An American sickness: how healthcare became big business and how you can take it back.* New York: Penguin Books.

Roy, A. (2011, April 29). Why Switzerland has the world's best health care system. *Forbes.*

Roy, A., van der Weijden, T., & de Vries, N. (2017). Predictors and consequences of rural clients' satisfaction level in the district public-private mixed health system of Bangladesh. *Global Health Research and Policy, 2*(1), 31.

Rozensky, R. H., & Janicke, D. M. (2012). Commentary: Healthcare reform and psychology's workforce: Preparing for the future of pediatric psychology. *Journal of Pediatric Psychology,* *37*(4), 359–368. doi:10.1093/jpepsy/jsr111 PubMed

Russo, L., Campagna, I., Ferretti, B., Pandolfi, E., Carloni, E., D'Ambrosio, A., ... Tozzi, A. E. (2017). What drives attitude towards telemedicine among families of pediatric patients? A survey. *BMC Pediatrics, 17*(1), 21. doi:10.118612887-016-0756-x PMID:28095894

Salas, E., Sims, D. E., & Burke, C. S. (2005). Is there a "Big Five" in teamwork? *Small Group Research, 36*(5), 555–599. doi:10.1177/1046496405277134

Savedoff, D. W. (2004). 40th Anniversary: Kenneth Arrow and the Birth of Health Economics. *Bulletin of the World Health Organization, 82*(2), 139–140. PMID:15042237

Schneider, E., Sarnak, D., Shah, A., & Doty, M. (2017). *Mirror, Mirror 2017: International Comparison Reflects Flaws and Opportunities for Better U.S. Health Care.* Retrieved from https://interactives.commonwealthfund.org/2017/july/mirror-mirror/

Schneider, M. (2017, July 19). *Google spent 2 years studying 180 teams. The most successful ones shared these 5 traits.* Retrieved from https://www.inc.com/michael-schneider/google-thought-they-knew-how-to-create-the-perfect.html

Schuetz, B., Mann, E., & Everett, W. (2010). Educating Health Professionals Collaboratively For Team-Based Primary Care. *Health Affairs, 29*(8), 1476–1480. doi:10.1377/hlthaff.2010.0052 PubMed

Schwantes, M. (2016). Science Says 92 Percent of People Don't Achieve Their Goals. Here's How the Other 8 Percent Do. *Inc.* Available from: https://www.inc.com/marcel-schwantes/science-says-92-percent-of-people-dont-achieve-goals-heres-how-the-other-8-perce.html

Schweitzer, J., & Synowiec, C. (2010). The economics of eHealth. *Health, 29*(2), 235–238.

Scott Kruse, C., Karem, P., Shifflett, K., Vegi, L., Ravi, K., & Brooks, M. (2018). Evaluating barriers to adopting Telemedicine worldwide: A systematic review. *Journal of Telemedicine and Telecare, 24*(1), 4–12. doi:10.1177/1357633X16674087 PMID:29320966

Scott, R. E., & Mars, M. (2013). Principles and framework for eHealth strategy development. *Journal of Medical Internet Research, 15*(7), e155. doi:10.2196/jmir.2250 PMID:23900066

Selladurai, R., & Carraher, S. (2014). Lead like the greatest leader! Case Study. In R. Selladurai & S. Carraher (Eds.), *Servant leadership: Research and Practice* (pp. 350–355). Hershey, PA: IGI Global. doi:10.4018/978-1-4666-5840-0.ch026

Senge, P. (1990). *The Fifth Discipline: The Art & Practice of the Learning Organization.* New York, NY: Doubleday Currency.

Simon, S. (2019, January 8). *Facts & Figures 2019: US Cancer Death Rate has Dropped 27% in 25 Years.* American Cancer Society. Retrieved from https://www.cancer.org/latest-news/facts-and-figures-2019.html

Simonet, D. (2010). Healthcare Reforms and Cost Reduction Strategies in Europe: The Cases of Germany, UK, Switzerland, Italy, and France. *International Journal of Health Care Quality Assurance, 23*(5), 470–488. doi:10.1108/09526861011050510 PMID:20845678

Snider, M. (2018, January 30). Amazon, Berkshire Hathaway, JPMorgan Chase to tackle employee healthcare costs, delivery. *USA Today (Online).* Retrieved from https://www.usatoday.com/story/money/americasmarkets/2018/01/30/amazon-berkshire-hathaway-jpmorgan-chase-tackle-employee-health-care-costs-delivery/1077866001/

Sood, S., Mbarika, V., Jugoo, S., Dookhy, R., Doarn, C. R., Prakash, N., & Merrell, R. C. (2007). What is telemedicine? A collection of 104 peer-reviewed perspectives and theoretical underpinnings. *Telemedicine Journal and e-Health, 13*(5), 573–590. doi:10.1089/tmj.2006.0073 PMID:17999619

Sorwar, G., Rahamn, M. M., Uddin, R., & Hoque, M. (2016). Cost and time effectiveness analysis of a telemedicine service in Bangladesh. *Studies in Health Technology and Informatics, 231,* 127–134. PMID:27782024

Southerland, J. H., Webster-Cyriaque, J., Bednarsh, H., & Mouton, C. P. (2016). Interprofessional collaborative practice models in chronic disease management. Dental Clinics, 60(4), 789–809. doi: PubMed doi:10.1016/j.cden.2016.05.001

Stack, S. (2016). Health Care Reform in the United States: Past, Present, and Future Challenges. *World Medical Journal, 62*(4), 153–157.

Starmer, A. J., Spector, N. D., Srivastava, R., West, D. C., Rosenbluth, G., Allen, A. D., ... Lipsitz, S. R. (2014). Changes in medical errors after implementation of a handoff program. *The New England Journal of Medicine, 371*(19), 1803–1812. doi:10.1056/NEJMsa1405556 PubMed

Stein, S., & Book, H. (2003). *The EQ Edge: Emotional Intelligence and Your Success.* Toronto, Canada: Multi-Health Systems.

Stevens, M. J., & Campion, M. A. (1994). The knowledge, skill, and ability requirements for teamwork: Implications for human resource management. *Journal of Management, 20*(2), 503–530. doi:10.1177/014920639402000210

Swanson Kazley, A., McLeod, A. C., & Wager, K. A. (2012). Telemedicine in an international context: definition, use, and future. In *Health Information Technology in the International Context* (pp. 143–169). Emerald Group Publishing Limited. doi:10.1108/S1474-8231(2012)0000012011

Teichert, E. (2018, October 16). *Anthem to pay $16M in record data breach settlement.* Retrieved from https://www.modernhealthcare.com/article/20181016/NEWS/181019927

Tengs, T. O., Adams, M. E., Pliskin, J. S., Safran, D. G., Siegel, J. E., Weinstein, M. C., & Graham, J. D. (1995). Five-Hundred Life-Saving Interventions and Their Cost-Effectiveness. *Risk Analysis, 15*(3), 369–390. doi:10.1111/j.1539-6924.1995.tb00330.x PMID:7604170

Tesch, D., Kloppenborg, T. J., & Frolick, M. N. (2007). IT Project Risk Factors: The Project Management Professionals Perspective. *Journal of Computer Information Systems, 47*(4), 61–69.

The U.S. Health Care System: An International Perspective. (n.d.). Retrieved from https://dpeaflcio. org/programs-publications/issue-fact-sheets/the-u-s-health-care-system-an-international-perspective/

The White House. (2019, October 3). *President Donald J. Trump's healthcare agenda puts seniors and American patients first.* Retrieved from https://www.whitehouse.gov/briefings-statements/president-donald-j-trumps-healthcare-agenda-puts-seniors-american-patients-first/?utm_source=ods&utm_medium=email&utm_campaign=1600d

Thomas, E. J., Sherwood, G. D., & Helmreich, R. L. (2003). Lessons from aviation: Teamwork to improve patient safety. *Nursing Economics*, *21*(5), 241. PubMed

Thom, K. A., Heil, E. L., Croft, L. D., Duffy, A., Morgan, D. J., & Johantgen, M. (2016). Advancing interprofessional patient safety education for medical, nursing, and pharmacy learners during clinical rotations. *Journal of Interprofessional Care*, *30*(6), 819–822. doi:10.1080/1356 1820.2016.1215972 PubMed

Thornton, G. C. III, & Rupp, D. E. (2006). *Assessment centers and human resource management.* Mahwah, NJ: Lawrence Erlbaum. doi:10.4324/9781410617170

Timsina, P., Liu, J., & El-Gayar, O. (2016). Advanced analytics for the automation of medical systematic reviews. *Information Systems Frontiers*, *18*(2), 237–252. doi:10.100710796-015-9589-7

Tracy, C. S., Bell, S. H., Nickell, L. A., Charles, J., & Upshur, E. G. (2013). Innovative Model of interprofessional primary care for elderly patients with complex health care needs. *Canadian Family Physician Medecin de Famille Canadien*, *59*(3), e148–e155. PubMed

Tsai, J.-M., Cheng, M.-J., Tsai, H.-H., Hung, S.-W., & Chen, Y.-L. (2019). Acceptance and resistance of telehealth: The perspective of dual-factor concepts in technology adoption. *International Journal of Information Management*, *49*, 34–44. doi:10.1016/j.ijinfomgt.2019.03.003

Tuzkaya, G., Sennaroglu, B., Kalender, Z. T., & Mutlu, M. (2019). Hospital service quality evaluation with IVIF-PROMETHEE and a case study. *Socio-Economic Planning Sciences*, *68*, 100705. doi:10.1016/j.seps.2019.04.002

Twachtman, G. (2019, May). CMS creates Primary Care First for small, solo practices. *Family Practice* , *49*(5), 1–4.

U.S. Health Care Spending Highest Among Developed Countries. (2019, January 7). Retrieved from https://www.jhsph.edu/news/news-releases/2019/us-health-care-spending-highest-among-developed-countries.html

United States: Swiss Health System offers Key Lessons. (2008, July 5). *Oxford Analytics Daily Brief Service*.

Van Dyk, L. (2013). *The development of a telemedicine service maturity model.* Stellenbosch: Stellenbosch University.

Van Dyk, L. (2014). A review of telehealth service implementation frameworks. *International Journal of Environmental Research and Public Health, 11*(2), 1279–1298. doi:10.3390/ijerph110201279 PMID:24464237

Vanderbilt University. (2019). About the Program. Retrieved from https://medschool.vanderbilt.edu/vpil/about-the-program/

Vanderbilt University. (2019). Vanderbilt Program in Interprofessional Learning: About the Program. Retrieved from https://medschool.vanderbilt.edu/vpil/

Venkatesh, V. (2000). Determinants of perceived ease of use: Integrating control, intrinsic motivation, and emotion into the technology acceptance model. *Information Systems Research, 11*(4), 342–365. doi:10.1287/isre.11.4.342.11872

Venkatesh, V., & Davis, F. D. (2000). A theoretical extension of the technology acceptance model: Four longitudinal field studies. *Management Science, 46*(2), 186–204. doi:10.1287/mnsc.46.2.186.11926

Venkatesh, V., Morris, M. G., Davis, G. B., & Davis, F. D. (2003). User acceptance of information technology: Toward a unified view. *Management Information Systems Quarterly, 27*(3), 425–478. doi:10.2307/30036540

Vermeeren, D. (2007). *365 Lessons from Amazing Success*. Business Boost SUCCESS.

Veterans Health Administration Patient Aligned Care Team. (2019). Retrieved from https://www.pcpcc.org/initiative/veterans-health-administration-patient-aligned-care-team-pact

Viscusi, W. K., & Aldy, J. E. (2003). The Value of a Statistical Life: A Critical Review of Market Estimates throughout the World. *Journal of Risk and Uncertainty, 5*(1), 5–76. doi:10.1023/A:1025598106257

Vishwanath, A., & Scamurra, S. D. (2007). Barriers to the adoption of electronic health records: Using concept mapping to develop a comprehensive empirical model. *Health Informatics Journal, 13*(2), 119–134. doi:10.1177/1460458207076468 PMID:17510224

Wachter, R. M., & Gupta, K. (2019). *Understanding Patient Safety* (3rd ed.)., Retrieved from https://accessmedicine-mhmedical-com.ezproxy.rosalindfranklin.edu/book.aspx?bookid=2203

Wagner, E. H. (1998). Chronic disease management: What will it take to improve care for chronic illness? *Effective Clinical Practice, 1*(1), 2–4. PubMed

Wakefield, M. (2000). To err is human: An Institute of Medicine report. *Professional Psychology, Research and Practice, 31*(3), 243–244. doi:10.1037/h0092814

Waller, M., & Stotler, C. (2018). Telemedicine: A primer. *Current Allergy and Asthma Reports, 18*(10), 54. doi:10.100711882-018-0808-4 PMID:30145709

Walshe, K., & Smith, J. (2011). *Healthcare management* (2nd ed.). Maidenhead, UK: Open University Press.

Wang, Y., Kung, L. A., & Byrd, T. A. (2018). Big data analytics: Understanding its capabilities and potential benefits for healthcare organizations. *Technological Forecasting and Social Change*, *126*, 3–13. doi:10.1016/j.techfore.2015.12.019

Weinstein, R. S., Krupinski, E. A., & Doarn, C. R. (2018). Clinical Examination Component of Telemedicine, Telehealth, mHealth, and Connected Health Medical Practices. *The Medical Clinics of North America*, *102*(3), 533–544. doi:10.1016/j.mcna.2018.01.002 PMID:29650074

Weinstein, R. S., Lopez, A. M., Joseph, B. A., Erps, K. A., Holcomb, M., Barker, G. P., & Krupinski, E. A. (2014). Telemedicine, telehealth, and mobile health applications that work: Opportunities and barriers. *The American Journal of Medicine*, *127*(3), 183–187. doi:10.1016/j.amjmed.2013.09.032 PMID:24384059

Weiss, K. B., Passiment, M., & Riodan, L. (n.d.). Wagner R for the National Collaborative for Improving the Clinical Learning Environment IP-CLE Report Work Group. *Achieving the Optimal Interprofessional Clinical Learning Environment: Proceedings From an NCICLE Symposium.* Retrieved from http://ncicle.org

Weld, H. (2015, June). Professional Identity (Trans)Formation in Medical Education. *Academic Medicine*, *90*(6), 701–706. doi:10.1097/ACM.0000000000000731 PMID:25881651

Werling, J., Keehan, S., Nyhus, D., Heffler, S., Horst, R., & Meade, D. (2014). The supply side of health care. *Survey of Current Business.*

West Virginia University. (2017). *Privacy Program Maturity Template.* Retrieved from: https://library.educause.edu/resources/2017/8/privacy-program-maturity-template

What can payers do to reduce costs? (n.d.). Retrieved from https://medcitynews.com/2019/08/what-can-payers-do-to-reduce-costs-start-by-simplifying-how-they-verify-provider-data/?rf=1

Whittaker, A. A., Aufdenkamp, M., & Tinley, S. (2009). Barriers and facilitators to electronic documentation in a rural hospital. *Journal of Nursing Scholarship*, *41*(3), 293–300. doi:10.1111/j.1547-5069.2009.01278.x PMID:19723278

Winnefeld, J. A., Jr., Kirchhoff, C., & Upton, D. M. (2015). Cybersecurity's Human Factor: Lessons from the Pentagon. *Harvard Business Review*, *93*(9), 86–17.

Woodside, A. G., Frey, L. L., & Daly, R. T. (1989). Linking sort/ice anlity, customer satisfaction, and behavioral intention. *Journal of Health Care Marketing*, *9*(4), 5–17. PMID:10304174

World Health Organization. (2010). The WHO Framework for Action. *Journal of Interprofessional Care*, *24*(5), 475–478. doi:10.3109/13561820.2010.504134 PubMed

World Health Organization. (2019). *Framework for action on interprofessional education and collaborative practice.* Geneva, Switzerland: World Health Organization.

World Health Organization's Ranking of the World's Health Systems. (n.d.). Retrieved from http://thepatientfactor.com/canadian-health-care-information/world-health-organizations-ranking-of-the-worlds-health-systems/

Yallah, A. (2014). *A Correlational Study of the Technology Acceptance Model and Georgia Behavioral Healthcare Provider Telemedicine Adoption.* ERIC.

Zamosky, L. (2018, Dec. 18). *Healthcare sharing ministries: A leap of faith?* Retrieved from https://www.healthinsurance.org/other-coverage/healthcare-sharing-ministries-a-leap-of-faith/

Zamosky, L. (2018, December 18). *Healthcare sharing ministries: A leap of faith?* Retrieved from https://www.healthinsurance.org/other-coverage/healthcare-sharing-ministries-a-leap-of-faith/

Zeithaml, V. A., Berry, L. L., & Parasuraman, A. (1996). The behavioral consequences of service quality. *Journal of Marketing, 60*(2), 31–46. doi:10.2307/1251929

Zobair, K. M. (2019). *Barriers, facilitators and expectations of telemedicine healthcare services adoption in rural public hospital settings in Bangladesh* (Unpublished Thesis). Retrieved from http://hdl.handle.net/10072/388646

Zobair, K. M., Sanzogni, L., & Sandhu, K. (2019). Expectations of telemedicine health service adoption in rural Bangladesh. *Social Science & Medicine, 238,* 112485. doi:10.1016/j.socscimed.2019.112485 PMID:31476664

Zorek, J., & Raehl, C. (2012). Interprofessional education accreditation standards in the USA: A comparative analysis. *Journal of Interprofessional Care, 27*(2), 123–130. doi:10.3109/13561 820.2012.718295 PMID:22950791

Zuvekas, S. H., & Cohen, J. W. (2016). Fee-For-Service, While Much Maligned, Remains The Dominant Payment Method For Physician Visits. *Health Affairs, 35*(3), 411–414. doi:10.1377/hlthaff.2015.1291 PMID:26953294

Zwarenstein, M., Goldman, J., & Reeves, S. (2009). Interprofessional collaboration: Effects of practice-based interventions on professional practice and healthcare outcomes. *Cochrane Database of Systematic Reviews.* https://doi-org.proxynw.uits.iu.edu/10.1002/14651858.CD000072

About the Contributors

Raj Selladurai is an Associate Professor of Management in the School of Business and Economics at Indiana University Northwest. He also serves as Small Business Institute (SBI) Director for the School of Business and Economics. He has owned and managed a consulting business in the energy industry and other related areas. His research interests focus on the areas of servant leadership, business-healthcare collaboration, leadership effectiveness, operations and supply chain management, and high-speed rail and supply chain management. He is currently leading a project team as the Lead Project Director, working on a book project, "Challenges and Opportunities for Healthcare Reform." The team consists of two business professors (Dr. Raj Selladurai and Dr. Charlie Hobson (Professors, Indiana University Northwest), and two physicians, (Dr. Roshini Selladurai MD, In His Image, OK, and Dr. Adam Greer (DO, Ascension St John, OK)), and they are working collaboratively on the healthcare project to be completed in 2020 and to be published by IGI Global, Inc. Healthcare Reform in the US is an ongoing, significant national initiative with strategic policy implications, which would affect several millions of stakeholders in the US, especially in the coming election year. He has published several papers, chapters, and case studies in various management and operations management related business publications and journals, including co-editing (with Shawn Carraher) a book on "Servant Leadership: Research and Practice." He also co-edited with Peggy Daniels Lee and George VandeWerken, his other recent book, "Emerging Challenges and Opportunities of High Speed Rail on Business and Society," which was published by IGI Global, Inc. Both of his innovative books are being actively promoted on social media like Twitter, with impressive results with around 33,000 impressions per month and growing! He has over 30 years of academic and professional business experience, including completing a Professional Certificate in "Servant Leadership: Path to High Performance" Executive Education Seminar at the prestigious Darden School of Business, University of Virginia. He also completed another Certificate in Organizational Behavior at Harvard Business School, Harvard University. He has also taught business management courses as Visiting Professor at universities in Austria and Switzerland. He has diverse leadership and administrative experiences in various organizations, including serving as a finance deacon at Bethel Church, Crown Point, Indiana, as a Group Leader at Bible Study Fellowship (BSF), and in other roles at the university, community, business, and other professional service organizations.

* * *

Scott Davis is the Chief Growth Officer of Prophet, a leading strategic growth firm. In over 25 years of brand and marketing strategy consulting, he has worked across an array of clients, including, GE, Allstate, Hershey's, Microsoft, Boeing, Sara Lee, NBC Universal, the NBA, Target, Gulfstream, United Airlines, the City of Chicago. His work in healthcare includes Johnson & Johnson, the Blue Cross Blue Shield Association, Mayo Clinic, Novant Health and an array of provider systems in the US and across the globe. Scott is a frequent guest lecturer at MBA programs across the country and served as an adjunct professor at the Kellogg School of Management at Northwestern University. Scott began his career at Procter & Gamble. Scott is a contributing columnist at forbes.com, and is the author of 3 previous books, including The Shift: The Transformation of Today's Marketers into Tomorrow's Growth Leaders.

Barry A. Doublestein, DSL, has spent the entirety of his vocational career serving various positions in undergraduate and postgraduate medical education. Currently, he serves as President of the Osteopathic Institute of the South, a medical education foundation, Adjunct Professor of healthcare leadership in the School of Business & Leadership at Regent University, former Clinical Associate Professor at the Kiram Patel College of Osteopathic Medicine at Nova Southeastern University, former Chief of Government Affairs for the Georgia Osteopathic Medical Association, and Adjunct Instructor of Healthcare Administration at Belhaven University. He earned his doctorate in strategic leadership from the School of Business & Leadership at Regent University with emphasis on strategic leadership in medicine. His research interests focus on physician professionalism development.

Jeff Gourdji is a Partner and co-leader of the healthcare practice at Prophet. With over 20 years of leading high-impact marketing & strategy projects, Jeff brings a breadth of experience that comes from working across many industries as marketing practitioner, management consultant and political strategist. Jeff has worked extensively across the health care value chain across an array of growth challenges. His current and past clients include Mayo Clinic, Northwestern Medicine, Encompass Health, Anthem, Eli Lilly & Company and several Blue Cross Blue Shield plans. Jeff is a frequent speaker and writer on healthcare topics, and has been published or cited in Becker's Hospital Review, Modern Healthcare, Medical Marketing & Media (MM&M), PM 360 and MediaPost. Jeff received his B.A. from the University of Michigan and his M.B.A. from the University of Chicago Booth School of Business.

Mike Gregory is an information security professional with over 30 years of experience in Information Technology, 15 of those years in healthcare. He is also a retired U.S. Air Force Officer with 33 years of meritorious service. His leadership focuses on digital transformation, educating the corporate culture in adopting technologies that promote security, compliance, and business opportunities. A high-energy individual with excellent team-building and partnering skills. A key influence in organizational committees, promotes innovation through customer advisory boards, speaking engagements, and literature. Mike is a graduate from the University of Puerto Rico and a current candidate of an MBA program from Indiana University Northwest.

Sean Haas is an undergraduate student at The University of Texas at Dallas studying finance and economics. His research covers the topics of macroeconomics and financial markets. He aspires to pursue a doctoral degree in finance in the fall of 2020.

Md. Jahirul Islam completed his Ph.D. from Griffith University, Australia. His research focus includes intimate partner violence and its physical and mental health contexts, gender and inequality, maternal and child health, and reproductive and environmental health issues.

Sanjana Janumpally is an undergraduate student attending The University of Texas at Dallas. She is majoring in Healthcare Management and Biology. She aspires to attend medical school and pursue her Master's in Public Health in the future.

Abburi Kumar is a Professor of Electrical and Computer Engineering at Prairie View A&M University, a Member of the Texas A&M University System. He has received and managed more than $1 million in research grants as a PI/Co-PI, and has contributed extensively to the production of research in a variety of disciplines, including education, manufacturing, radiation and community and economic development with specific emphasis on workforce development. For his work in public education and his achievements in research, he was one of five faculty members in the TAMU System to have received the Distinguished Achievement Award from the Board of Regents in 2004, the Thurgood Marshall College Fund's Outstanding Achievement Award for School Reform in 2008 and Harmony Schools Public Servant Award in 2012. He travelled to China, Malaysia, Singapore and Ghana to visit universities, schools and government organizations to explore how education and research are conducted in those countries. Prior to joining Prairie View A&M University, he worked as research associate in England, Belgium, Canada and Texas A&M University. Over the past few years he has been studying organizational principles and nature of work in the developing realm of artificial intelligence. Of particular interest to him is the organizational reform of healthcare institutions.

Walter T. Lee, MD, is Associate Professor of Otolaryngology-Head & Neck Surgery at Duke University Medical Center, Co-Director of the Head and Neck Program, Duke Cancer Institute and Staff Surgeon at the Durham VA Medical Center. He earned a BA in Philosophy (ethics) and an MD from George Washington Medical School. Dr. Lee completed his residency and subsequent fellowship at the Cleveland Clinic. His areas of research include professional formation and integrating a virtue-based approach to healthcare delivery. He also is involved with medical student and resident education as well as global health education and development.

April Newton is the Director of Interprofessional Practice Development at Indiana University's Interprofessional Education and Practice Center. She is a fellow in the National Academies of Practice, a founding member in the American Interprofessional Healthcare Collaborative, and a board member of the Academy of Physical Therapy Education.

Chidiebele Constance Obichi is an assistant professor at the Indiana University Northwest School of Nursing. She facilitates learning for graduate and undergraduate nursing students in mental health, nursing management, and public health. She has been teaching in multiple academic settings for over 20 years. Her educational background in linguistics, healthcare management, and nursing has given her a broad base from which she can approach many topics. Dr. Obichi has been working to organize faculty and students to launch an interprofessional students' organization to take on projects that address social determinants of health in Lake County, Indiana. Her research interests include health disparities, health promotion, risk reduction, and prevention in Cardiovascular Disease. She especially enjoys activities that promote community engagement in collaboration with other health professionals and faith-based organizations. Learn more about her at https://www.linkedin.com/in/chidiebele-obichi-phd-msn-rn-aa154425.

Ukamaka Oruche is an Associate Professor at the Indiana University School of Nursing. A nationally recognized expert in psychiatric nursing, Dr. Oruche has made sustained and exemplary contributions to our understanding of the challenges experienced by families of adolescents with Disruptive Behavior Disorders. Her cutting-edge research ensures that the mental health needs of family caregivers are given full clinical consideration. Dr. Oruche facilitated an interdisciplinary team in the development of the state of Indiana's largest integrated primary and behavioral health program. Dr. Oruche's work with underserved populations has had an international impact. She is the founder of Providence Community Health Initiative, which has conducted weekly clinics for diabetes, hypertension, and malaria in southern Nigeria since 2004. Her contributions to clinical practice and research have resulted in expanded scope and reach through leadership on boards that influence mental health policy in Indiana, US, and globally. She is a fellow of the American academy of Nursing.

Andrea Pfeifle is Associate Dean and Director for the Indiana University Interprofessional Practice and Education Center, Associate Professor of Family Medicine, and Adjunct Associate Professor in the School of Health and Human Sciences Department of Physical Therapy.

Richard M. Pfohl, DSL, is an anticipatory thought leader recognized for transforming organizations through his strategy, innovation, and leadership solutions. Presently, he is President of Leadership Peaks, LLC, an Adjunct Professor of Organizational Behavior & Leadership as well as a Course Writer with LeTourneau University, and an entrepreneur, aligned with SCORE, helping small to medium-sized businesses start, grow, and succeed. He earned his Doctorate in Strategic Leadership from the School of Business & Leadership at Regent University with an emphasis on Anticipatory Leadership in Healthcare. His research and practice is currently focused on anticipatory leadership, coaching, entrepreneurship, healthcare transformation, and healthcare professionalism development.

Cynthia Roberts is a Professor of Organizational Behavior and Leadership and Dean of the School of Business and Economics at Indiana University Northwest. Her teaching and research interests include leadership development and team building. She received her BS degree in medical technology from Northern Illinois University and worked in the healthcare field as a medical laboratory specialist, manager, and educator. Roberts received MS degrees in Organizational Development and Training and Development from Loyola University in Chicago and her Ph.D. in Organization Development from Benedictine University. As a registered organization development consultant (RODC), she founded Strategic Learning Partners, Inc. a consulting practice dedicated to improving the effectiveness of leadership through staff and systems development. Roberts has authored 22 publications and 21 academic presentations related to leadership development, ethics, organizational change, and women's advancement. She has also served as a professional speaker on numerous occasions.

Kuldeep Sandhu is a Senior Lecturer in the Department of Business Strategy and Innovation. He holds the positions of Program Director, Masters of International Business, Master of Information Systems, Graduate Certificate in International Business and Graduate Certificate in Information Systems for the Griffith Business School and Discipline Leader (Information Systems), Department of Business Strategy and Innovation. His research expertise includes financial management information systems, human resource business intelligence, information systems, database modelling and management, e-government, e-business, e-commerce, e-health and mobile technology.

Louis Sanzogni is a member of Faculty at Griffith University in Brisbane Australia where he currently lectures in Management and Management Information System. His research interests are in the areas of Diffusion of Innovation and Technology Adoption. In his more recent publications, Dr Sanzogni explored the effects of user perceptions on the adoption of innovations proposing a number of successful variations in pre-established as well as newly developed adoption models.

George Vande Werken is a retired community banker, having served as the Regional President of Providence Bank & Trust, a Chicago area community bank, for the last 10 years of his career. He has worked in a variety of different roles in community banking for over forty years. George has also served on numerous civic and charitable organization boards during his long career in banking. He holds undergraduate degrees in both history and accounting, and an advanced degree in theology, and has been an interested advocate for improved public services for many years. He has served on the boards of Pine Rest Christian Mental Health Services (the fourth largest U.S. behavioral health services provider, located in West Michigan), Providence Life Services (a multi-campus continuum of care/senior living services organization with locations in Illinois, Indiana and Michigan) and Chicago Christian Counseling Center (a multi-location counseling/mental health services provider in the greater Chicago area). He is co-editor of and contributor to the book entitled Evaluating Challenges and Opportunities for Healthcare Reform (IGI Global, 2020) and also Emerging Challenges and Opportunities of High Speed Rail Development on Business and Society (IGI Global, 2016). In 2015 he and his wife, Gayle, relocated from the Chicago area to the greater Austin, Texas area. George and Gayle have four married children and twelve grandchildren.

Khondker Zobair is a Sessional Lecturer, Department of Business Strategy and Innovation, Griffith Business School, Nathan Campus, Griffith University, Queensland, Australia.

Index

Recommended Reference Books

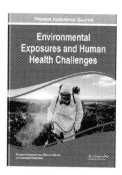

ISBN: 978-1-5225-7635-8
© 2019; 449 pp.
List Price: $255

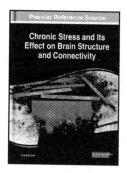

ISBN: 978-1-5225-7513-9
© 2019; 318 pp.
List Price: $225

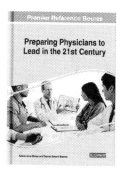

ISBN: 978-1-5225-7576-4
© 2019; 245 pp.
List Price: $245

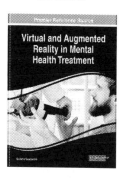

ISBN: 978-1-5225-7168-1
© 2019; 329 pp.
List Price: $265

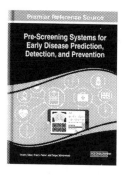

ISBN: 978-1-5225-7131-5
© 2019; 395 pp.
List Price: $245

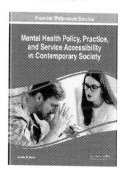

ISBN: 978-1-5225-7402-6
© 2019; 323 pp.
List Price: $245

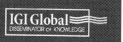

Ensure Quality Research is Introduced to the Academic Community

Become an IGI Global Reviewer for Authored Book Projects

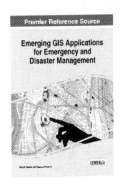

Premier Reference Source

Emerging GIS Applications for Emergency and Disaster Management

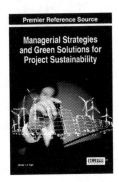

Premier Reference Source

Managerial Strategies and Green Solutions for Project Sustainability

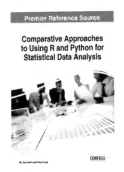

Premier Reference Source

Comparative Approaches to Using R and Python for Statistical Data Analysis

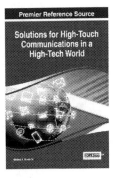

Premier Reference Source

Solutions for High-Touch Communications in a High-Tech World

The overall success of an authored book project is dependent on quality and timely reviews.

In this competitive age of scholarly publishing, constructive and timely feedback significantly expedites the turnaround time of manuscripts from submission to acceptance, allowing the publication and discovery of forward-thinking research at a much more expeditious rate. Several IGI Global authored book projects are currently seeking highly-qualified experts in the field to fill vacancies on their respective editorial review boards:

Applications and Inquiries may be sent to:
development@igi-global.com

Applicants must have a doctorate (or an equivalent degree) as well as publishing and reviewing experience. Reviewers are asked to complete the open-ended evaluation questions with as much detail as possible in a timely, collegial, and constructive manner. All reviewers' tenures run for one-year terms on the editorial review boards and are expected to complete at least three reviews per term. Upon successful completion of this term, reviewers can be considered for an additional term.

If you have a colleague that may be interested in this opportunity, we encourage you to share this information with them.

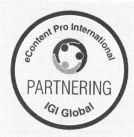

IGI Global Proudly Partners With eContent Pro International

Receive a 25% Discount on all Editorial Services

Editorial Services

IGI Global expects all final manuscripts submitted for publication to be in their final form. This means they must be reviewed, revised, and professionally copy edited prior to their final submission. Not only does this support with accelerating the publication process, but it also ensures that the highest quality scholarly work can be disseminated.

English Language Copy Editing

Let eContent Pro International's expert copy editors perform edits on your manuscript to resolve spelling, punctuaion, grammar, syntax, flow, formatting issues and more.

Scientific and Scholarly Editing

Allow colleagues in your research area to examine the content of your manuscript and provide you with valuable feedback and suggestions before submission.

Figure, Table, Chart & Equation Conversions

Do you have poor quality figures? Do you need visual elements in your manuscript created or converted? A design expert can help!

Translation

Need your documjent translated into English? eContent Pro International's expert translators are fluent in English and more than 40 different languages.

Email: customerservice@econtentpro.com **www.igi-global.com/editorial-service-partners**

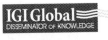

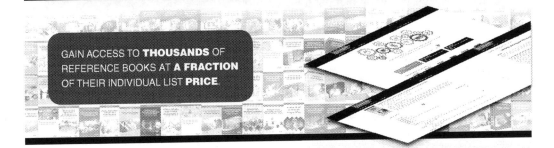

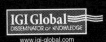

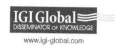
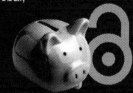

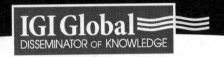
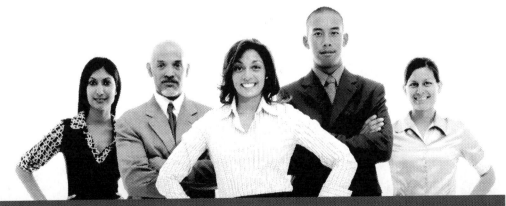

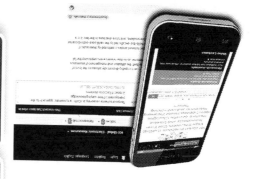
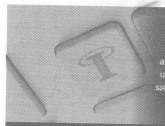